Managing Chronic Obstructive Pulmonary Disease

Edited by

LAURA BLACKLER RN, BSc, MSc
Guy's and St Thomas' Hospital, London

CHRISTINE JONES RN, Clinical Nurse Specialist – Respiratory
King's College Hospital, London

CAROLINE MOONEY RN, Community Nurse Specialist – Respiratory
Luton Treatment Centre, Luton

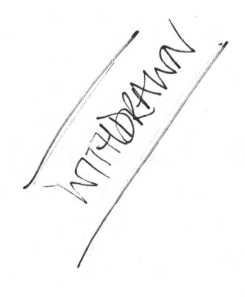

BICENTENNIAL
1807
WILEY
2007
BICENTENNIAL

John Wiley & Sons, Ltd

Other Wiley Editorial Offices

John Wiley & Sons Inc., 111 River Street, Hoboken, NJ 07030, USA

Jossey-Bass, 989 Market Street, San Francisco, CA 94103-1741, USA

Wiley-VCH Verlag GmbH, Boschstr. 12, D-69469 Weinheim, Germany

John Wiley & Sons Australia Ltd, 42 McDougall Street, Milton, Queensland 4064, Australia

John Wiley & Sons (Asia) Pte Ltd, 2 Clementi Loop #02-01, Jin Xing Distripark, Singapore 129809

John Wiley & Sons Canada Ltd, 6045 Freemont Blvd, Mississauga, ONT, L5R 4J3

Wiley also publishes its books in a variety of electronic formats. Some content that appears in print may not be available in electronic books.

Anniversary Logo Design: Richard J. Pacifico

Library of Congress Cataloging-in-Publication Data

Managing chronic obstructive pulmonary disease / [edited by] Laura Blackler, Christine Jones, Caroline Mooney.
    p. ; cm.
  Includes bibliographical references.
  ISBN 978-0-470-02718-9 (alk. paper)
  1. Lungs–Diseases, Obstructive.   I. Blackler, Laura.   II. Jones, Christine, RN.   III. Mooney, Caroline.
  [DNLM: 1. Pulmonary Disease, Chronic Obstructive – nursing.   2. Pulmonary Disease, Chronic Obstructive – therapy.   3. Quality of Life.   4. Self Care. WY 163 M266 2007]
  RC776.O3M366 2007
  616.2'4 – dc22

                                                                              2007011290

A catalogue record for this book is available from the British Library

ISBN 13: 978-0-470-02718-9

Typeset in 10/12 pt Times by SNP Best-set Typesetter Ltd, Hong Kong
Printed and bound in Great Britain by TJ International Ltd, Padstow, Cornwall

This book is printed on acid-free paper responsibly manufactured from sustainable forestry in which at least two trees are planted for each one used for paper production.

Contents

List of Contributors

Paul Bains, Lead Pharmacist, Hammersmith Hospital, NHS Trust, London

Claudia Bausewein, The Cicely Saunders Foundation Research Training Fellow, King's College London School of Medicine, London, and Interdisciplinary Centre for Palliative Medicine, University Hospital Munich

Jacqui Fenton, Senior Respiratory Clinical Nurse, King's College Hospital, London

Linda Fisher, Dept of Health Training Fellow, Cognive Behaviour Therapist, Dept of Psychological Medicine, King's College Hospital, London

Sue Foxley, Nurse Consultant – Continence, King's College Hospital, London

Amy Grant, Senior Respiratory Physiotherapist, Lambeth and Southwark Pulmonary Rehabilitation Team

Sunny Kaul, lecturer in Palliative Care, King's College Hospital, London

William D.C. Man, Specialist Registrar in Respiratory Medicine, Royal Brompton Hospital

Tracey Mathieson, Lead Physiotherapist, King's College Hospital, London

Andrew Menzies-Gow, Consultant in Respiratory Medicine, Royal Brompton Hospital

Lauren Moore, Senior Respiratory Physiotherapist, Lambeth and Southwark Pulmonary Rehabilitation Team

Fliss Murtagh, Research Training Fellow, King's College Hospital, London

Tanya Navarro, Occupational Therapist, King's College Hospital, London

Mary Preston, Clinical Nurse Specialist – Palliative Care, King's College Hospital, London

Vijay A. Selvan, Medical Care Group and A&E Link Pharmacist, King's College Hospital, London

Patrick White, GP and Clinical Senior Lecturer, King's College School of Medicine, London

Richard C. Wilson, Senior Dietician, King's College Hospital, London

Patricia Yerbury, Pharmacy Team Leader for General Medicine Care Group, King's College Hospital, London

Preface

COPD is on the increase worldwide, and it is predicted that by 2020, it will be the third leading cause of death. It has been recognised that there is a need to improve the care offered, to ensure an early diagnosis and raise the public profile of the disease. Health care providers are at the forefront of this, and can have a huge impact on improving an individual's quality of life; through health education, early diagnosis, and better management through all stages of the disease.

COPD is a chronic, progressive debilitating disease, which not only affects the individual, but also has consequences for family members. These individuals come into frequent contact with health care providers in both primary and secondary care sectors. Therefore it is important that the care given is evidence-based and seamless, supporting the individual and their family through the various stages of the disease. To promote this, the NICE guidelines *Management of Chronic Obstructive Pulmonary Disease in Adults in Primary and Secondary Care* (2004) will be referred to throughout the book.

This book is written for nurses and allied health professionals caring for patients with COPD at all stages of their disease. It is about the patient's journey including: diagnosis, management of acute episodes, living with the disease, and end of life issues. The aim is to develop nurses' and allied health care professionals' knowledge and skills in caring for the individual with COPD.

The book takes the reader on a journey from initial diagnosis, through to end of life. The opening chapter provides the reader with an insight into the growth of the disease, the pathophysiology of COPD, and interventions that can have an impact on its progression. It is written to follow the patients' journey using an MDT approach that can be utilised by all health care professionals involved in caring for this group of patients. Throughout the book, direct quotes from patients with COPD are highlighted in bold. It is an opportunity to provide an insight into this debilitative disease; focusing upon the psychological, physical and social components, and uses quotes from patients to highlight these.

Contributions to the book have been obtained from different health care specialists who care for this group of patients. Each chapter is evidence-based and fully referenced and there is a glossary at the end of the book which explains the terms used throughout the book. The term is indicated in bold on its first occurrence.

Introduction

LAURA BLACKLER
Guy's and St Thomas' Hospital, London

CHRISTINE JONES
King's College Hospital, London

CAROLINE MOONEY
Luton Treatment Centre, Luton

FACTS AND FIGURES

EPIDEMIOLOGY

Chronic obstructive pulmonary disease (COPD) is a growing problem throughout the world and in the report *Global Burden of Disease* (2006) undertaken for the World Health Organisation (WHO) and the World Bank it was estimated that the prevalence of COPD was:

11.6/1000 – men
8.77/1000 – women

It was estimated that there were 2.75 million deaths as a result of COPD; however, this could well be underestimated due to COPD being seen as a contributory factor rather than the primary cause of death. WHO have estimated that, in 2005, approximately 80 million people had moderate to severe COPD and there were 3 million deaths.

In the UK, the British Thoracic Society commissioned a report *Burden of Lung Disease* (Gupta & Limb 2006) and this showed that, in 2004, there were over 27,000 deaths due to COPD, there is an almost 50:50 split between men and women. This is 23 per cent of all deaths due to respiratory disease, and, overall, 20 per cent of all deaths in 2004 were due to respiratory disease.

COST OF COPD IN THE UK

There is a significant cost to the NHS of the 845,000 inpatient admissions with respiratory diseases during 2004/2005 and this represents 7 per cent of all admissions. COPD accounted for nearly 10 per cent of all hospital bed days – 5.2 million bed days were used for patients with respiratory disease and COPD accounted for 21 per cent of these.

In 2004, in England, 51 million prescriptions were dispensed for respiratory diseases, 49 per cent of these were for bronchodilators and 26 per cent for corticosteroids. This figure accounts for 7 per cent of all drug prescriptions dispensed.

RISK OF DEVELOPING COPD

A study by Løkke et al. (2006) followed over 8000 people, who at the beginning of the study had normal lung function, over a period of 25 years. They found that those who stopped smoking, particularly in the early part of the study, decreased their risk of developing COPD substantially but that for the continuous smokers there is at least a 25 per cent risk of developing COPD; this figure is higher than what had previously been estimated.

Smoking cessation is the key to the prevention of COPD and there are now a number of health education initiatives focusing on this. There has been an overall drop in the number of people who smoke in the UK: between 1998/99 and 2004/05 the prevalence of people over the age of 16 years smoking fell from 28 per cent to 25 per cent (Office of National Statistics 2006). Cigarette smoking continues to be more common in people aged between 20–34 years, and it is this group that should be targeted to be encouraged to stop. In the General Household Survey (GHS) (Office of National Statistics 2005), the gap between the number of men and women who smoke is very close – 26 per cent men and 23 per cent women (Figure 0.1).

However, in the past 30 years, there has been a decrease of about 50 per cent in the number of adults who smoke. In 2004, the government set a target to reduce the number of smokers to 21 per cent or less by 2010, and it would appear, based on the current trend, that this is achievable.

A large number of smokers would like to give up: 73 per cent of smokers stated this in the GHS (Office of National Statistics 2006), and in 2004/05 around 530,000 people set a date to quit through the NHS stop smoking services in England. In a follow-up, 56 per cent were still not smoking and the success rate was greater in those over the age of 60. The most common reason for wanting to give up smoking was health-related and nearly 9 out of ten smokers stated this (Office of National Statistics 2006).

The GHS also showed that there is an increased awareness of the health risks due to smoking and 51 per cent of respondents thought that smoking was the main cause of premature death in the UK. The effects of second-hand smoking were also known by most respondents and an increased number of non-smokers stated that they would mind if people smoked near them. An increasing number of people supported smoking restrictions in public places; the largest increase was for restrictions in pubs with 65 per cent supporting this.

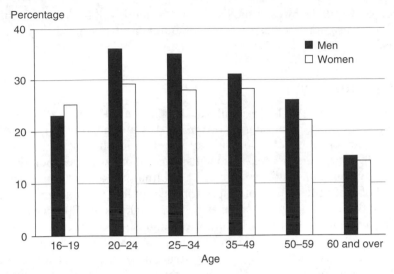

Figure 0.1. Percentage of UK adults who smoke cigarettes, by age and gender, Office of National Statistics (2004)

In 2004, enclosed workplaces became smoke-free by law in Ireland; the primary aim was to protect workers from exposure to the harmful effects of second-hand smoke (Agnew et al. 2005; McCaffrey et al. 2005). The Office of Tobacco Control carried out a review a year later to look at compliance and the health benefits derived from this ban. They found that compliance with the legislation was high, over 95 per cent, and that the majority of people, both smokers and non-smokers, supported it. Prior to the implementation of the law there had been fears raised that this would affect profits. Although there is a decline in bar sales of 4.4 per cent in 2004, this was not different to 2003 when there was a decline of 4.2 per cent (Central Statistics Office 2005).

The air quality in 24 pubs was measured before and a year after the smoke ban came into force and it showed significant reduction in particulate particles (McCaffrey et al. 2005). This result is further supported by another study that looked at the ultra-fine particles in 12 pubs which showed a dramatic decrease with levels similar to those found in non-smoking homes (Kelleher & McLaughlin 2005). Another study carried out by Agnew et al. (2005) looked at the breath carbon monoxide of bar workers and found that there was a substantial fall in carbon monoxide levels in both smokers and non-smokers at the end of the year following the ban.

Following on from this, the Health Bill proposes smoke-free premises with the government planning to implement the regulations in the summer of 2007. Consultations were sought and the results published by the Department of Health on 18 December 2006. At the time of writing the proposed date for implementation was 1 July 2007 and it will be interesting to see how this impacts on COPD. However, the likelihood is that it will be some time before there is any significant decrease in the number of people diagnosed with COPD.

ILLICIT DRUG USE

Cannabis is the most widely used illegal drug in the UK across all ages; about 11 per cent of the population used this in 2004 (Eaton et al. 2005). There have been a number of studies looking at the relationship between cannabis and COPD; however, there is no conclusive evidence whether there is a link. There is evidence of long-term effects of habitual use of cannabis having significantly higher prevalance of respiratory symptoms in comparison to non-smokers (Bloom et al. 1987; Tashkin et al. 1987; Taylor et al. 2000). The problem with most studies is that they have not distinguished between smoking only cannabis, and smoking cannabis and tobacco together. It has been suggested that 3–4 cannabis cigarettes a day is equivalent to 20 or more tobacco cigarettes in terms of damage to bronchial mucosa (British Lung Foundation 2007). More research into this area is needed before a consensus can be achieved.

REFERENCES

Agnew M, Goodman P G, Clancy L (2005) Evaluation of the lung function of bar workers in Dublin, pre and post the induction of the workplace ban on smoking in Ireland. Paper presented at scientific symposium 'The health impacts of smoke-free workplaces in Ireland', Dublin: March.

Bloom J W, Kaltenborn W T, Paoletti P, et al. (1987) Respiratory effects of non-tobacco cigarettes. *British Medical Journal* **295**: 1516–1518.

British Lung Foundation (2007) A smoking gun? The impact of cannabis smoking on respiratory health. Available at: www.britishlungfoundation.org/downloads/A_Smoking_Gun (accessed 9 Jan. 2007).

Central Statistics Office (2005) National Retail Index. Available at: www.cso.ie/releasespublications/pr_services.htm (accessed 21 April 2006).

Department of Health (2006) Smoke-free premises and vehicles: consultation of the proposed regulations to be made under powers in the Health Bill – an analysis on consultation responses. Available at: www.doh.gov.uk (accessed 9 Jan. 2007).

Eaton G, Morelo M, Lodwick A, Bellis M, McVeigh J (2005) *United Kingdom Drug Situation: Annual Report to European Monitoring Centre for Drugs and Drug Addiction (EMCDDA)*. Available at: www.doh.gov.uk (accessed 28 Jan. 2007).

Gupta R, Limb E (2006) *Burden of Lung Disease*. 2nd edn. Available at: www.brit-thoracic.org.uk (accessed October 2006).

Kelleher K, McLaughlin J (2005) Ultrafine airborne particle measurements in Dublin before and after the smoking ban. Paper presented at scientific symposium 'The health impacts of smoke-free workplaces in Ireland', Dublin: March.

Løkke A, Lange P, Scharling H, Fabrious P, Vestbo J (2006) Developing COPD – a 25 year follow up study of the general population. *Thorax* **61**: 935–939.

McCaffrey M, Goodman P G, Clancy L (2005) Particulate pollution levels in Dublin pre and post induction of the workplace smoking ban. Paper presented at scientific symposium 'The health impacts of smoke-free workplaces in Ireland', Dublin: March.

NICE Guidelines (2004) *Chronic Obstructive Pulmonary Disease: Management of Chronic Obstructive Pulmonary Disease in Adults in Primary and Secondary Care. Clinical Guideline.* London: HSMO.

Office of National Statistics (ONS) (2005) General Household Survey: Smoking and Drinking among Adults. Available at: www.statistics.gov.uk/StatBase/Product. asp?vink=5756 (accessed 9 Jan. 2007).

Office of National Statistics (ONS) (2006) Smoking: Smoking habits in Great Britain. Available at: www.statistics.gov.uk/statbase/Product.asp?vink=1638 (accessed 21 April 2006).

Office of Tobacco Control (2005) *Smoke-free Workplaces in Ireland: A One-year Review.* Dublin: Office of Tobacco Control.

Tashkin D P, Coulson A H, Clark V A, et al. (1987) Respiratory symptoms and lung function in habitual, heavy smokers of marijuana alone, smokers of marijuana and tobacco, smokers of tobacco alone and nonsmokers. *American Review of Respiratory Disease* **135**: 209–216.

Taylor D R, Poulton R, Moffitt T E, et al. (2000) The respiratory effects of cannabis dependence in young adults. *Addiction* **95**: 1669–1677.

World Health Organization (2006) Global Burden of Disease. Available at: www.who. int/respiratory/burden/copd/en/ (accessed 1 Oct. 2006).

1 Pathophysiology

SUNNY KAUL
King's College Hospital, London

COPD: DEFINITION

The definition of COPD that is recognised by both the American Thoracic Society and the European Respiratory Society is that it is a preventable and treatable disease characterised by airflow limitation that is not fully reversible and does not change markedly over several months (American Thoracic Society 1962; 2005). The airflow limitation is usually progressive and is associated with an abnormal inflammatory response of the lungs to noxious particles or gases, primarily caused by cigarette smoking.

COPD is an umbrella term that covers many well-known smoking-related lung diseases. They include **chronic bronchitis**, **emphysema** and some cases of chronic asthma. Chronic bronchitis is defined clinically as chronic productive **cough** for three months in each of two successive years in a patient in whom other causes of productive chronic cough have been excluded (American Thoracic Society 1962). Emphysema is defined pathologically as the presence of permanent enlargement of the airspaces distal to the **terminal bronchioles**, accompanied by destruction of their walls and without obvious fibrosis (Snider et al. 1985). Patients with COPD have features of both conditions, although one may be more prominent than the other.

RISK FACTORS

SMOKING

Smoking is the main cause of COPD, but other environmental and industrial pollutants can also result in COPD in people who have never smoked. Passive exposure to cigarette smoke also can contribute to respiratory symptoms and COPD.

POLLUTION

Indoor air pollution from some fuels used for cooking and heating in poorly vented dwellings may contribute to airflow limitation.

Managing Chronic Obstructive Pulmonary Disease, Edited by L. Blackler, C. Jones and C. Mooney
© 2007 John Wiley & Sons Ltd

With respect to outdoor pollution, studies have shown a relationship between levels of atmospheric pollution and respiratory problems in both adults and children. Therefore, outdoor air pollution adds to the burden of inhaled particles, although to what degree is unknown. It is mainly comprised of **particulates** and gases. The particulates mainly originate from the incomplete combustion of solid fuels and diesel, ash and fine dusts. The main gaseous components are the various oxides of sulphur, nitrogen and carbon, again from the combustion of fossil fuels, **hydrocarbons** and **ozone**. The role of outdoor air pollution in the evolution of COPD remains controversial.

OCCUPATION

Any occupation in which the local environment is polluted with gases and particles increases the risk of developing COPD. There is evidence that cadmium and silica also increase the risk of COPD particularly in smokers. At-risk occupations include coal miners, metal workers, grain handlers, cotton workers and workers in paper mills.

INFECTION

The role of viral infections of the upper and lower respiratory tract in the pathogenesis of COPD is still unclear. Respiratory infections in early childhood also are associated with reduced lung function and increased respiratory problems in adulthood, which may lead to COPD. Once COPD is established, repeated infective exacerbations of airflow obstruction, either viral or bacterial, may accelerate the decline in lung function.

INHERITED

There also is a rare, inherited form of emphysema known as **alpha-1-antitrypsin deficiency**, which causes COPD. This mainly results in **panacinar emphysema** that largely affects the lower lobes.

GENDER

It is frequently stated that COPD is more prevalent in men. However, when smoking and occupational exposure are taken into account, the relative risk of developing COPD is not significantly higher in men than women.

SOCIO-ECONOMIC STATUS

In studies conducted in the UK in the 1950s and the 1960s, there is a clear social class gradient for COPD with a higher prevalence in the lower socio-economic groups. There is also a higher prevalence of smoking in the lower socio-economic strata, and they are more likely to be employed in jobs where they may be at risk from occupational exposure. Poorer housing conditions and use of fossil fuels for heating without adequate ventilation may also be important contributory factors.

PATHOLOGY

The pathogenic mechanisms causing COPD are not clear but are likely to be diverse. The increased number of activated **polymorphonuclear leukocytes** and **macrophages** release **elastases** in a manner that cannot be counteracted effectively by **antiproteases**, resulting in lung destruction. Pathological changes in COPD occur in the large (central) airways, the small (peripheral) **bronchioles**, lung **parenchyma** and **pulmonary vasculature**. These will now be described in turn.

CENTRAL AIRWAYS

The central airways include the **trachea, bronchi,** and bronchioles greater than 2–4 mm in internal diameter. In patients with chronic bronchitis, the **epithelium** and associated ducts are infiltrated with an inflammatory exudate of fluid and cells (Mullen et al. 1985; O'Shaughnessy et al. 1997). The predominant cells in this inflammatory exudate are macrophages and CD8+ T **lymphocytes** (Sactta et al. 1993; O'Shaughnessy et al. 1997).

Chronic inflammation in the central airways is also associated with an increase in the number of **goblet** and **squamous cells**; dysfunction, damage, and/or loss of **cilia**; enlarged **submucosal** mucus-secreting glands (Reid 1960); an increase in the amount of smooth muscle and connective tissue in the airway wall (Jamal et al. 1984); degeneration of the airway **cartilage** (Thurlbeck et al. 1974; Haraguchi et al. 1999); and mucus hypersecretion. The various pathological changes in the central airways are responsible for the symptoms of chronic cough and sputum production, which identify people at risk for COPD and may continue to be present throughout the course of the disease.

PERIPHERAL AIRWAYS

The peripheral airways include small bronchi and bronchioles that have an internal diameter of less than 2 mm. The early decline in lung function in COPD is correlated with inflammatory changes in the peripheral airways, similar to those that occur in the central airways: exudate of fluid and cells in the airway wall and lumen, goblet and squamous cell metaplasia of the epithelium (Cosio et al. 1978), oedema of the airway mucosa due to inflammation, and excess mucus in the airways due to goblet cell **hyperplasia**.

However, the most characteristic change in the peripheral airways of patients with COPD is airway narrowing. Inflammation initiated by cigarette smoking (Niewoehner et al. 1974) and other risk factors (Pride & Burrows 1995) leads to repeated cycles of injury and repair of the walls of the peripheral airways. Injury is caused either directly by inhaled toxic particles and gases such as those found in cigarette smoke, or indirectly by the action of **inflammatory mediators**; this injury then initiates repair processes. It seems likely that disordered repair processes can lead to tissue remodelling with altered structure and function. Cigarette smoke may impair lung repair mechanisms, thereby further contributing to altered lung structure (Laurent et al. 1983; Osman et al. 1985; Nakamura et al. 1995). Even normal lung repair mechanisms can lead to airway remodelling because tissue repair in the airways, as elsewhere in the body, may involve scar tissue formation. This injury and repair process results in increasing **collagen** content and scar tissue formation that narrows the lumen and produces fixed airways obstruction (Matsuba & Thurlbeck 1972).

The peripheral airways become the major site of airways obstruction in COPD, and direct measurements of **peripheral airways resistance** (Hogg et al. 1968) show that the structural changes in the airway wall are the most important cause of the increase in peripheral airways resistance in COPD.

Inflammatory changes such as airway oedema and mucus hypersecretion also contribute to airway narrowing in COPD as does the loss of elastic recoil, but **fibrosis** of the small airways plays the largest role (Figure 1.1).

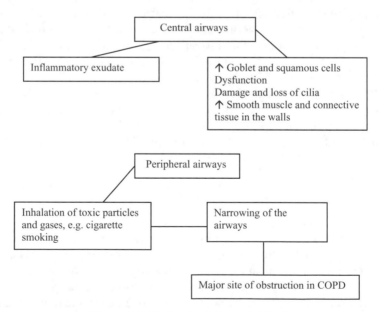

Figure 1.1. Pathophysiology of COPD

LUNG PARENCHYMA

The lung parenchyma includes the gas-exchanging surface of the lung (respiratory bronchioles and alveoli) and the pulmonary capillary system.

The most common type of parenchymal destruction in COPD patients is the **centrilobular** form of emphysema, which involves dilatation and destruction of the respiratory bronchioles (Leopold & Geoff 1957). These lesions occur more frequently in the upper lobes. In advanced disease they may appear diffusely throughout the entire lung and also involve destruction of the pulmonary capillary bed.

Panacinar emphysema, which extends throughout the **acinus**, is the characteristic lesion seen in alpha-1 antitrypsin deficiency and involves dilatation and destruction of the alveolar ducts and sacs as well as the respiratory bronchioles. It tends to affect the lower more than upper lung regions. Because this process usually affects all of the acini in the secondary lobule, it is also referred to as **panlobular emphysema**. The primary mechanism of lung parenchyma destruction, in both smoking-related COPD and alpha-1 antitrypsin deficiency, is thought to be an imbalance of **endogenous** proteinases and antiproteinases in the lung.

PULMONARY VASCULATURE

Pulmonary vascular changes in COPD are characterised by a thickening of the vessel wall that begins early in the natural history of the disease, when lung function is reasonably well maintained and pulmonary vascular pressures are normal at rest (Wright et al. 1983). Endothelial dysfunction of the pulmonary arteries occurs early in COPD (Peinado et al. 1998). Since **endothelium** plays an important role in regulating **vascular tone** and **cell proliferation**, it is likely that endothelial dysfunction might initiate the sequence of events that results ultimately in structural changes. Thickening of the **intima** is the first structural change (Wright et al. 1983), followed by an increase in vascular **smooth muscle** and the infiltration of the vessel wall by inflammatory cells, including macrophages and CD8[+] T lymphocytes (Peinado et al. 1999).

These structural changes are correlated with an increase in pulmonary vascular pressure that develops first with exercise and then at rest. As COPD progresses, greater amounts of smooth muscle and collagen (Riley et al. 1977) further thicken the vessel wall. In severe disease, the changes in the muscular arteries may be associated with emphysematous destruction of the pulmonary capillary bed.

PATHOPHYSIOLOGY

Pathological changes in COPD lead to corresponding physiological abnormalities that usually become evident first on exercise and later also at rest.

Physiological changes characteristic of the disease include: mucus hypersecretion, ciliary dysfunction, airflow limitation, pulmonary hyperinflation, gas exchange abnormalities, **pulmonary hypertension**, and **cor pulmonale**, and they usually develop in this order over the course of the disease. In turn, the various physiological abnormalities contribute to the characteristic symptoms of COPD – chronic cough and **sputum** production and **dyspnoea**.

MUCUS HYPERSECRETION AND CILIARY DYSFUNCTION

Mucus hypersecretion in COPD is caused by the stimulation of the enlarged mucus-secreting glands and increased number of goblet cells by inflammatory mediators such as **leukotrienes**, proteinases, and neuropeptides. Ciliated epithelial cells undergo squamous **metaplasia** leading to impairment in mucociliary clearance mechanisms. These changes are usually the first physiological abnormalities to develop in COPD, and can be present for many years before any other physiological abnormalities develop.

AIRFLOW LIMITATION AND PULMONARY HYPERINFLATION

Expiratory airflow limitation is the hallmark physiological change of COPD. The airflow limitation characteristic of COPD is primarily irreversible, with a small reversible component. Several pathological characteristics contribute to airflow limitation and changes in pulmonary mechanics.

The irreversible component of airflow limitation is primarily due to remodelling (Hogg et al. 1968; Matsuba & Thurlbeck 1972; Cosio et al. 1978; Mullen et al. 1985; Matsuba et al. 1989; Kuwano et al. 1993), fibrosis and narrowing of the small airways that produces fixed airways obstruction and a consequent increase in airways resistance. The sites of airflow limitation in COPD are the smaller conducting airways, including bronchi and bronchioles less than 2 mm in internal diameter.

Parenchymal destruction (emphysema) plays a smaller role in this irreversible component but contributes to expiratory airflow limitation and the increase in airways resistance in several ways. Destruction of alveolar attachments inhibits the ability of the small airways to maintain patency (Dayman 1951). Alveolar destruction is also associated with a loss of elastic recoil of the lung (Butler et al. 1960; Mead et al. 1967), which decreases the intra-alveolar pressure driving **exhalation**.

Although both the destruction of alveolar attachments to the outer wall of the peripheral airways and the loss of lung elastic recoil produced by emphysema have been implicated in the pathogenesis of peripheral airways obstruction (Dayman 1951; Lane et al. 1968), direct measurements of peripheral airways resistance show that the structural changes in the airway wall are the most important cause of the increase in peripheral airways resistance in COPD.

Airway smooth muscle contraction, ongoing airway inflammation, and **intra-luminal** accumulation of mucus and plasma exudate may be responsible for the small part of airflow limitation that is reversible with treatment. Inflammation and accumulation of mucus and exudate may be particularly important during **exacerbations** (Burnett & Stockley 1981).

Airflow limitation in COPD is best measured through **spirometry**, which is key to the diagnosis and management of the disease. The essential spirometric measurements for diagnosis and monitoring of COPD patients are the **forced expiratory volume in one second (FEV$_1$)** and **forced vital capacity (FVC)**. As COPD progresses, with increased airway wall thickness, loss of alveolar attachments, and loss of lung **elastic recoil**, both FEV$_1$ and FVC decrease. A decrease in the ratio of FEV$_1$ to FVC is often the first sign of developing airflow limitation. FEV$_1$ declines naturally with age, but the rate of decline in COPD patients is generally greater than that in normal subjects.

With increasing severity of airflow limitation, **expiration** becomes flow-limited during **tidal breathing**. Initially, this occurs only during exercise, but later it is also seen at rest. In parallel with this, **functional residual capacity (FRC)** increases due to the combination of the decrease in the elastic properties of the lungs and premature airway closure.

As airflow limitation develops, the rate of lung emptying is slowed and the interval between **inspiratory** efforts does not allow expiration to the relaxation volume of the respiratory system; this leads to **dynamic** pulmonary **hyperinflation**. The increase in FRC can impair inspiratory muscle function.

These changes occur as the disease advances but are almost always seen first during exercise, when the greater metabolic stimulus to ventilation stresses the ability of the ventilatory pump to maintain gas exchange.

AIRFLOW RESISTANCE

Resistance is defined as the pressure required to produce flow. In emphysema, the destruction of collagen and **elastin** fibres leads to a reduction in the radial traction of the airways, which in turn leads to a reduced airway calibre. Chronic bronchitis is associated with a chronic inflammatory process that consists of cellular infiltration and airway wall oedema; this along with the mucus in the lumen leads to a further reduction in airway calibre. Chronic inflammatory process develops into **granulation** tissue and peribronchial fibrosis. These irreversible changes initially start in the small airways but can and often do progress into the larger airways. Consequently the reduced airway calibre results in increased airways resistance and therefore airflow resistance. During expiration there is increased pressure around the airways that increases the tendency for the airways to collapse. Increased airways resistance is indicated by a reduced forced expiratory volume **FEV$_1$/FVC** ratio and increased expiratory time. In the normal lung, resistance of the smaller airways makes up a small percentage of the total airways resistance (Hogg et al. 1968). But in patients with COPD the total lower airways resistance approximately doubles, and most of the increase is due to a large increase in peripheral airways resistance (Hogg et al. 1968). There is wide agreement that the peripheral airways become the major site of obstruction in COPD.

COMPLIANCE

Lung compliance is defined as change in volume per unit change in pressure. This measurement represents the relationship between the volume of the respiratory system and the recoil pressures of the lungs and chest wall. **Lung recoil pressure** comprises two components:

1 Tension of the elastic fibres and connective tissue network of the lungs.
2 Surface tension at the air–liquid interface in the alveoli; at FRC the lung recoil pressure is equal to the outward recoil pressure of the chest wall.

Low compliance infers that the lungs are stiff in that for a given pressure a small volume change is achieved; a high value of compliance indicates that the lungs inflate easily as for a given pressure there is a large volume change. The pressure–volume relationship of the respiratory system is shown in Figure 1.2.

In health, breathing occurs over the linear part of the curve, i.e. between FRC and FRC + 500 mls, where the compliance values are high and the work of breathing least.

PEEP

Dynamic airway collapse and insufficient tidal expiratory time result in the end-expiratory lung volume rising above the FRC, leading to dynamic **hyper-inflation**. This in turn means that due to end-expiratory elastic recoil the alveo-

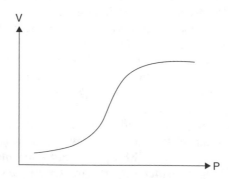

Figure 1.2. The pressure–volume curve

lar pressure remains positive at the end of expiration. Therefore before the inspiratory muscles can create a negative pressure in the central airways and produce inspiratory flow, they must overcome this **positive end expiratory pressure (PEEP)** in the alveoli, termed **intrinsic PEEP (IPEEP)**.

GAS EXCHANGE ABNORMALITIES

In advanced COPD, the combination of peripheral airways obstruction, parenchymal destruction, and pulmonary vascular abnormalities reduces the lung's capacity for gas exchange, producing **hypoxaemia** and in advanced disease, also **hypercapnia**. The correlation between routine lung function tests and arterial blood gases is poor, but significant hypoxaemia or hypercapnia is rare when FEV_1 is greater than $1.00 L$ (Lane et al. 1968). Hypoxaemia is initially only present during exercise, but as the disease continues to progress it is also present at rest.

Inequality in the **ventilation/perfusion ratio (V_A/Q)** is the major mechanism behind hypoxaemia in COPD, regardless of the stage of the disease. Chronic hypercapnia usually reflects inspiratory muscle dysfunction and **alveolar hypoventilation**.

PULMONARY HYPERTENSION AND COR PULMONALE

Pulmonary hypertension develops late in the course of COPD usually after the development of severe hypoxaemia ($PaO_2 < 8.0 kPa$ or $60 mmHg$) and often hypercapnia as well. It is the major cardiovascular complication of COPD and is associated with the development of cor pulmonale and with a poor prognosis (MacNee 1994). However, even in patients with severe disease, pulmonary arterial pressure is usually only modestly elevated at rest, though it may rise markedly with exercise. Pulmonary hypertension in COPD is believed to progress rather slowly even if left untreated. Further studies are required to firmly establish the natural history of pulmonary hypertension in COPD.

Factors that are known to contribute to the development of pulmonary hypertension in patients with COPD include **vasoconstriction**; remodelling of pulmonary arteries, which thickens the vessel walls and reduces the lumen; and destruction of the pulmonary capillary bed by emphysema, which further increases the pressure required to perfuse the pulmonary vascular bed.

In advanced COPD, **hypoxia** plays the primary role in producing pulmonary hypertension, both by causing vasoconstriction of the pulmonary arteries and by promoting remodelling of the vessel wall.

Pulmonary hypertension is associated with the development of cor pulmonale. Cor pulmonale is defined as right ventricular failure resulting from diseases affecting the function and/or structure of the lungs, except when these pulmonary alterations are due to diseases that primarily affect the left side of the heart, as in congenital heart disease.

The prevalence and natural history of cor pulmonale in COPD are still to be clarified. Pulmonary hypertension and reduction of the vascular bed due to emphysema can lead to right ventricular **hypertrophy** and right heart failure, but right ventricular function appears to be maintained in some patients despite the presence of pulmonary hypertension (Biernacki et al. 1988). Right heart failure is associated with **venous stasis** and thrombosis that may result in pulmonary embolism and further compromise the pulmonary circulation.

Severe stable COPD is associated with severe derangement in respiratory mechanics and abnormal V/Q ratios. During an exacerbation the inflammatory process in the airways further impairs the respiratory mechanics as well as further challenging the gas exchange process.

During an exacerbation the increase in airflow resistance results in an increase in the work of breathing of the inspiratory muscles and also reduces the rate of lung emptying. The presence of expiratory flow limitation means that there is insufficient tidal expiration time to empty the lungs; consequently the end-expiratory lung volume rises above the FRC, leading to dynamic hyperinflation. This in turn means that due to end-expiratory elastic recoil, the alveolar pressure remains positive at the end of expiration. Therefore, before the inspiratory muscles can create a **negative pressure** in the central airways and produce inspiratory flow, they must overcome this positive end-expiratory pressure in the alveoli, termed intrinsic peep (IPEEP). This intrinsic PEEP adds to the resistive load. So an acute exacerbation of COPD is associated with an increase in the resistive and elastic loads by an increase in the inspiratory workload. Additionally, dynamic hyperinflation decreases the overall pressure generating capacity by the inspiratory muscles. This is due in part to the shortening of the inspiratory muscles and the alteration in the geometric interaction between the muscle groups.

In patients with chronic obstructive pulmonary disease, a thorough understanding on the clinician's part of the pathophysiologic basis of airflow limitation greatly enhances decisions regarding patient care.

REFERENCES

American Thoracic Society (1962) Chronic bronchitis, asthma and pulmonary emphysema: a statement by the Committee on Diagnostic Standards for Nontuberculous Respiratory Diseases. *American Review of Respiratory Disease* **85**: 762–768.

American Thoracic Society (2005) COPD Guidelines. Available at: http://www.thoracic.org/sections/copd/for-health-professionals/definition-diagnosis-and-staging/definitions.html (accessed 5 March 2006).

Biernacki W, Flenley D C, Muir A L, MacNee W (1988) Pulmonary hypertension and right ventricular function in patients with COPD. *Chest* **94**: 1169–1175.

Burnett D, Stockley R A (1981) Serum and sputum alpha 2 macroglobulin in patients with chronic obstructive airways disease. *Thorax* **36**: 512–516.

Butler J, Caro C, Alkaler R, Dubois A B (1960) Physiological factors affecting airway resistance in normal subjects and in patients with obstructive airways disease. *Journal of Clinical Investigations* **39**: 584–591.

Cosio M, Ghezzo H, Hogg J C, Corbin R, Loveland M, Dosman J, et al. (1978) The relations between structural changes in small airways and pulmonary-function tests. *New England Journal of Medicine* **298**: 1277–1281.

Dayman H (1951) Mechanics of airflow in health and emphysema. *Journal of Clinical Investigations* **30**: 1175–1190.

Haraguchi M, Shimura S, Shirato K (1999) Morphometric analysis of bronchial cartilage in chronic obstructive pulmonary disease and bronchial asthma. *American Journal of Respiratory Critical Care Medicine* **159**: 1005–1013.

Hogg J C, Macklem P T, Thurlbeck W M (1968) Site and nature of airway obstruction in chronic obstructive lung disease. *New England Journal of Medicine* **278**: 1355–1360.

Jamal K, Cooney T P, Fleetham J A, Thurlbeck W M (1984) Chronic bronchitis. Correlation of morphologic findings to sputum production and flow rates. *American Review of Respiratory Disease* **129**: 719–722.

Kuwano K, Bosken C H, Pare P D, Bai T R, Wiggs B R, Hogg J C (1993) Small airways dimensions in asthma and in chronic obstructive pulmonary disease. *American Review of Respiratory Disease* **148**: 1220–1225.

Lane D J, Howell J B, Giblin B (1968) Relation between airways obstruction and CO_2 tension in chronic obstructive airways disease. *British Medical Journal* **3**: 707–709.

Laurent P, Janoff A, Kagan H M (1983) Cigarette smoke blocks cross-linking of elastin in vitro. *Chest* **83**: 63S–65S.

Leopold J G, Geoff J (1957) Centrilobular form of hypertrophic emphysema and its relation to chronic bronchitis. *Thorax* **12**: 219–235.

MacNee W (1994) Pathophysiology of cor pulmonale in chronic obstructive pulmonary disease. Part two. *American Journal of Respiratory Critical Care Medicine* **150**: 1158–1168.

Matsuba K, Thurlbeck W M (1972) The number and dimensions of small airways in emphysematous lungs. *American Journal of Pathology* **67**: 265–275.

Matsuba K, Wright J L, Wiggs B R, Pare P D, Hogg J C (1989) The changes in airways structure associated with reduced forced expiratory volume in one second. *European Respiratory Journal* **2**: 834–839.

Mead J, Turner J M, Macklem P T, Little J B (1967) Significance of the relationship between lung recoil and maximum expiratory flow. *Journal of Applied Physiology* **22**: 95–108.

Mullen J B, Wright J L, Wiggs B R, Pare P D, Hogg J C (1985) Reassessment of inflammation of airways in chronic bronchitis. *British Medical Journal* (Clinical Research Edition) **291**: 1235–1239.

Nakamura Y, Romberger D J, Tate L, Ertl R F, Kawamoto M, Adachi Y, et al. (1995) Cigarette smoke inhibits lung fibroblast proliferation and chemotaxis. *American Journal of Respiratory Critical Care Medicine* **151**: 1497–1503.

Niewoehner D E, Kleinerman J, Rice D B (1974) Pathologic changes in the peripheral airways of young cigarette smokers. *New England Journal of Medicine* **291**: 755–758.

O'Shaughnessy T C, Ansari T W, Barnes N C, Jeffery P K (1997) Inflammation in bronchial biopsies of subjects with chronic bronchitis: inverse relationship of CD8+

T lymphocytes with FEV$_1$. *American Journal of Respiratory Critical Care Medicine* **1155**: 852–857.

Osman M, Cantor J O, Roffman S, Keller S, Turino G M, Mandl I (1985) Cigarette smoke impairs elastin resynthesis in lungs of hamsters with elastase-induced emphysema. *American Review of Respiratory Disease* **132**: 640–643.

Peinado V I, Barbera J A, Abate P, Ramirez J, Roca J, Santos S, et al. (1999) Inflammatory reaction in pulmonary muscular arteries of patients with mild chronic obstructive pulmonary disease. *American Journal of Respiratory Critical Care Medicine* **159**: 1605–1611.

Peinado V I, Barbera J A, Ramirez J, Gomez F P, Roca J, Jover L, et al. (1998) Endothelial dysfunction in pulmonary arteries of patients with mild COPD. *American Journal of Physiology* **274**: L908–913.

Pride N B, Burrows B (1995) Development of impaired lung function: natural history and risk factors. In: Calverley P M, Pride N B (eds) *Chronic Obstructive Lung Disease*. London and Glasgow: Chapman and Hall Medical.

Reid L (1960) Measurement of the bronchial mucous gland layer: a diagnostic yardstick in chronic bronchitis. *Thorax* **15**: 132–141.

Riley D J, Thakker-Varia S, Poiani G J, Tozzi C A (1977) Vascular remodeling. In: Crystal R G, West J B, Barnes P J, Weibel E R (eds) *The Lung: Scientific Foundations*. Philadelphia, PA: Lippincott-Raven.

Saetta M, Di Stefano A, Maestrelli P, Ferraresso A, Drigo R, Potena A, et al. (1993) Activated T-lymphocytes and macrophages in bronchial mucosa of subjects with chronic bronchitis. *American Review of Respiratory Disease* **147**: 301–306.

Snider G L, Kleinerman J, Thurlbeck W M, Bengali Z K (1985) The definition of emphysema: report of a National Heart, Lung and Blood Institute, Division of Lung Diseases, Workshop. *American Review of Respiratory Disease* **132**: 182–185.

Thurlbeck W M, Pun R, Toth J, Frazer R G (1974) Bronchial cartilage in chronic obstructive lung disease. *American Review of Respiratory Disease* **109**: 73–80.

Wright J L, Lawson L, Pare P D, Hooper R O, Peretz D I, Nelems J M, et al. (1983) The structure and function of the pulmonary vasculature in mild chronic obstructive pulmonary disease: The effect of oxygen and exercise. *American Review of Respiratory Disease* **128**: 702–707.

2 Diagnosing COPD

WILLIAM D.C. MAN
Royal Brompton Hospital, London

INTRODUCTION

COPD is by far the commonest respiratory cause of mortality and morbidity in adults in the UK. Although diagnosis is relatively straightforward, it is dependent on having a high index of suspicion for COPD in middle-aged or elderly patients with breathlessness, cough or exercise limitation. The diagnosis requires careful history taking and a thorough physical examination, supported by spirometry. The majority of patients are diagnosed in primary care, but many will come to the attention of respiratory specialists, especially as COPD is a progressive disease. This chapter summarises the important symptoms and physical signs that should be sought in the initial diagnosis of COPD, as well as the value of relevant investigations including spirometry. Ways of distinguishing COPD from other respiratory disorders, such as asthma, will also be discussed. Finally, the chapter will describe clinically relevant situations when referral to a specialist would be indicated. Many of the points in this chapter are based upon the recommendations of the National Clinical Guidelines on the management of COPD (NICE Guidelines 2004).

CLINICAL FEATURES

SYMPTOMS

COPD should be considered in any patient over the age of 35 (especially a current or ex-smoker) presenting with one or more of the following symptoms:

- cough
- dyspnoea (breathlessness), particularly on exertion
- wheeze
- regular sputum production
- frequent episodes of 'bronchitis' or 'chest infections', particularly in winter months.

Managing Chronic Obstructive Pulmonary Disease. Edited by L. Blackler, C. Jones and C. Mooney
© 2007 John Wiley & Sons Ltd

The two main symptoms of COPD are cough and breathlessness. *Cough* may be dry or productive of clear or purulent sputum. It is usually worse in the mornings, but bears no relationship to the severity of the disease. A history of persistent productive cough or *recurrent chest infections*, particularly during the winter months, is common. Excessive purulence or volume of sputum is unusual and may suggest an alternative diagnosis such as **bronchiectasis**.

"I knew what emphysema was and the world fell out of me."

"The doctor told me I had emphysema. I had never heard of it before, he told me it would cut 10 years off my life."

Breathlessness is commonly seen, particularly during an infective exacerbation, and is often the primary reason for seeking medical advice. Breathlessness progresses gradually, and if a patient leads an inactive lifestyle, many patients will have lost significant amounts of lung function before breathlessness becomes problematic. It is important to objectively characterise the severity of breathlessness as this provides a simple indicator to the effect upon a patient's quality of life, and a method of assessing the effects of treatments. Breathlessness should be assessed using the Medical Research Council (MRC) Dyspnoea Scale (Fletcher et al. 1959) (Figure 2.1).

"Not being able to breathe properly is frightening, absolutely terrifying, you feel like you are never going to breathe normally again."

"I used to climb Snowdon every year: it was like going for a stroll, now I can't walk to my front door like without being out of breath."

Grade	Degree of Breathlessness
1	Breathless only on strenuous exercise.
2	Breathless on hurrying or walking up a slight hill.
3	Walk slower than similar aged people because of breathlessness, or need to stop for breath when walking at own pace.
4	Breathless after walking about 100 metres or a few minutes on the flat.
5	Too breathless to leave the house, or breathless when dressing or undressing

Figure 2.1. The MRC Dyspnoea Scale. *Source*: Modified from Fletcher et al. (1959)

Wheeze is often an accompanying feature of breathlessness. However, significant day-to-day or **diurnal variability** and night-time waking with wheeze are more suggestive of asthma.

The degree of breathlessness will partly determine *functional capacity*. An estimate of exercise capacity should always be made; the distance a patient can walk on the flat or uphill without stopping, the ability to manage stairs to their home or any stairs within their home, and most importantly, any effects upon activities of daily living.

Patients with presumed COPD should also be asked about symptoms that may indicate alternative diagnoses. **Haemoptysis** is relatively rare in COPD, and is more commonly seen in lung cancer or bronchiectasis. Chest pain, likewise, is uncommon in COPD, and alternative diagnoses such as angina, lung cancer, **pulmonary embolism** or **pneumothorax** must be considered. Ankle swelling, **orthopnoea**, fatigue and **paroxysmal nocturnal dyspnoea** are symptoms associated with congestive cardiac failure, but can occur in COPD patients with cor pulmonale. Weight loss occurs in patients with malignancy, but is in fact quite common in patients with COPD. Approximately 20 per cent of patients with moderate and severe disease (without evidence of lung cancer) experience weight loss and loss of fat-free body mass, known as **cachexia** (Scholes et al. 1993). Early morning headaches are characteristic of hypercapnia, which occurs in severe respiratory failure.

About 90–95 per cent of patients with COPD are smokers or ex-smokers, and a careful smoking history must always be taken. The number of smoking pack-years should be calculated; 20 cigarettes a day for one year is one pack-year, 40 cigarettes a day for 30 years is 60 pack-years. The smoking history of a partner or close household contact should also be considered. Other risk factors for COPD are a strong family history and an occupational history (for example, coal mining or contact with inhaled chemical fumes). There is also increasing evidence that indoor air pollution, such as wood-burning ovens in poorly ventilated dwellings, is a major risk factor. As many patients with COPD are smokers, they often have other medical problems. A careful past medical history must be taken, particularly of heart disease, as this may contribute to breathlessness and poor exercise tolerance.

CLINICAL SIGNS

It should be noted that physical examination alone is insufficient to diagnose COPD; indeed, some patients with COPD will have no abnormal physical signs. Possible abnormal physical signs may include:

- an increased respiratory rate
- cyanosis
- pursed-lip breathing

- flapping tremor ('asterixis') due to carbon dioxide retention
- use of the accessory muscles of the neck and shoulder girdle
- reduced **crico–sternal distance** (due to hyperinflation of the lungs)
- paradoxical retraction of the lower rib interspaces during inspiration (Hoover's sign)
- hyperinflated chest that is hyperresonant on percussion
- wheeze
- reduced breath sounds
- cachexia
- raised jugular venous pressure, enlarged tender liver, ankle swelling with cor pulmonale.

Clinical examination should include the measurement of weight and height, and calculation of the body mass index – weight (in kilos) divided by height (in metres) squared. Recent research suggests that body mass index is an important predictor of morbidity and mortality in COPD (Celli et al. 2004).

COPD is a diagnostic label given to a group of diseases characterised by airway obstruction. It encompasses conditions such as 'chronic bronchitis' (a history of productive cough that produces sputum for three months or more in at least two consecutive years) and 'emphysema' (a histological diagnosis characterised by abnormal permanent enlargement of air spaces distal to the terminal bronchioles, accompanied by the destruction of the walls). Traditionally these patients were often distinguished in terms of their clinical appearance. 'Blue bloaters' (chronic bronchitis) were centrally cyanosed at rest, obese with signs of right heart failure, complained of large volumes of sputum and were often in respiratory failure with cor pulmonale. Despite the respiratory failure, blue bloaters were only moderately breathless, presumably due to poor **respiratory drive**. 'Pink puffers' (emphysema), in comparison, were often underweight, with high respiratory drive and respiratory rate, pursed-lip breathing but no evidence of right heart failure or cyanosis. Although there is some truth in these clinical descriptions, it is recognised that most patients with COPD have characteristics of both.

INVESTIGATIONS

SPIROMETRY

Spirometry is essential in the diagnosis of COPD. The diagnosis is dependent on the demonstration of airflow obstruction, which can only be measured confidently with spirometry. Health-care professionals involved in the management of COPD patients should be able to obtain maximal reproducible results from patients, and be confident in the interpretation of results. All should have easy access to spirometry, particularly as accurate handheld

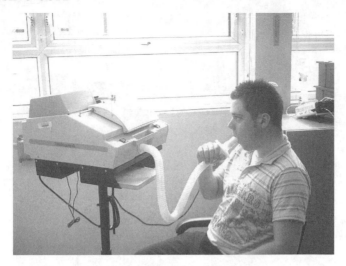

Figure 2.2. Spirometry
Reproduced by permission of Daniel Cox

spirometers (Figure 2.2) have become cheaper in recent years. Peak flow meters are cheaper and more available than spirometers, but **peak expiratory flow** (PEF) rates have not been validated for the diagnosis of COPD. No national or international guidelines advocate the use of PEF for diagnostic purposes; furthermore, a normal PEF does not exclude significant airflow obstruction (Nolan & White 1999). However, serial PEF measurements may be useful in the diagnosis of asthma; there is often a greater than 20 per cent diurnal or day-to-day variability.

The forced expiratory volume in one second (FEV_1) is the most important spirometric variable for assessment of airflow obstruction. It represents the volume of air exhaled in the first second of the forced vital capacity (FVC) manoeuvre. The FVC is the maximal volume of air exhaled with maximally forced effort from a position of maximal inspiration, and is dependent on the expiratory time in severe COPD. The flow–volume Loop (also called a spirogram) is a plot of inspiratory and expiratory flow (on the Y-axis) against volume (on the X-axis) during the performance of maximally forced inspiratory and expiratory manoeuvres.

The FEV_1 is easily measurable and has less variability than other measurements of airways dynamics. Its normal value is predictable from age, gender, and height, and the measured FEV_1 is usually expressed as a percentage of the predicted normal value. All published guidelines use the percentage predicted FEV_1 to determine the degree of airflow obstruction as it declines in direct and linear proportion with clinical worsening of airways obstruction, and is a good predictor of prognosis (see Figure 2.3).

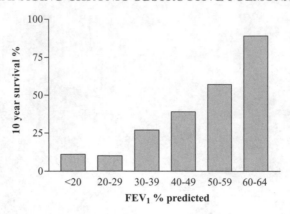

Figure 2.3. Ten-year survival rates in COPD patients who are under the age of 65. *Source*: Adapted from Traver et al. (1979)

The FVC is also easily measured, but is dependent on the expiratory time. The slow or relaxed vital capacity (VC) is the maximal volume of air slowly exhaled from the point of maximal inhalation. In normal subjects these two values are similar, but the FVC is usually lower than the VC in subjects with airways obstruction. In severe COPD, VC values may be larger than FVC values by as much as 1 litre, and some experts advocate the routine use of the VC rather than the FVC. The FEV_1/FVC ratio is the fraction (or the percentage, when multiplied by 100) of the vital capacity that can be exhaled in the first second. As a rough guideline in middle-aged patients, 70 per cent is the lower limit of normal for the FEV_1/FVC ratio. In the mildest degree of airflow obstruction, the FEV_1/FVC ratio falls below 70 per cent and the FEV_1 percentage predicted is normal. However, once a patient has been identified with airways obstruction, the FEV_1/FVC ratio becomes less useful in estimating disease severity, since the FVC also tends to fall with increasing obstruction. Hence, the FEV_1, not the FEV_1/FVC ratio, should be used for following patients with COPD.

The flow–volume loop should always be examined before interpreting spirometric data. Non-reproducible results or poorly performed manoeuvres are easily detected by looking at the flow–volume loop, whilst patients with COPD have a characteristic abnormal contour of the loop. The normal expiratory part of the flow–volume curve consists of a rapid rise to the peak flow rate, followed by a nearly linear fall in flow as the patient exhales out (see Figure 2.4). The inspiratory curve, in contrast, is a relatively symmetrical, saddle-shaped curve. Patients with COPD have a 'scooped-out' or 'concave upwards' pattern in their expiratory loop (see Figure 2.4). Maximal expiratory flow rates during the latter two-thirds of an expiratory manoeuvre are not usually effort-dependent, and are determined more by elastic recoil of the lung and inversely

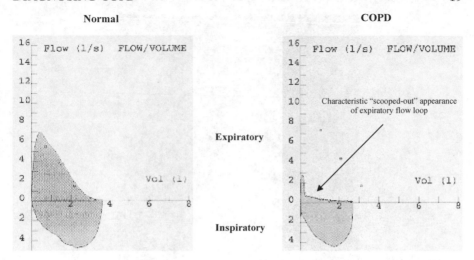

Figure 2.4. Flow–volume loops for a normal subject and a COPD patient

by airway resistance. The characteristic pattern of the flow–volume loop is principally due to reduced elastic recoil of the lung because of destruction to lung parenchyma, and increased airways resistance due to secretions, **broncho-spasm**, or loss of small airways.

RADIOLOGY

All patients with suspected COPD should have a plain chest X-ray at initial diagnostic evaluation. This may show characteristic features of emphysema such as flattened hemi-diaphragms, widened rib spaces, large volume lungs, reduced peripheral vascular markings ('black lungs') and a narrow, long heart shadow. A typical example is seen in Figure 2.5. It must be remembered that the chest X-ray is insensitive in diagnosing COPD, particularly in mild and moderate cases. The principal reason for performing a chest X-ray is to exclude other pathologies, such as bronchiectasis, pulmonary fibrosis or lung cancer. The presence of an abnormal shadow on the X-ray should prompt an urgent referral to a respiratory physician.

Computed tomography (CT) scans, especially high resolution CT (HRCT), have greater sensitivity and specificity than plain chest X-rays for the diagnosis of emphysema. However, in view of the increased cost and larger radiation dose associated with CT scanning compared with plain X-rays, CT scanning is not recommended in the initial routine evaluation of patients with COPD. Respiratory specialists may organise CT or HRCT scans of the thorax in certain situations:

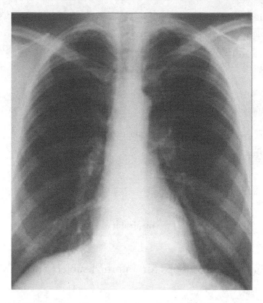

Figure 2.5. A chest X-ray of a patient with COPD

- to further investigate abnormalities seen on a chest X-ray, such as a mass lesion;
- to investigate symptoms out of proportion to spirometric impairment;
- to assess suitability of patient for surgery (**bullectomy**/lung volume reduction surgery). The recent NETT study has demonstrated survival benefits with lung volume reduction surgery in patients with predominantly upper-lobe emphysema and low exercise capacity (Fishman et al. 2003).

OTHER INVESTIGATIONS

A full blood count should be measured in the initial diagnostic evaluation of all patients with suspected COPD (NICE 2004). This is to identify any patients with **anaemia** (a low haemoglobin level) or **polycythaemia** (a high haemoglobin level). Recent evidence suggests that **anaemia** may be associated with a poorer prognosis, with up to 10–15 per cent of severe COPD patients being affected (Similowski et al. 2006). However, there is scanty evidence that blood transfusions are helpful. The prevalence of polycythaemia increases as arterial partial pressure of oxygen falls, and indicates the need for assessment for long-term oxygen therapy. Other blood tests that may be helpful include an alpha-1-antitrypsin level, particularly in patients with early onset disease or with a strong family history. Alpha-1-antitrypsin (AAT) deficiency is a genetically acquired disorder affecting the lung, liver, and rarely skin. The abnormalities in the lungs are indistinguishable from emphysema.

Lung function tests, other than spirometry, may be helpful in cases where diagnosis is unclear or where symptoms appear out of proportion to the abnormalities seen on spirometry. COPD patients tend to be hyperinflated with increased lung volumes (total lung capacity, functional residual capacity and **residual volume**). The **transfer factor** and coefficient for carbon monoxide (T_LCO and **KCO**) are usually reduced in COPD. Pure asthmatics may have obstructive spirometry and increased lung volumes, but have near normal (or even increased) T_LCO and KCO. Highly symptomatic COPD patients with disproportionately low transfer factor and coefficient in relation to spirometry should raise suspicion of a concomitant disease, such as pulmonary fibrosis.

Pulse oximetry is a simple, non-invasive test that is becoming increasingly available in the primary care setting. It should primarily be used as a screening tool; patients with **oxygen saturations** below 93 per cent on room air at rest should be referred for domiciliary long-term oxygen therapy assessment. Patients who show a significant drop in oxygen saturation on exercise should be referred for ambulatory oxygen assessment. Arterial blood gas sampling occurs in the secondary and tertiary care setting, and is commonly used in the management of hospital admissions for COPD. It is also essential in the assessment for suitability for domiciliary long-term oxygen therapy.

The clinical presence of cor pulmonale should prompt further cardiac investigations, such as an electrocardiogram (ECG) and an echocardiogram. An echo can give an estimate of pulmonary artery pressures and right heart function that can be used to assess the severity of cor pulmonale. It must be remembered that a significant proportion of patients with COPD may also have concomitant ischaemic heart disease, and an ECG is an appropriate screening investigation.

Sputum microscopy and culture are rarely helpful in the management of acute exacerbations of COPD as they are relatively insensitive, and a good proportion of exacerbations are secondary to viral infections (Wedzicha 2004). Sputum examination may be helpful in patients who have persistent purulent sputum. The most frequent bacteria found in the sputum are *Streptococcus pneumoniae* and *Haemophilus influenzae*. Other oropharyngeal flora such as *Moraxella catarrhalis* have been shown to cause exacerbations. Persistently positive sputum cultures should alert the health-care professional to a diagnosis of bronchiectasis.

DISTINGUISHING COPD FROM OTHER DISORDERS

A variety of rare disorders may be indistinguishable from COPD in terms of symptoms, signs and spirometry, but are often treated in a similar manner.

Bronchiectasis is a respiratory disorder that can present with cough, shortness of breath, wheeze and chronic sputum production; furthermore, spirometry is often obstructive. The characteristic feature in bronchiectasis is a history of chronic production of large volumes of purulent sputum. There may often be a history of childhood illness (such as measles, whooping cough, pneumonia) or tuberculosis, and symptoms usually start at a slightly earlier age than in COPD. Bronchiectasis is associated with congenital syndromes such as cystic fibrosis, and can sometimes co-exist with COPD. The investigation of choice is a HRCT scan as bronchiectasis has a characteristic appearance.

Differentiating asthma from COPD may also occasionally be difficult, but is a worthwhile exercise, given that the disease processes vary in their response to inhaled corticosteroids. Table 2.1 summarises clinical features that may be used to distinguish between asthma and COPD. Although these features are helpful in untreated patients presenting for the first time, some patients present having been treated with bronchodilators and steroids for many years. Furthermore, chronic asthma that is poorly treated may develop over time into fixed, or poorly reversible, airways obstruction, which is strictly classified as COPD.

A controversial issue in distinguishing COPD from asthma is the value of spirometric reversibility testing following bronchodilator therapy or corticosteroids. In past guidelines, reversibility testing was promoted in the diagnostic process because asthma is deemed a fully reversible disease whilst COPD is only partially reversible. However, there are several problems with this approach. First, it has been recognised that there is natural variability in within-occasion and between-occasion FEV_1 measurements, and it is unknown what level of change in FEV_1 is deemed clinically significant. Second, there is between-occasion variability in bronchodilator response within individuals (Calverley et al. 2003). Finally, the long-term clinical response to bronchodilators or corticosteroids cannot be predicted from acute reversibility testing (Burge et al. 2003; Man et al. 2004). Consequently, the NICE Guidelines do

Table 2.1. Clinical features distinguishing asthma from COPD

Feature	COPD	Asthma
Smoker or ex-smoker	Almost always	Possibly
Symptoms before age 35	Very rare	Often
Breathlessness	Progressive	Variable
Chronic productive cough	Common	Uncommon
Nocturnal waking with wheeze	Uncommon	Common
Significant day-to-day variability	Possibly	Common
Significant diurnal variability of symptoms	Uncommon	Common
Marked response to inhaled steroids	Uncommon	Common

Source: Adapted from the NICE Guidelines (2004)

not recommend routine spirometric reversibility testing in the initial diagnostic process nor in the planning of initial therapy (NICE 2004). Although asthmatic patients can usually be distinguished from the clinical features described in Table 2.1, reversibility testing may be useful in cases of diagnostic difficulty. A diagnosis of COPD is unlikely if there is a very large response in FEV_1 (i.e. over 400 ml) to bronchodilators or corticosteroids, or if FEV_1 and the FEV_1/ FVC ratio return to normal following treatment. If uncertainty remains, other investigations such as transfer factor or CT imaging may be helpful, as previously discussed.

ASSESSING SEVERITY OF COPD

Most national and international guidelines have used spirometry to assess the severity of COPD because FEV_1 is known to predict prognosis (Traver et al. 1979). However, given the heterogeneity of the disease process, it is not surprising to see that FEV_1 is a poor predictor of health status and disability (Jones 2001). Nevertheless, spirometry is readily accessible, easily performed and remains the best objective guide to severity of airflow obstruction. Although the international GOLD guidelines (Pauwels et al. 2001) and the UK NICE Guidelines (2004) vary in the definition of mild, moderate and severe disease, the thresholds of FEV_1 30 per cent predicted and 50 per cent predicted are common to both as they have implications with regard to therapy.

Recently, a multidimensional index (the BODE index) was developed to further assess the risk of death from COPD in an individual patient (Celli et al. 2004). The index comprised four factors:

- **B**ody mass index (BMI)
- **O**bstruction of airways, as measured by FEV_1 per cent predicted
- **D**yspnoea, as measured by the modified MRC Dyspnoea Scale
- **E**xercise capacity, as measured by the 6-minute walk test.

The BODE index was superior to the FEV_1 at predicting the risk of death from any cause and from respiratory causes among patients with COPD. Furthermore, the index was a better predictor of hospitalisation than FEV_1 or the GOLD COPD staging system.

A 6-minute walk test is not practical in the clinical setting, but the BMI, spirometry and the MRC Dyspnoea Scale should be measured routinely in the assessment of disease severity.

SPIROMETRY IN ALL SMOKERS?

As discussed previously, symptoms may not occur in patients until considerable lung function has been lost. Opportunistic case-finding studies in primary care have demonstrated that more than 25 per cent of smokers or ex-smokers over the age of 35 with a chronic cough have a reduced FEV_1 (Van Schayck et al. 2002). Knowledge of abnormal lung function motivates patients sufficiently to improve their smoking cessation rates (Risser & Belcher 1990). The National Clinical Guidelines have recommended opportunistic case-finding in primary care linked with smoking cessation services as a cost-effective strategy. Spirometry should therefore be performed in all current or ex-smokers over 35 years of age, with a chronic cough.

WHEN TO REFER FOR SPECIALIST ADVICE

Many patients come to the attention of specialists either when their disease has progressed to such an extent that symptoms are having a significant impact upon activities of daily living, or patients are hospitalised due to an infective

Table 2.2. When to refer to a respiratory specialist

Reason	Purpose
Diagnosis of COPD suspected or uncertain	Make a diagnosis and optimise treatment
Suspicion of severe disease/rapid worsening of symptoms	Assess severity and optimise treatment
Symptoms out of proportion to spirometry	Look for other explanations, identify additional or alternative pathology
Patient requests second opinion	Make a diagnosis, patient education and optimise treatment
Smoking cessation	Assess and referral to specialist smoking cessation clinic
Suspicion of cor pulmonale	Appropriate investigations and optimise treatment
Assessment for domiciliary oxygen	Optimise therapy, measure arterial blood gases
Assessment for home nebuliser therapy	Optimise therapy, assess inhaler technique, stop unnecessary prescriptions, assess patient
Assessment for surgical intervention	Identify patients suitable for lung transplantation, lung volume reduction surgery, or bullectomy
Diagnosis of COPD in patient younger than forty or with strong family history	Check α-1 antitrypsin deficiency; consider screening family
Pulmonary rehabilitation referral	Identify and assess appropriate candidates
Frequent infections/purulent sputum	Exclude bronchiectasis
Haemoptysis/weight loss	Exclude carcinoma of the bronchus

Source: Adapted from the NICE Guidelines (2004)

exacerbation. In both scenarios, patients will have usually lost a significant amount of lung function such that they are classified as severe. However, a specialist opinion may be helpful at any stage of disease, and not restricted to the management of severe COPD. For example, referral may be required when diagnosis is uncertain, or for accessing specialist treatments such as long-term domiciliary oxygen, pulmonary rehabilitation, domiciliary non-invasive ventilation, and lung volume reduction surgery or lung transplantation. A particular situation where urgent referral is required is in the exclusion of lung cancer, especially when symptoms such as haemoptysis are present. It is important to emphasise that a specialist opinion need not always come from a respiratory physician; other members of the multidisciplinary team with the appropriate training and expertise are often more appropriate for certain referrals, such as in the assessment for pulmonary rehabilitation. Table 2.2 shows possible reasons for specialist referral.

REFERENCES

Burge P S, Calverley P M, Jones P W, Spencer S, Anderson J A (2003) Prednisolone response in patients with chronic obstructive pulmonary disease: results from the ISOLDE study. *Thorax* **58**(8): 654–658.

Calverley P M, Burge P S, Spencer S, Anderson J A, Jones P W (2003) Bronchodilator reversibility in chronic obstructive pulmonary disease. *Thorax* **58**(8): 659–664.

Celli B R, Cote C G, Marin J M, Casanova C, Montes de Oca M, Mendez R A, et al. (2004) The body mass index, airflow obstruction, dyspnea and exercise capacity index in chronic obstructive pulmonary disease. *New England Journal of Medicine* **350**(10): 1005–1012.

Fishman A, Martinez F, Naunheim K, Piantadosi S, Wise R, Ries A, et al. (2003) A randomised trial comparing lung-volume-reduction surgery with medical therapy for severe emphysema. *New England Journal of Medicine* **348**(21): 2059–2073.

Fletcher C M, Elmes P C, Fairbairn A S, Wood C H (1959) The significance of respiratory symptoms and the diagnosis of chronic bronchitis in a working population. *British Medical Journal* **5147**: 257–266.

Jones P W (2001) Health status measurement in chronic obstructive pulmonary disease. *Thorax* **56**(11): 880–887.

Man W D, Mustfa N, Nickoletou D, Kaul S, Hart N, Rafferty G F, et al. (2004) Effect of salmeterol on respiratory muscle activity during exercise in poorly reversible COPD. *Thorax* **59**(6): 471–476.

NICE (2004) National Clinical Guidelines on management of chronic obstructive pulmonary disease in adults in primary and secondary care. *Thorax* **59** Suppl. 1: 1–232.

Nolan D, White P (1999) FEV1 and PEF in COPD management. *Thorax* **54**(5): 468–469.

Pauwels R A, Buist A S, Calverley P M, Jenkins C R, Hurd S S (2001) Global strategy for the diagnosis, management and prevention of chronic obstructive pulmonary disease. NHLBI/WHO Global Initiative for Chronic Obstructive Lung Disease

(GOLD) Workshop Summary. *American Journal of Respiratory and Critical Care Medicine* **163**(5): 1256–1276.

Risser N L, Belcher D W (1990) Adding spirometry, carbon monoxide and pulmonary symptom results to smoking cessation counselling: a randomised trial. *Journal of General Internal Medicine* **5**(1): 16–22.

Scholes A M, Soeters P B, Dingemans A M, Mosteri R, Frantzen P J, Wouters E F (1993) Prevalence and characteristics of nutritional depletion in patients with stable COPD eligible for pulmonary rehabilitation. *American Review of Respiratory Disease* **147**(5): 1151–1156.

Similowski T, Agusti A, MacNee W, Schonhofer B (2006) The potential impact of anaemia of chronic diseases in COPD. *European Respiratory Journal* **27**(2): 390–396.

Traver G A, Cline M G, Burrows B (1979) Predictors of mortality in chronic obstructive pulmonary disease: a 15-year follow-up study. *Review of Respiratory Disease* **119**(6): 895–902.

Van Schayck C P, Loozen J M, Wagena E, Akkermans R P, Wesseling G J (2002) Detecting patients at a high risk of developing chronic obstructive pulmonary disease in general practice: cross-sectional case finding study. *British Medical Journal* **324**(7350): 1370.

Wedzicha J A (2004) Role of viruses in exacerbations of chronic obstructive pulmonary disease. *American Thoracic Society* **1**(2): 115–120.

3 Symptom Management

3.1 PHARMACOLOGICAL MANAGEMENT

PATRICIA YERBURY
King's College Hospital, London

PAUL BAINS
Hammersmith Hospital, London

VIJAY A. SELVAN
King's College Hospital, London

Section 3.1 will highlight the key pharmacological priorities and stepwise management of Chronic Obstructive Pulmonary Disease (COPD) as outlined in the NICE Guidelines (2004). The staging systems for COPD, the objectives and stepwise pharmacological approach to COPD management as well as the importance of patient and device assessment are also addressed. The effects of the various medications will be discussed, including their mechanisms of action, side effect profile, formulations and devices available. The importance of risk management and the need for routine vaccination as well as patient education will also be discussed.

Awareness of COPD as an important chronic disease worldwide has increased due to the publication of international guidelines for both the diagnosis and its management (Ohri and Steiner 2004). The NICE Guideline encompasses all aspects of COPD management across both primary and secondary care, from diagnosis through to the management of exacerbations and complications (NICE 2004). NICE recommendations are graded based on the level of evidence to support their implementation.

NICE have identified key priorities for implementation. The recommendations that specifically relate to drug management include:

- *Use of effective inhaled therapy* – emphasises the role of *long-acting* bronchodilators (**beta$_2$ [B$_2$] agonists** and **anticholinergics**) for the symptomatic relief and improvement in exercise capacity in patients who continue to experience problems despite the use of *short-acting* bronchodilators (B$_2$ agonists and anticholinergics). Inhaled corticosteroids should be added to long-acting bronchodilators to reduce exacerbation frequency in those with an FEV$_1$ of ≤50 per cent predicted who have had two or more exacerbations

Managing Chronic Obstructive Pulmonary Disease. Edited by L. Blackler, C. Jones and C. Mooney
© 2007 John Wiley & Sons Ltd

requiring treatment with antibiotics or oral corticosteroids in the preceding 12-month period.

• *Management of exacerbations* – addresses the appropriate use of inhaled corticosteroids, bronchodilators and vaccinations to help reduce the frequency of exacerbations. Self-management advice on responding promptly to symptoms of an exacerbation with appropriate oral steroids and/or antibiotics are emphasised to minimise the impact of exacerbations.

The NICE Guideline on COPD updates the 1997 British Thoracic Society guidelines (BTS 1997) with a move to treatment decisions being based more on patient symptoms rather than on spirometry readings, since trial results that have shown subjective improvement in breathlessness have not necessarily translated into better spirometry scores. Nevertheless spirometry is still recommended for the diagnosis and assessment of COPD.

STAGING SYSTEMS

Simple staging systems are used to categorise the severity of COPD according to a reduction in FEV_1 (NICE 2004; GOLD 2005). The NICE Guideline defines the severity of airflow obstruction according to the FEV_1 as a percentage of the anticipated normal value as shown in Table 3.1.1.

Such definitions are limited in that they do not describe the disabilities of COPD. Other factors such as patient symptoms including breathlessness, reduced exercise tolerance, frequency and severity of exacerbations, respiratory complications, co-morbidities and general health may prove more significant in reflecting how well patients feel and their quality of life.

OBJECTIVES OF MANAGEMENT

The objectives of COPD management are to do the following:

• prevent disease progression
• relieve symptoms
• improve exercise tolerance, activities of daily living, health status and achieve optimal quality of life
• prevent and treat exacerbations and complications
• reduce morbidity, disability and mortality.

Table 3.1.1. Assessment of severity of airflow obstruction according to FEV_1 as a percentage of the predicted normal value

Severity of airflow obstruction	FEV_1 % predicted
Mild	50–80
Moderate	30–49
Severe	≤30

These should be achieved with minimal adverse effects from treatment. However, this can be difficult since many patients with COPD suffer from co-morbidities that are also increasingly prevalent with age and can be exacerbated by the medications used to treat COPD.

STEPWISE APPROACH IN THE PHARMACOLOGICAL MANAGEMENT

Although there is no cure for COPD, various pharmacological therapies are available for its management. Due to the progressiveness of this chronic condition, a stepwise management plan is inevitably required. It is most important to ensure that all medicines are appropriate according to the guidelines and are efficacious to the patient. Treatment should be monitored closely and adjusted accordingly so as to achieve the goals of the individualised management plan. Choice of drugs should take into account patient preference and ability to use the chosen device, response and efficacy of the drug, side effects experienced as well as cost. Thorough questioning of the patient, in addition to lung function tests, should assess the efficacy of the therapy. All patients should have their therapy and device technique checked prior to initiation and whenever an adjustment is made to therapy, since an inadequate **inhalation** technique may be mistaken for a lack of response to the drug.

Although none of the existing treatments for COPD have been shown to modify the long-term decline in lung function, drug therapy is used to achieve the objectives of COPD management. Long-term oxygen and smoking cessation are the only therapies that have been shown to have a long-term effect on mortality (NICE 2004; BNF 2007). Although COPD is characterised by irreversible airflow obstruction, many patients show clinical benefit from bronchodilators. For this reason the mainstay of treatment is inhaled bronchodilator therapy – B$_2$ agonists and anticholinergics. Patients vary in their response to different therapeutic agents and failure to respond to one should not exclude a trial of another. If no impact on the patient's condition is evident with a particular therapy, then a review with the aim of stopping is essential.

DRUG DELIVERY DEVICES

Drug delivery, for many of the therapies used for the management of COPD, is by inhalation. This is the preferred route of administration since it allows:

- direct drug delivery to the airways;
- smaller doses of medicines being required, leading to fewer systemic side effects;
- fast onset of action.

There are a number of different inhaler devices available and choice will be determined by patient dexterity, preference and acceptability so as to ensure treatment is delivered easily, reliably and consistently. Spacer devices (e.g.

Aerochamber®, Volumatic® and Nebuhaler®) improve drug delivery and deposition to the lungs when used with metered dose inhalers (MDIs) by reducing the need to co-ordinate between the actuation and the inhalation thus allowing more time for the evaporation of the propellant, so allowing a larger proportion of the drug particles to be inhaled and deposited in the lungs. A spacer device also reduces the velocity of the aerosol from the MDI and its impact on the oropharynx, thereby causing less deposition of the drug at the back of the throat (Figure 3.1.1). Spacers are useful for patients with a poor inhaler technique due to poor co-ordination and those prone to **candidiasis**, commonly seen in those on higher doses of inhaled corticosteroids (BNF 2007). The size of the spacer is important, the larger ones with a one-way valve (Volumatic®) being most effective (BNF 2007). It is essential to prescribe a spacer device that is compatible with the chosen MDI. Spacers should be washed monthly for optimal care, and should be replaced every 6–12 months. Haleraids® (placed over MDIs) are available to assist patients who have manual difficulty in actuating the canister (BNF 2007). Breath-actuated aerosol inhalers and dry powder devices (both of which are activated by the patient's inhaled breath) are an option if patients find the MDIs (+/− spacer) difficult to use. On switching from a MDI to a dry powder device, patients may notice a lack of sensation in the mouth and throat previously associated with each actuation of the MDI and coughing may also occur (BNF 2007).

Devices used to deliver inhaled medications are as important as the drug. Effectiveness of therapy will be determined by the correct use of their inhaler device. Patient education as well as the documentation of the use of a variety of inhaler devices should be undertaken so as to ensure selection of the most appropriate device type for the individual. A faulty technique should be rem-

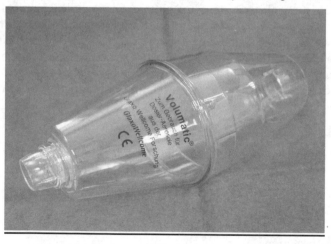

Figure 3.1.1. An example of a Volumatic®. *Source*: Reproduced with permission of GlaxosmithKline. Ventolin, Volumatic, Accuhaler and the Accuhaler device shape are registered trademarks of the GlaxosmithKline group of companies

edied or the patient switched to an alternative device. Dexterity as well as mental ability can limit the efficacy of a chosen device. Most patients will have the ability to acquire and maintain adequate technique, providing they have been given appropriate instructions. Regular assessment and reinstruction are essential from members of the multidisciplinary team.

A nebuliser converts a solution of a drug into an aerosol for inhalation. It allows higher drug doses to be delivered than standard inhalers. The routine use of nebulisers in stable COPD is generally discouraged. They are often the choice when optimal inhaled treatments have failed to achieve therapeutic goals, so are preferable in those who require regular high dose treatment, those with severe or advanced disease with distressing symptoms or for the management of acute exacerbations. In COPD, nebuliser solutions must be driven by air (not oxygen) or by means of a compressor. Nebulisers should be continued only if there is one or more of the following: (1) reduction in symptoms; (2) increase in activities of daily living; (3) increase in exercise capacity; or (4) improvement in lung function.

EFFECTS OF DRUGS IN COPD

The mainstay of drug management of COPD is bronchodilator therapy; bronchodilators relieve breathlessness, cough and wheeze. The main classes of bronchodilator therapy are B_2 agonists and anticholinergics.

Beta₂ (B_2) agonists

This class comprises two types: short- and long-acting B_2 agonists. The most commonly prescribed short-acting B_2 agonists are salbutamol and terbutaline. They work by acting on the **B_2 receptors** in the airway smooth muscle. This leads to relaxation of the airway smooth muscle and subsequent bronchodilation. They are also believed to enhance muco-ciliary clearance. There is no evidence to suggest that one short-acting agent is more effective than another. They have an onset of action of 5–15 minutes and their effects usually last for 3–5 hours (BNF 2007). As their effects are short-lived, they need to be given at least four times a day if used on a regular basis, and, if wheeziness occurs, used additionally as required. Short-acting B_2 agonists are used as relievers providing instant symptomatic relief.

Long-acting B_2 agonists (LABAs) include formoterol and salmeterol. They usually take longer to work than the shorter-acting B_2 agonists and therefore should not be used as relievers. They have a duration of action of approximately 12 hours and so are used twice a day. LABAs are useful and convenient for patients who require regular bronchodilators as their effects last longer and are more effective.

The main adverse effects of B_2 agonists include tremor (particularly affecting the hands), nervous tension, headache, muscle cramps and tachycardia.

These side effects are minimal when the drugs are inhaled at their recommended dose. Plasma potassium should be monitored as these agents may cause potentially serious **hypokalaemia**. Particular caution is required if they are used in high doses, when nebulised or used with concomitant theophylline or its derivatives, corticosteroids (especially oral), diuretics or during a hypoxic episode. Due to the risk of tachycardia, patients' heart rate should also be monitored.

The B_2 agonists are available in a wide variety of formulations and devices including MDIs, breath-actuated aerosol inhalers (Easi-Breathe®), dry powder inhalers (Accuhaler® (Figure 3.1.2), Clickhaler®, Diskhaler®, Turbohaler®) as well as a hard capsule formulation for inhalation (Cyclocaps® for use with the Cyclohaler®), nebuliser solutions, tablets, capsules, liquid and injections (BNF 2007).

Anticholinergics

As with the B_2 agonists there are two main types of anticholinergics – short and long acting. The only short-acting anticholinergic is ipratropium. Anticholinergics work by blocking the cholinergic receptors in the airways. This leads to reduced cholinergic activation of the airway smooth muscle and subsequent bronchodilation. They are also believed to reduce mucus secretion in the airway. They are as effective as B_2 agonists. They have a slower onset of action than the B_2 agonists with a maximum effect 30–60 minutes after use of the

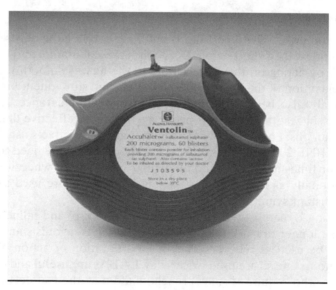

Figure 3.1.2. An example of a breath actuater inhaler. *Source*: Reproduced with permission of GlaxosmithKline. Ventolin, Volumatic, Accuhaler and the Accuhaler device shape are registered trademarks of the GlaxosmithKline group of companies

aerosol inhalation and duration of action of 3–6 hours (BNF 2007). Ipratropium effects are short lived and so it needs to be given three to four times a day if needed on a regular basis. The only long-acting anticholinergic available is tiotropium: due to its long duration of action, it is inhaled once daily.

The main adverse effects of anticholinergics are dry mouth, blurred vision, headache, urinary retention, nausea and constipation. These side effects are minimal and the overall safety profile is favourable when they are inhaled at the recommended dose. When ipratropium is given via a nebuliser, a mouthpiece is preferable to the mask. If a nebuliser mask is used, it must be fitted carefully and used in a well-ventilated environment, since nebulised ipratropium can cause or worsen glaucoma on contact with the eyes.

Anticholinergics are available in a wide variety of formulations and devices (BNF 2007). Ipratropium is available as a MDI, dry powder capsules for inhalation (Aerohaler®) and a nebuliser solution. Tiotropium is only available for inhalation via a dry powder inhaler – HandiHaler®. This device allows the drug to be incorporated into a capsule for inhalation.

Inhaled corticosteroids

Corticosteroids have been shown to be effective in reducing the frequency of exacerbations in patients with severe COPD (GOLD 2005). Inhaled corticosteroids are the preferred delivery route to minimise the adverse effect profile. The NICE Guideline states that inhaled corticosteroids should be added to long-acting bronchodilators to decrease exacerbation frequency in patients with a FEV_1 less than or equal to 50 per cent of the predicted normal value who have had two or more exacerbations requiring treatment with antibiotics or oral corticosteroids in the preceding 12-month period. In such cases, they will usually be combined with a LABA, the combination of which has been shown to be more effective than either drug alone (GOLD 2005). Currently there are two inhalers available which combine a LABA with an inhaled corticosteroid – Symbicort® and Seretide®. Symbicort® is a combination of budesonide and formoterol whereas Seretide® combines fluticasone and salmeterol. These combinations provide greater control of breathlessness so their use is reserved for patients who are still symptomatic despite optimal bronchodilator therapy (see Figure 3.1.3 on p. 36). COPD patients require a higher dosage of inhaled corticosteroids compared to those used for asthma (BNF 2007). Daily doses of 1000 micrograms of fluticasone are often used for COPD patients. Patients on high doses of inhaled corticosteroids should be given a steroid treatment card due to the potential risk of **adrenal suppression**.

Inhaled corticosteroids have considerably fewer systemic adverse effects than oral corticosteroids. The main local adverse effects of inhaled corticosteroids include vocal hoarseness and oral candidiasis, which can be minimised by recommending patients rinse their mouth with water after inhalation and/or by using a spacer device. Systemic adverse effects include adrenal suppression, reduced bone mineral density predisposing to **osteoporosis**, weight gain and oedema. Plasma potassium should be monitored as corticosteroids (especially when given orally) can cause hypokalaemia, which is potentiated when given concomitantly with B_2 agonists, theophylline and its derivatives, diuretics and during hypoxia (BNF 2007).

Of the combination products, Symbicort® is available as a dry powder inhaler (Turbohaler®) while Seretide® is available as a MDI (Evohaler®) and as a dry powder inhaler (Accuhaler®). There are five inhaled corticosteroids currently available (beclometasone, budesonide, ciclesonide, fluticasone and mometasone) none of which are licensed for monotherapy in COPD. They are available in a variety of formulations and devices including MDIs (Becotide®, Becloforte®), breath-actuated inhalers (AeroBec®, Beclazone Easi-Breathe®, Qvar Autohaler®, Qvar Easi-Breathe®), dry powder inhalers (Turbohaler®, Asmabec Clickhaler®, Becodisks®), nebuliser solutions (Budesonide Respules® or Fluticasone Nebules®) and as hard capsules for inhalation via a Cyclohaler® device (BNF 2007).

Oral corticosteroids

Oral steroids (usually prednisolone) are recommended for the management of COPD exacerbations in those patients with a significant increase in breathlessness which affects daily activities and in all hospitalised patients, unless contra-indicated. The recommended dose is 30 mg prednisolone every morning for 7 to 14 days (NICE 2004). Thereafter, the dose is then either stopped abruptly or tapered slowly depending on patients' clinical status, number of previous exacerbations or whether the patient was previously taking maintenance oral steroids. The dose is given once daily in the morning to minimise adrenal suppression and is best given with or after breakfast to reduce gastrointestinal adverse effects. Maintenance doses of oral corticosteroids are not recommended but may be necessary in those patients with advanced disease unable to withdraw from oral steroids following an exacerbation. In such cases, the dose of the corticosteroid should be kept to a minimum and patients over the age of 65 years should be prescribed an osteoporosis prophylactic agent due to the adverse effects of corticosteroids reducing bone mineral density (NICE 2004). Patients on maintenance doses of corticosteroids should be given a steroid card due to the potential risk of adrenal suppression.

Theophylline

Theophylline is a **methylxanthine**. Theophylline acts as a weak bronchodilator and is also thought to increase muco-ciliary clearance and increase diaphragmatic strength. Theophylline has a narrow therapeutic index. This means that usually below a plasma drug level of 10 mg/L, the therapeutic effect may be minimal. Likewise, a plasma drug level greater than 20 mg/L increases the risk of toxicity. Therefore when theophylline is used, the measurement of blood (plasma) theophylline levels is essential, especially when toxicity is suspected. This is known as therapeutic drug monitoring (TDM). TDM is also useful when compliance is questionable and can also be useful when the patient is taking additional medicines that interact with theophylline. Theophylline is generally reserved for patients who are still symptomatic despite optimisation of previously discussed treatments (see Figure 3.1.3 on p. 36).

Theophylline is given by injection as aminophylline, a mixture of 80 per cent theophylline and 20 per cent ethylenediamine; the latter confers greater solubility in water thus making aminophylline twenty times more soluble than theophylline (BNF 2005).

The main adverse effects of theophylline include nausea, gastrointestinal disturbances, headache, insomnia, tachycardia, palpitations, arrhythmias and convulsions, especially if given rapidly by intravenous injection. Adverse effects to ethylenediamine include **urticaria**, **erythema** and exfoliative dermatitis.

Plasma potassium should be monitored as theophylline can cause hypokalaemia which is potentiated when given concomitantly with B_2 agonists, corticosteroids, diuretics and during hypoxia (BNF 2007). Patients' heart rate should also be monitored due to the possibility of tachycardia and arrhythmias.

Theophylline is available as modified release tablets (Nuelin SA®, Uniphyllin Continus®) and capsules (Slo-Phyllin®) (BNF 2007). Aminophylline is also available as modified release tablets (Phyllocontin Continus®, Amnivent® and Norphyllin®) (BNF 2007). It is important that theophylline and aminophylline are prescribed by their respective brand names due to differences in the bioavailability of the various brands available. Aminophylline injection is reserved for acute severe exacerbations of COPD. If the patient is currently taking an oral form of theophylline, a plasma theophylline level must be obtained before administering intravenous aminophylline. Doses will be determined according to plasma levels and patient symptoms.

Mucolytics

This class appears for the first time in UK clinical guidelines. Oral mucolytic drugs (BNF 2007) include carbocisteine (Mucodyne®) and mecysteine (Visclair®) that have been shown to reduce the number of exacerbations in patients with COPD and a chronic productive cough. They work by reducing sputum viscosity. They are reserved for those who have a chronic productive cough, but should be discontinued after a one-month trial if there is no symptomatic improvement of their cough and sputum production. Patients should monitor the quantity of sputum production, colour, ease of expectoration and amount of coughing. Adverse effects are rare but include gastrointestinal irritation and skin rashes. This class of drug should be avoided in patients with active peptic ulcer disease.

Antibiotics

Antibiotics are used to treat exacerbations of COPD associated with a history of more purulent sputum or clinical evidence of **pneumonia**.

NICE GUIDELINES

NICE outlines an algorithm for the pharmacological management of COPD based upon breathlessness and exercise limitation as well as frequent exacerbations. This is summarised in Figure 3.1.3. The co-administration of tiotro-

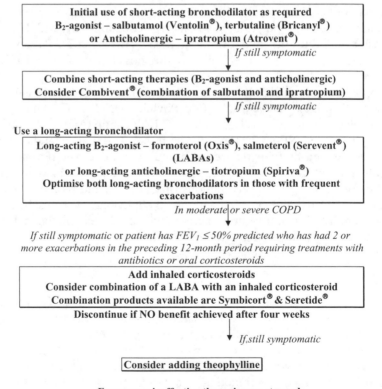

Figure 3.1.3. Summary of stepwise pharmacological approach to COPD treatment

pium (unless contra-indicated) with ipratropium should be avoided as they are within the same therapeutic class of drugs.

VACCINATIONS AND ANTI-FLU TREATMENTS

The Department of Health (DoH) advocates that all patients with chronic respiratory disease (unless contra-indicated) are vaccinated with the annual influenza vaccine as well as the pneumococcal vaccine which have been shown to reduce health-care use and may prevent exacerbations (DoH 2003; BNF 2007). Within their licensed indications, zanamivir and oseltamivir are recommended for at-risk patients who present with influenza-like illness within 48 hours of onset of symptoms. Patients with COPD should have a short-acting bronchodilator (e.g. salbutamol) available when using zanamivir because of the risk of bronchospasm (NICE 2004).

PATIENT EDUCATION AND ADVICE

Patient education plays a major role in the management of COPD and should incorporate thorough counseling and explanation of the medication regimen to enhance patients' overall knowledge and compliance to treatment. It can help improve patients' ability to cope with their illness and health status as well as improve their understanding of COPD and its progression. Patients should be advised to manage their symptoms associated with an exacerbation by promptly starting appropriate rescue treatment with oral steroids and/or antibiotics, as well as adjusting their bronchodilator therapy that may prevent hospital admissions.

"I forgot which inhaler does what and they keep changing them."

CONCLUSION

Overall management of COPD is a challenge to all involved. COPD causes considerable morbidity and mortality. It is important to identify patients at risk at an early stage and reduce their risk factors such as smoking. Management of COPD aims to control symptoms with the expectation that a stepwise increase in therapy will occur resulting in multiple therapies to achieve therapeutic goals. To date, none of the drug therapies alter the long-term decline in lung function or underlying disease process. At each stage a clinical assessment should be undertaken, addressing effects of drug therapy as well as inhaler technique. Treatments should be optimised accordingly so as to achieve the patient's individual goals, and discontinued if proven ineffective after a reasonable assessment period. Patient education and self-management advice are paramount and should be given to patients to ensure they have an understanding of their illness so they can improve their overall compliance to therapy and respond promptly to an exacerbation to help prevent potential hospital admissions.

3.2 ADHERENCE/CONCORDANCE

CAROLINE MOONEY
Luton Treatment Centre, Luton

The terms 'compliance and adherence' are generally used interchangeably in the literature (Kettler et al. 2002). However, it is argued that there is an important difference between them (Meichenbaum & Turk 1987). Compliance is defined as 'the extent to which patients are obedient and follow the instructions, proscriptions and prescriptions of health care professionals' (Meichenbaum & Turk 1987), while adherence is defined as 'the extent to which a person's behaviour (in terms of taking medications, following diets or executing lifestyle changes) coincides with medical and health advice' (Haynes 1979).

Patient non-adherence is one of the best documented but least understood health-related behaviours (George et al. 2005). There are many factors in the literature identified as risk factors for non-adherence:

- *Disease*
- *Marital status*
- *Age*
- *Patients' belief*: Patients are more likely to adhere to treatments when they perceive that treatment makes sense, in light of their personal beliefs (with past illness and/or current symptoms) (Leventhal et al. 1992). They often evaluate their treatments by weighing up the benefits against costs (Pound et al. 2005). Benefits, in terms of symptom relief, relapse avoidance, or disease progression are compared against the side effects of the treatment regimen, and consequences on daily living.
- *Co-morbidities*: These are common among patients with COPD. For this, they are often prescribed complex medication regimens by multiple routes for both respiratory and non-respiratory conditions (Dolce et al. 1991).
- *Depression*: Depression is a common co-morbidity in patients with COPD (Van Mannen et al. 2002) and is a known risk factor for non-adherence (Di Matteo et al. 2000).

CONSEQUENCES OF NON-ADHERENCE

The consequences of poor adherence are significant (Abbott & Gee 1998). Cluss and Epstein (1985) cited 'exacerbation of disability, progression of disease, more frequent medical emergencies, unnecessary prescriptions of more potent and toxic drugs and ultimately, failure of treatment' as consequences of poor adherence to medical regimens and treatments.

Among COPD patients, poor adherence to drug therapy and disease management programmes has been identified as the major factor resulting in emergency hospital admissions (Col et al. 1990). However, the EFRAM study (Garcia-Aymerich et al. 2001) did not find an association in COPD patients between poor compliance and risk of admission.

Several factors predispose COPD patients to non-adherence (George et al. 2005). Management of COPD is complex, with patients needing to make behavioural and lifestyle changes such as stopping smoking and adherence to exercise therapy along with optimal medication adherence (Pauwels et al. 2001).

ADHERENCE AND MEDICATION

Dolce et al. (1991) state that it is quite common for patients to be prescribed as many as 5–8 oral and inhaled medications to be taken at different intervals, either regularly or as needed. Rand et al. (1995) suggest that four times a day dosing leads to diminished compliance. It is suggested that, wherever possible, regimens should be simplified (Mellins et al. 1992).

Many researchers have reported that the inhaler technique in patients with obstructive lung disease is inadequate, with the percentage of patients using their inhalers therapeutically ranging between 10–85 per cent (van der Palen et al. 1995). With incorrect inhaler technique, much of the medication never reaches the lungs, leading to reduced medication effectiveness, excessive medication use and increased costs (National Heart, Lung and Blood Institute 1997).

Patients may also rely on inaccurate methods of determining whether a pressurised metered-dose inhaler (PMDI) canister is empty, such as by shaking the inhalers or estimating the weight of the canisters. In one such study (Ogren et al. 1995), 54 per cent of patients surveyed were unaware of the maximum number of actuations listed by the manufacturer for the PMDIs they were using, and only 8 per cent reported counting the number of actuations used.

Rubin et al. (2004) state that patients are rarely instructed to count the number of doses used throughout the life of a PMDI inhaler and to discard the inhaler once the stated maximum number of puffs are used, even though this is the only accurate method to tell when a canister should be discarded. However, in practice, for inhaled medications that are taken 'as required' counting doses is difficult and is often inaccurate. For this reason, they state that devices with built-in dose counters will have a great impact in the effectiveness of the inhaled drug delivery.

The NCCCC Guidelines suggest that most patients can learn to use an inhaler of some sort, if they receive adequate instruction. The exception to this is patients with cognitive impairment (Allen 1992). The use of a spacer could overcome difficulties with co-ordination, however due to the size there may be problems with portability and it can be seen as inconvenient. It is therefore argued that a small volume spacer (e.g. Aero chamber or Able-spacer) or a dry powder inhaler can be a useful and effective alternative (Booker 2003).

Patients need to be able to use the inhaler effectively and it needs to fit in with their lifestyle. Technique must be taught and regularly checked by a competent health-care professional (NCCCC 2004). Interiano and Guntupalli (1993) found that respiratory care practitioners were the most knowledgable of health-care providers in teaching people how to use inhalers.

The NCCCC (2004) has made several recommendations for the use of placebo inhaler devices in clinical practice:

• Patients should be reminded to bring all of their inhaler devices with them to each review.
• Placebo and spacer devices should never be used for different patients where there is a known infection control risk.
• As far as reasonably practicable, all devices should be single patient use.
• However, if placebo devices are used for more than one patient, they must be decontaminated each time they are used.

ADHERENCE AND NEBULISERS

Patients with COPD who are given domiciliary nebulisers are those who are experiencing high levels of morbidity and whose symptoms are not fully controlled by medications delivered by handheld devices. Despite this, Bosley et al. (1996) found that they are no more likely than other patient groups to take their medications as often as prescribed. They found that increased impairment in quality of life was associated with poor adherence to treatment; they suggest that adherence is not consequent on previous experience of illness but is related to current problems.

SELF-MANAGEMENT

The NICE Guidelines (NCCCC 2004) suggest that patients at risk of exacerbations should be given self-management advice to enable them to respond promptly in the event of exacerbations by:

• starting oral corticosteroids if their increased breathlessness interferes with their normal activities of living;
• starting antibiotics if their sputum becomes purulent;
• adjusting their bronchodilator therapy to control their symptoms.

However, a Cochrane review of educating patients with COPD on self-management did not find any effect on the number of hospital admissions, A&E attendances, days of work, and lung function (Monninkhof et al. 2003).

It found that self-management plans may result in greater use of short courses of oral corticosteroids and antibiotics for exacerbations and less use of short-acting bronchodilators for relief of acute symptoms (Monninkhof et al. 2003).

METHODS TO IMPROVE ADHERENCE

The Medicines Partnership (Carter 2003) drew a number of conclusions about non-adherence. One of the main reasons for non-adherence was a complex regimen. Van der Palen et al. (1999) carried out a study on the influence of the use of different types of inhalers. They recommend that 'whenever possible, only one type of inhaler should be prescribed'.

The aim of multicompartment medication compliance devices is to improve patient adherence to oral medication. They are designed to improve easy access to medication, to organise treatment regimens as well as to remind patients. McGraw (2004) carried out a review on the effectiveness of multi-compartment compliance devices and compliance. She found that there was limited evidence of effect, as a single focus intervention for people with poor adherence.

Education alongside adherence aids such as medicating lists and dossette boxes are also methods to improve compliance (George et al. 2005).

CONCLUSION

COPD is a disease that predisposes patients to non-adherence with treatment. The consequences of non-adherence are significant.

It is suggested that when prescribing, health-care professionals should address adherence as a vital part of their consultation. Health-care profession-als should ensure that treatment regimens are simplified as much as possible. They should also provide a high standard of patient education about their treatment regimens (Rand et al. 1995), in order to improve adherence. The importance of checking inhaler technique has been discussed, and it is impera-tive that individuals are taught by a competent health-care professional, to ensure therapeutic administration of inhaled medication. Whenever possible, aids to improve adherence should also be adopted.

3.3 NEBULISED THERAPY AT HOME

CHRISTINE JONES
King's College Hospital, London

Nebuliser treatments are frequently used in hospital during an acute exacerba-tion of COPD but also used at home where patients are unable to use an inhaler device effectively.

The indications for nebulised therapy and its use in the treatment of chronic airflow limitation will be discussed in this section. A suggested protocol for a nebuliser trial will be given and the care and management of the nebuliser system, with guidelines for follow-up for clinicians, will be presented. This section lays down a suggested protocol for the prescribing of nebulised therapy drawing on the recommendations contained in the British Thoracic Society Guidelines (BTS 1997).

WHAT IS A NEBULISER?

A nebuliser allows the patient to administer a therapeutic dose of a drug in the form of fine aerosol mist, which is penetrated into the lungs through inhalation over a short period of time, usually 5–10 minutes (BTS 1997).

The term 'nebuliser' simply refers to the small plastic chamber in which the drug is placed; however, the word is used loosely to describe the compressor, mouthpiece and facemask. There are many types of nebulisers available in the United Kingdom and all are given in a paper entitled 'Selecting and using nebuliser equipment' on pages S92–S101 (Kenderick et al. 1997), but all systems have four main parts to the unit (Figure 3.3.1):

- the compressor: this is the power source which supplies the nebuliser with the gas or air to convert the drug into a fine mist;
- the nebuliser chamber holds the medicine and changes it into a fine mist;
- the mouthpiece and/or facemask;
- the oxygen tubing.

CLINICAL INDICATIONS FOR NEBULISER THERAPY

Nebulisers are prescribed when:

- patients with severe airflow limitation require high doses of bronchodilator therapy;
- inhaled antibiotics and other medicines cannot be delivered by other means;
- patients are unable to use inhaler devices.

NEBULISERS VERSUS INHALERS – WHICH IS BETTER?

Jenkins et al. (1987) studied a group of patients with severe airflow limitation comparing equivalent doses of nebulised salbutamol and salbutamol administered by a metered dose inhaler. The results demonstrated no clear advantage of nebulisers over metered dose inhalers and Gunawardena (1986) produced similar findings. Although taking 12–50 actuations via a hand-held device is equivalent to a nebulised dose, patients and health professionals prefer nebulised treatment particularly in the acute situation. This is for a number of

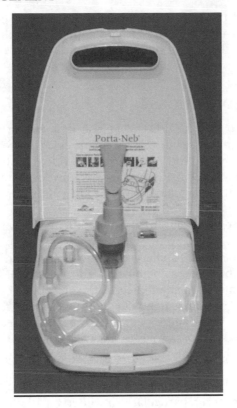

Figure 3.3.1. An example of a nebuliser. © Picture courtesy of Respironics (UK) Ltd

reasons. First, it provides reassurance to the staff that even with tidal breathing the entire drug will be inhaled and no extra demands are placed on the patient (Muers 1997). Second, it is not only time saving but it frees the practitioner to undertake other duties instead of having to stand and supervise each actuation by administering multiple doses from a pressurised metered dose inhaler and spacer. Therefore it is generally accepted that the bronchodilation obtained is largely a reflection of the dose of the bronchodilator administered rather than the mode of administration (Mestitz et al. 1989).

THE USE OF NEBULISED BRONCHODILATOR THERAPY IN ACUTE EXACERBATION OF COPD

BTS guidelines recommend that nebulised bronchodilators should be administered on arrival to the accident and emergency (A&E) department at 4–6-hourly intervals. This should be continued for 24–48 hours until the patient has improved clinically, and once the patient has recovered from the acute episode, nebulised therapy should be stopped. Inhaler technique should be assessed and the patient converted to the appropriate delivery device.

It is advised that the patient should be observed for a period of 24–48 hours using an inhaler prior to discharge (BTS 1997).

SPECIAL CONSIDERATIONS

Some patients who have COPD are at risk of hypercarbia or acidosis and should have their nebuliser driven by compressed air, or via an air-driven nebuliser system. This will prevent carbon dioxide retention that is sensitive to high levels of oxygen. Patients can receive low levels of oxygen, 1–2 litres, via nasal equipment during nebulisation. This will prevent the fall in oxygen while using the nebuliser (BTS 1997).

When **anticholinergic** agents are used in patients known to have glaucoma, there is a risk that, if the ipratropium bromide gets into the eye, there is a possibility that prolonged papillary dilatation can occur. The risk increases when ipratropium bromide is combined with salbutamol. Therefore it is suggested for all patients that a mouthpiece is the preferable option. If a facemask is to be used, then it should be tightly sealed to the face so that the mist doesn't go directly into the eyes (Kenderick et al. 1997). It is advised that a mouthpiece is used for nebulised corticosteroids as this will reduce the risk of skin and eye exposure. Rinsing the mouth will prevent soreness and oral candidiasis from developing.

Ischaemic heart disease is commonly found among the elderly population. Hypokalaemia can occur particularly in elderly patients who have a poor dietary intake and are on diuretics. Oral theophylline can also cause hypokalaemia and the level of theophylline must be monitored. The health-care professional needs to be aware that delivering a high dose of a beta$_2$ agonist via a nebuliser may cause dysrhythmias and tremor in the elderly. The BTS Guidelines suggest that high doses of B$_2$ agonist should be avoided unless absolutely necessary (Pounsford 1997).

NEBULISER ASSESSMENT

O'Driscoll (1997) recommends that before the individual is supplied with a nebuliser system, they should be fully assessed by a respiratory specialist or general practitioner (GP).

The first step is to confirm the diagnosis and severity of COPD by undertaking lung function tests, asking the patient to record their baseline level of symptoms: see the nebuliser assessment chart (Box 3.3.1). This involves the patient monitoring their peak expiratory flow, using a peak flow meter, and the symptoms they experience. The individual's ability to use a spacer and metered dose inhaler should be assessed, as well as the use of any hand-held device. Optimising existing inhaled therapy is strongly recommended prior to a nebuliser trial.

A suggested protocol is:

Week 1: high dose bronchodilator with volumatic
Week 2: 2.5–5 mg salbutamol or terbutaline 5–10 mg four times a day
Week 3: nebulised anticholinergic.

In week 1, the high doses of bronchodilator therapy should be administered via a dry powdered device metered dose inhaler and spacer with 1 mg terbutaline or 400 ug salbutamol and 160 ug ipratropium bromide four times a day.

In the second week a formal trial of a home nebuliser should be undertaken. The guidelines suggest for example 2.5–5 mg salbutamol or 5–10 mg terbutaline four times a day, or ipratropium bromide 0.25–0.5 mg four times a day or a combination of these treatments (O'Driscoll 1997).

The clinician then assesses the patient's response to these treatments and decides whether the individual has received adequate subjective and objective benefit to justify the cost of issuing a machine (O'Driscoll et al. 1990; Goldman et al. 1992).

MAINTENANCE OF NEBULISER MACHINE AT HOME

If a nebuliser and compressor machine have been given for long-term use, then the patient and carer need to be instructed in how to set up the nebuliser, in the cleaning of equipment, and local arrangements for servicing and replacements. All written instructions should also include telephone numbers for emergency replacement.

Instructions to be given to the patient and carer include:

- It is recommended that the nebuliser system should be kept on a firm surface: if kept on the floor, cold dusty air will be drawn into the machine and is liable to cause a chest infection.
- The compressor and unit can be kept clean by wiping the inside and outside about once a week with a damp cloth, making sure the compressor is disconnected from the mains. The compressor and tubing must never be immersed in water.
- A practical demonstration on how to keep the delivery system clean should include how to disassemble the nebuliser. This should be immersed in warm soapy water on a daily basis and should be rinsed and dried thoroughly.
- The facemask or mouthpiece should also be washed in warm water, rinsed and left to dry about 2–3 times a week. The tubing does not need to be washed. After drying the nebuliser, reassemble it by connecting it to the

compressor and turn it on for 10–15 seconds as this will blow air through the nebuliser, drying any excess residue.

- If the nebuliser or equipment is dirty or moist, this can allow bacteria to breed and cause the patient to develop an infection.
- It is advisable to change the nebuliser, tubing and facemasks/mouthpieces every three months: this is essential to ensure the nebuliser is working efficiently.
- A durable nebuliser lasts for 12 months and should be boiled for 5–10 minutes in water with a little detergent after every 30 uses.
- If the nebuliser is taking more than 15–20 minutes to deliver per treatment, then equipment is faulty. The patient should be advised to try a new nebuliser system; this includes the mask/mouthpiece, nebuliser pot and tubing.
- It is essential that the patient always keeps a spare set in reserve: if changing the nebuliser system does not help, then the patient will need to contact the respiratory department to have the compressor checked.
- Patients should have a spacer and a metered dose inhaler for emergency use. They should be educated in how to administer doses equivalent to a nebuliser dose.

There is no clear indication of when nebulisation has finished, therefore it is suggested that patients should be educated to nebulise until spluttering occurs and then to continue for a further minute, tapping the side of the nebuliser chamber so that large particles are encouraged to fall back into the nebuliser chamber (BTS 1997).

Each nebuliser system will have a filter, the aim is that the filter cleans the air as it is drawn into the machine. If the filter becomes blocked, the machine will be less efficient, therefore it is strongly recommended that the instruction manual be followed for the time of replacement.

The compressors should be serviced at least annually; this is the sole responsibility of the individual to return the machine to the hospital on the date marked for servicing.

HOW TO SET UP A NEBULISER

1 Connect the plastic tubing to the compressor, unscrew the two halves of the nebuliser chamber and pour the medication into the bottom half.
2 Screw the two halves back together and connect to the plastic tubing, and attach either the facemask or mouthpiece.
3 Plug the compressor into the mains and switch on the machine.
4 Hold the nebuliser in an upright position to prevent spilling. On some compressors there is an allotted slot on the compressor that the nebuliser can be attached to while the patient settles into a comfortable position.

PURCHASING A NEBULISER MACHINE

Patients should not be encouraged to purchase their own machines but if they wish to buy one, they need to discuss with their GP whether they would be willing to prescribe the drugs to put into the nebuliser. If this is the case, the GP or prescribing physicians need to ensure the patient is assessed in the same way before long-term treatment commences.

If the individual intends to buy a machine, the British Lung Foundation produces an information sheet with the names of suppliers in the UK, although the list is not exhaustive. They can also be bought via the internet; however, this should be done with caution.

In buying or choosing a suitable nebuliser, it is important to consider what the nebuliser system will be used for. High-powered nebuliser systems should be used for antibiotics, but steroids and bronchodilators can be delivered with medium- or high-powered systems.

TRAVEL

In the UK the compressors are designed to be used with 220–240 volts (v). In other parts of the world, including some parts of South America, the USA and Middle Eastern countries, the voltage is usually 100/110 v. Therefore, it is advisable to check with the travel agent the power source of the country one wishes to travel to. There are a few nebuliser systems that are multivolt and can run at 100/110 v or on a 12v DC source for use with car batteries (Kenderick et al. 1997). Portable compressors which run off batteries or a car cigarette lighter can be purchased or hired from some respiratory units that loan the individual the nebuliser system.

FOLLOW-UP ASSESSMENTS

The BTS Guidelines (1997) suggest that the patient should be reviewed in a clinic or in surgery within three months of starting the treatment and then at least annually to determine if the treatment is effective and necessary. This evaluation should include an assessment of breathlessness and symptoms, and whether the patient has experienced any side effects. It is a good opportunity to assess if the individual can demonstrate effective use of the nebuliser system (BTS 1997). Box 3.3.1 presents an example of an assessment form to be completed by the patient.

CONCLUSION

Patients with severe airflow limitation may benefit from nebulised therapy; however, every effort should be made to optimise existing therapy first and to ensure that the individual is able to use their hand-held devices correctly. Once

Box 3.3.1. Assessment form

NAME: ....

HOSPITAL

NO: ....

DOB: ....

START DATE: ....

INHALER OR NEBULISER: ....

		DAY	1	2	3
PEAK FLOW FILL IN EVERY MORNING AND EVENING 20 MINUTES AFTER INHALER OR NEBULISER	MORNING	DATE			
		BEST PEAK FLOW			
Perform the test three times in the morning and three times in the evening and record the best value out of the three each time	EVENING	BEST PEAK FLOW			
SYMPTOMS FILL IN EVERY EVENING	COUGH & WHEEZE AT NIGHT				
RECORD ONE NUMBER IN EACH BOX TO REPRESENT YOUR SYMPTOMS OVER THE LAST 24 HOURS 0–none 1–mild 2–moderate 3–severe	DAY-TIME COUGH				
	DAY-TIME WHEEZE				
	BREATHLESSNESS ON EXERCISE				
	PHLEGM PRODUCTION				
MEDICINE FOR ASTHMA/ AIRWAYS OBSTRUCTION	INHALER A				
FILL IN EVERY EVENING	INHALER B				
Record the total number of puffs or tablets of each drug taken in the last 24 hours.	NEBULISER				
e.g. If you took 2 puffs of an inhaler 4 times a day, then record 8	OTHER				
	OTHER				

all options have been explored, then a nebuliser trial should be considered as suggested with monitoring of the symptoms, and those with clear benefit should be considered for a nebuliser loan (Pearson 2001).

3.4 LONG-TERM OXYGEN THERAPY

LAURA BLACKLER
Guy's and St Thomas' Hospital, London

Long-term oxygen therapy (LTOT) is defined by the British Thoracic Society (BTS 2005) as 'the provision of oxygen therapy for the continuous use at home by patients with chronic hypoxaemia'. A large number of people with COPD will develop day-time hypoxaemia at rest as their disease progresses and this is related to a poor prognosis. There have been various studies looking at the processes that lead to the problems with gas exchange and these have led to the use of continuous oxygen to maintain the **PaO_2** above 8.0 kPa (Calverley 2000). In the 1980s there were two significant randomised control trials (RCTs) that looked at the effectiveness of continuous oxygen therapy for patients with severe hypoxaemia. A study carried out by the Nocturnal Oxygen Therapy Trial Group in 1980 compared the use of continuous oxygen with nocturnal oxygen and found that there was a substantial reduction in mortality in those who had continuous oxygen. A randomised controlled trial undertaken by the Medical Research Council (1981) showed that there was a significant reduction in mortality over 5 years in individuals with severe day-time hypoxaemia (PaO_2 5.3–8.0 kPa) who had at least 15 hours of oxygen therapy per day. Despite both studies being over 20 years old, the results are still the basis for evidence-based practice in the use of LTOT.

"I never used to sleep until I got the oxygen."

Other RCTs showed that there was no significant difference in mortality following the use of long-term domiciliary oxygen in those with mild to moderate hypoxaemia (Gorecka et al. 1997; Chaouat et al. 1999). However, in a pilot study carried out by Haidi et al. (2004), results showed that patients with reversible hypercapnia and mild hypoxaemia benefited from LTOT because it improved endurance and reduced dyspnoea after 1 year.

A systematic review was carried out by Cranston et al. (2005) and confirms that there have been no studies which have disproved the results above and home oxygen can improve the survival in patients with severe hypoxaemia.

LTOT is not recommended for those who still smoke, due to the fire hazard. Therefore, it is important to establish if the patient is still smoking or living with anyone who smokes and the health-care professional should discuss the safety aspects.

ADHERENCE TO LTOT

There have been discussions about the poor level of adherence to oxygen therapy despite the number of studies that have shown the benefits. Reasons for poor adherence have been suggested: the equipment is heavy, cumbersome and bulky; loss of taste and smell through the use of nasal equipment. However, there is a dearth of evidence about the rationale for non-adherence. In 2002, Earnest undertook a study to look at this and found that adhering to oxygen therapy was difficult and complex. Users evolved their level of adherence over time but the use of supplementary oxygen meant compromises in their lifestyle. This would suggest that while it has been proved clinically that LTOT improves quality of life through physiological measurements it is important to consider the impact of LTOT on an individual's life and how this may affect their adherence to the therapy.

OXYGEN PRESCRIPTION – LTOT

Oxygen must be prescribed and the following should be considered:

- What is the correct dose – oxygen concentration?
- Which is the most appropriate delivery system?
- Is humidification necessary?
- What type and frequency of monitoring are required – arterial blood gas, pulse oximetry?
- What are the parameters to be maintained/achieved?

ASSESSMENT PROCESS FOR LTOT

The following conditions are necessary:

- confident diagnosis of a disorder associated with chronic hypoxaemia;
- optimal medical management and clinical stability for at least 5 weeks;
- arterial blood gas – PaO_2 is consistently at or below 7.3 kPa:
  - measured on two occasions at least three weeks apart;
  - measured after breathing air for at least 30 minutes if they have had any supplementary oxygen.

The patient must be referred to a service directed by a consultant physician with an interest in respiratory medicine for arterial blood gas measurement and assessment for LTOT (BTS 2005).

EQUIPMENT

From 1 February 2006, a new home oxygen therapy service is available 24 hours a day to streamline the provision of oxygen and equipment. There are now 10 oxygen 'regions' which each have a single contractor to provide an

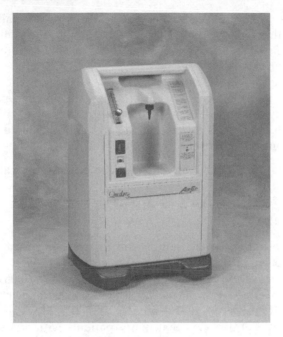

Figure 3.4.1. An example of an oxygen concentrator. *Source*: Photo courtesey of AirSep Corporation

integrated service for patients, clinicians and primary care trusts. The following equipment is used:

- *Oxygen cylinders*: for use by those who only require intermittent oxygen.
- *Oxygen concentrator*: if an individual requires oxygen for more than 8 hours per day (or 21 cylinders per month), it is more cost-effective to provide a concentrator (Figure 3.4.1).
- *Conserver*: a conserver device is essentially a machine that is attached to an oxygen cylinder. However, the benefit of having this device is that it only releases oxygen when a person inhales. Therefore, there is less wastage, so cylinders can last between 3–5 times longer.
- *Liquid oxygen*: this does not need a power source to operate it; therefore it is useful in locations where the power supply can be intermittent. It is less bulky than the equivalent capacity of high-pressure gaseous storage – 1 litre of liquid oxygen = 860 gaseous litres.

OXYGEN DELIVERY SYSTEMS

The following pieces of equipment are used:

- *Nasal cannulae*: patients with COPD often prefer to wear these rather than a mask, because they are comfortable to use over long periods and patients can still continue to have oxygen whilst eating, drinking and talking. The FiO_2 depends on the flow rate and will vary according to the ventilatory minute volume. The flow rate should not be any more than 4 l/minute because it can cause irritation in the nasal passage.

• **Venturi valve and mask** (low-flow mask): the equipment valves use the principle of jet mixing. Oxygen passes through the narrow opening, creating a high-velocity stream that draws a constant proportion of room air through the base of the valve; this means that the amount of inspired oxygen can be accurately controlled between 24–60 per cent.

Most people requiring LTOT can manage with either the nasal equipment or a low-flow mask.

AMBULATORY OXYGEN THERAPY

This is the provision of oxygen therapy during exercise and activities of daily living. It can be prescribed for those patients on LTOT who are mobile and need to or can leave the house on a regular basis (BTS 2005). Studies have shown that it is effective in increasing the exercise capacity and reducing breathlessness (Leach et al. 1992; Eaton et al. 2002). However, surveys have shown (McDonald et al. 1995) that many patients with ambulatory oxygen therapy do not spend much time outside their home and use it infrequently, therefore it is important to ascertain the level of outside activity so that the most effective and economical device is provided (BTS 2005).

Under the new procedures for providing ambulatory oxygen therapy patients' requirements have been divided into three categories:

1 Grade 1 – LTOT low activity: This group of patients is mainly housebound, requires LTOT up to 24 hours per day, and only requires ambulatory oxygen occasionally (Figure 3.4.2). The flow rate will be the same as used with LTOT at home.
2 Grade 2 – LTOT active group: This is for patients who require LTOT but are mobile and need to leave home on a regular basis (Figure 3.4.3). An assessment will determine the flow rate and type of device suitable.
3 Grade 3 – Non-LTOT: This group of patients should only be considered for ambulatory oxygen if there is evidence that there is:
   (a) exercise oxygen desaturation
   (b) improvement in exercise capacity
   (c) less breathlessness.

An assessment will determine the flow rate and type of device suitable.

ASSESSMENT PROCESS FOR AMBULATORY OXYGEN THERAPY

A hospital specialist should only prescribe ambulatory oxygen therapy after an assessment. At present, the assessment is designed to look at the short-term

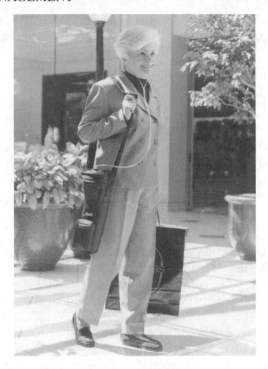

Figure 3.4.2. An example of portable oxygen. *Source*: Photo courtesey of AirSep Corporation

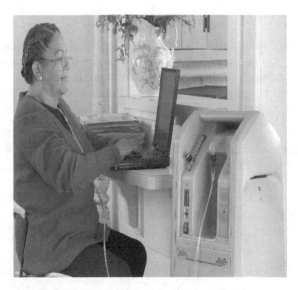

Figure 3.4.3. Living with long-term oxygen therapy. *Source*: Photo courtesey of AirSep Corporation

response to supplementary oxygen therapy, where the patient does an exercise test, e.g. six-minute walking test – see Chapter 5 for more information about this test (NCCCC 2004)

PATIENT EDUCATION

When a decision has been made to provide LTOT or ambulatory oxygen, it is essential that the patient and relative/carer are given both written and verbal information about the reason for the use of oxygen at home and the principles of oxygen therapy. This can be provided by anyone within the MDT (nurse, doctor, physiotherapist, contractor, etc.) in relation to the individual and should include the following:

- reason for LTOT/ambulatory oxygen;
- length of time it should be used and why;
- flow rate and explanation of the principles behind this;
- principles of the use of ambulatory oxygen;
- explanation of how the oxygen concentrator/cylinder works;
- demonstration of the method of refilling and maintenance of portable equipment;
- home service agreements and electricity reimbursement;
- dangers of smoking in the presence of the oxygen equipment;
- contact number of the nurse specialist/physiotherapist/technician;
- advice on travel with oxygen therapy – see Chapter 6 in this volume.

PATIENT FOLLOW-UP

Under the clinical standards (NCCCC 2004), formal arrangements should be made to follow up patients using home oxygen therapy to ensure that it is adequately correcting hypoxaemia, to review compliance, to detect any clinical deterioration and to ensure there is a continued need for home oxygen. The following arrangements should be made:

- *four weeks after initial prescription*: visited at home by health-care professional to provide further education and support, record SaO_2;
- *three months after initial prescription*: all patients should be reviewed by an appropriate specialist;
- *six monthly*: visited at home to measure SaO_2 on air and on LTOT;
- *annually*: arterial blood gas check and if there is a clinical deterioration, they should be referred to the hospital specialist.

HOME OXYGEN ORDERS (HOOF)

A hospital specialist will initiate most prescriptions and any patients who may require LTOT should be referred to a designated hospital specialist, who will be supported by a multidisciplinary team trained in the assessment of home oxygen provision. Prescriptions will be made on the Home Oxygen Service Order form which is then faxed to the contractor who will organise delivery of the appropriate equipment.

PATIENT CONSENT

Consent must be obtained from the patient prior to any arrangements for the delivery of oxygen to the home and a copy of the consent must be sent to the contractor when the first order is placed.

HOME OXYGEN RECORD (HOR)

The HOR form consists of three parts:

1 LTOT order
2 ambulatory oxygen order
3 short burst oxygen order.

There is also information about:

- diagnosis
- arterial blood gas measurement
- recommended hours of use
- type of oxygen administration device
- provision of humidifier and back-up cylinder if appropriate.

A copy of the HOR should be kept in the patient's hospital notes and also one is sent to the patient's GP.

SAFETY ADVICE

Patients and health-care practitioners using oxygen should be aware of the correct handling procedures for oxygen, as shown in Box 3.4.1.

CONCLUSION

LTOT has been proved to have many benefits for patients with COPD and severe hypoxaemia; however, adherence to the therapy is important if it is to have any impact on an individual's quality of life. It is important that patients and their relatives/carers have an understanding about the principles of oxygen therapy and the benefits it could have on their health. Communication with hospital and primary care is essential, and community nurses should be aware of when to make prompt referrals for reassessment and/or deliver safe levels of oxygen whilst waiting for emergency services (Edwards 2005).

Box 3.4.1. Safety issues for patients using oxygen

1 As materials burn easier in oxygen than in air, patients should not smoke, or use oxygen equipment near open fires or flames.
2 Only use and store oxygen in a well-ventilated area.
3 Patients should be advised not to use oils or grease on their oxygen equipment.
4 Whilst using oxygen, patients should be advised not to use aerosol sprays.

Safety advice for storing oxygen cylinders at home:

1 Store lying down unless there is a stand provided.
2 Do not store near direct heat.
3 Do not switch the oxygen cylinder on near naked flames.

In February 2006, a new procedure for prescribing and monitoring home oxygen therapy was introduced and it is crucial that health-care professionals, both in hospital and the community, are familiar with these standards and have developed strategies to meet them in order to provide the level of care required for these individuals. Community practitioners are in a prime position to provide the ongoing support to patients and their families/carers as they are likely to have other nursing needs and therefore should take every opportunity to encourage compliance with the therapy.

3.5   SURGICAL INTERVENTIONS

ANDREW MENZIES-GOW
Royal Brompton Hospital, London

In light of the relative paucity of effective pharmacological therapies for COPD, it is not surprising that surgical approaches to correct the underlying abnormality of airway physiology have been investigated. Emphysematous destruction of the lungs produces decreased **elastic recoil pressure**, which in turn means that at residual volume the lung requires less pressure than a normal lung to inflate and, once inflated, exerts less pressure to empty. Therefore, emphysematous lungs tend to be hyperinflated, with overexpansion of the rib cage and flattening of the **diaphragm**. This hyperinflation can compress areas of more normal lung, leading to V/Q mismatch and hypoxaemia. The main rationale of all the surgical procedures discussed below, except for transplantation, is an attempt to overcome this hyperinflation and compression of normal lung.

BULLECTOMY

Bullectomy for giant **bullae** is the one procedure that is based on sound physiological principles and has stood the test of time. Normally bullae in emphysematous lungs range from 1–4 cm in diameter; occasionally giant bullae can occupy a third or more of the hemithorax. These giant bullae may be compressing adjacent healthy lung tissue, reducing ventilation and perfusion to potentially functioning lung. Bullectomy can improve symptoms by allowing expansion of compressed lung (Gaensler et al. 1986) and improving elastic recoil and decreasing pulmonary vascular resistance (Mehran & Deslauriers 1995). Other indications for bullectomy include bullae that are associated with recurrent infection, haemoptysis or repeated pneumothorax. Pre-operative work up includes CT chest, full lung function and V/Q scanning. Chest CT is the most accurate method of determining bulla size and can also assess disease elsewhere in the lung as well as identify the presence of normal lung being compressed by the bulla. Pulmonary function testing and differential V/Q scanning help determine the volume of gas trapped in the bulla and the relative contribution of each lung to gas exchange respectively. The surgical approach for bullectomy is either lateral thoracotomy, midline sternotomy or video-assisted **thoracoscopy** with stapling of bullae.

LUNG VOLUME REDUCTION SURGERY

Given the improvement seen with bullectomy, the logical next step was lung volume reduction surgery (LVRS) in individuals with diffuse emphysema. It was hypothesised that removal of a portion of the emphysematous lung would have a beneficial effect on the remaining lung by increasing radial traction on the airways, improving expiratory flow and improving the mechanical function of the respiratory system, thereby reducing symptoms. The early pioneer of LVRS was Brantigan, who performed a stepwise procedure to remove 20–30 per cent of the most diseased appearing portion from both lungs via a thoracotomy (Brantigan & Mueller 1957). He documented subjective improvement in the majority of patients, however, the procedure was associated with a 16 per cent surgical mortality rate and never gained widespread acceptance.

The resurgence of interest in LVRS as a treatment modality for severe COPD took place in the 1990s with reports of LVRS conducted via video-assisted thoracoscopy with laser (Wakabayashi et al. 1991). In 1995, Cooper et al. published their findings on 20 patients who had undergone bilateral LVRS via median sternotomy, with resection of 20–30 per cent of each lung (Cooper et al. 1995). Their patients demonstrated a mean increase in FEV_1 of 82 per cent and FVC of 27 per cent with a concomitant fall in TLC and RV. Six-minute walk tests and quality of life indicators were both improved. The interest generated by this and other similar small studies led to the need for prospective, randomised, controlled trials to evaluate LVRS, the largest of which is the National Emphysema Treatment Trial (NETT).

The NETT is a randomised controlled trial of maximal medical therapy, including pulmonary rehabilitation, versus the same therapy plus LVRS (NETT Research Group 1995). The study was undertaken to answer outstanding questions on the risks, benefits and long-term outcomes of LVRS. The primary outcomes were mortality and exercise capacity. Secondary outcomes included quality of life, lung function and 6-minute walk distance. Of the 3,777 patients evaluated for entry into the study, 1,218 were enrolled; 608 into the surgical arm and 610 into the medical arm. Prior to completion of the study, a high-risk group of patients was identified who had a very high mortality rate and little chance of benefiting from LVRS (NETT Research Group 2001). Patients with a FEV_1 < 20 per cent predicted and either a low T_LCOc (<20 per cent predicted) or homogeneous emphysema on CT had a 16 per cent 30-day mortality rate. Analysis of the results revealed two factors that predicted different responses to LVRS: upper lobe distribution of emphysema and low exercise capacity at baseline (Fishman et al. 2003). Those patients with upper lobe emphysema and low exercise capacity had a high likelihood that LVRS would benefit their mortality, quality of life and exercise capacity. For those patients in the previously mentioned high-risk group and those with non-upper lobe emphysema and a high baseline exercise capacity, LVRS was associated with a higher mortality and little likelihood of quality of life or exercise improvement. Finally, for patients with upper lobe emphysema and high baseline exercise capacity and those with non-upper lobe disease and low exercise capacity, LVRS produced little likelihood of survival benefit, but a significant chance of improved quality of life and exercise capacity.

The demonstrated benefits of LVRS, in combination with the clear morbidity and mortality, have led investigators and medical equipment manufacturers to develop minimally invasive techniques to achieve lung volume reduction including bronchial occlusion devices inserted via fibreoptic bronchoscopy and bronchopulmonary fenestrations to enhance expiratory flow. One-way endobronchial valves have been developed, which promote **atelectasis** in emphysematous regions by preventing airflow into the bronchus while allowing outflow of air. The resulting atelectasis may decrease hyperinflation and dead space and thus allow expansion of previously compressed normal lung, thereby improving gas exchange. Even without atelectasis, the valve may decrease V/Q mismatching by shifting ventilation away from emphysematous regions of dead space to better perfused areas of lung. Early pilot studies have been reported with encouraging results with functional improvement in selected groups of patients with heterogeneous emphysema (Toma et al. 2003; Venuta et al. 2005). Although the early evidence is promising, large multi-centre randomised controlled trials with long-term follow-up are required.

BRONCHIAL FENESTRATION

The concept of bronchial fenestration was generated by the hypothesis that placement of stents between pulmonary parenchyma and large airways could effectively improve expiratory flow, because of the extensive collateral ventilation present in emphysematous lungs, thus reducing dynamic hyperinflation. The wall of a **segmental bronchus** is punctured under bronchoscopic guidance and a stent inserted, thereby creating an internal bronchopulmonary communication for expiration. The evidence for this technique is at an early stage, comprising mainly an experimental model (Lausberg et al. 2003) and a study of safety and efficacy in patients having lung transplantation or lobectomy for cancer (Rendina et al. 2003).

LUNG TRANSPLANTATION

Lung transplantation is an option for patients with severe COPD. Individuals with COPD who are candidates for transplantation are those who are predicted to have a survival of less than two years. Generally accepted criteria include a $FEV_1 < 25$ per cent when there is a rapid decline in lung function, hypoxaemia, hypercapnia and secondary pulmonary hypertension despite maximal medical therapy. Candidates for a single-lung transplant should be <65 years old and for a double-lung <60 years old. Both unilateral and bilateral transplantation are possible for patients with COPD. Functional exercise capacity is not significantly different between unilateral and bilateral transplant recipients, despite the fact that pulmonary function is nearly always better in those receiving bilateral transplants. Unilateral transplantation therefore tends to be the preferred option to best utilise the scarce resource of donor lungs (Lands et al. 1999). The main indication for a double-lung transplant in a patient with COPD is the presence of co-pathology, such as bronchiectasis, which would put the **allograft** at significant risk of infection by secretions from the native lung (Schulmann 2000).

Outcome data for COPD patients undergoing transplantation appear to be better than for patients with some other lung diseases (Hosenpud et al. 1999). One-year survival is approximately 90 per cent (Gaissert et al. 1996) and five-year survival 41–53 per cent (Sundaresan et al. 1996). It is not clear whether lung transplantation provides a survival benefit. The survival curve of patients with COPD following transplant is never greater than the curve for those that continue to wait on the transplant list (Hosenpud et al. 1998). Given the available information, the rationale for lung transplantation must therefore be to improve pulmonary function (Levine et al. 1994), exercise capacity (Pellegrino et al. 1998) and quality of life (Gross et al. 1995), for which there are clear data.

In summary, an ever-increasing range of surgical and minimally invasive modalities to treat severe COPD are being developed. Unfortunately, to date, none have been widely applicable for a variety of reasons, including only being of benefit to subsets of patients and the lack of availability of donor organs. In the future, minimally invasive techniques may well bring the benefit of older surgical techniques to a broader group of patients with COPD with a significantly improved morbidity and mortality profile.

REFERENCES

3.1 PHARMACOLOGICAL MANAGEMENT

British National Formulary No 53 – September 2007 Edition.

British Thoracic Society Standards of Care Committee (1997) The 1997 BTS Guidelines on the Management of COPD. *Thorax* **52**: (Suppl V).

Department of Health (1996) *Immunisation against Infectious Disease* ('The Green Book'). London: Department of Health.

Department of Health (2003) Pneumococcal. In *Immunisation Against Infectious Disease* ('The Green Book'). London: Department of Health.

Global Initiative for Chronic Obstructive Lung Disease (GOLD) Executive Committee (2005) *Global Strategy for the Diagnosis, Management and Prevention of Chronic Obstructive Pulmonary Disease*. Available at: www.guideline.gov/summary (accessed 21 Oct. 2005).

NICE (2004) *Clinical Guidance 12: Chronic Obstructive Pulmonary Disease – Management of Chronic Obstructive Pulmonary Disease in Adults in Primary and Secondary Care*. London: HMSO.

Ohri C M, Steiner M C (2004) COPD – the disease and non-drug treatment. *Hospital Pharmacist* **11**(9): 359–376.

3.2 ADHERENCE/CONCORDANCE

Abbott J, Gee L (1998) Contemporary psychosocial issues in cystic fibrosis: treatment and adherence and quality of life. *Disability Rehabilitation* 20: 662–671.

Allen S C (1992) Competence thresholds for the use of inhalers in people with dementia. *Age & Ageing* **26**: 83–86.

Booker R (2003) Life in the COPD straitjacket: Improving lives of sufferers. *British Journal of Nursing* **12**(18): 1061.

Bosley C, Corden Z, Rees P, Cochrane G (1996) Psychological factors associated with use of home nebulized therapy for COPD. *European Respiratory Journal* **9**(11): 2346–2350.

Carter M (2003) Review: evidence on the effectiveness of interventions to assist patients' adherence to prescribed medications is limited. *Evidence Based Nursing* **6**(3): 78.

Cluss P A, Epstein L H (1985) The measurement of medical compliance in the treatment of disease. In Karoly P (ed.) *Measurement Strategies in Health Psychology*. New York: Wiley and Sons.

Col N, Fanale J E, Kronholm P (1990) The role of medication on compliance and adverse drug reactions in hospitalisations of the elderly. *Archives of Internal Medicine* **150**: 841–845.

Di Matteo M R, Lepper H S, Croghan T W (2000) Depression is a risk factor for non-compliance with medical treatment: meta analysis of the effects of anxiety and depression on patient adherence. *Archives of Internal Medicine* **160**: 2102–2107.

Dolce J J, Crisp C, Manzella B, et al. (1991) Medication adherence patterns in COPD. *Chest* **99**: 837–841.

Garcia-Aymerich J, Monson E, Marrades R M, Escarrrabill J, Felez M A, Sunyer J, Anto J M, and the EFRAM investigators (2001) Risk factors for hospitalisation for COPD exacerbation. *American Journal of Respiratory Critical Care Medicine* **164**: 1002–1007.

George J, Kong D C M, Thoman R, Stewart K (2005) Factors associated with medication non-adherence in patients with COPD. *Chest* **128**(5): 3198–3204.

Haynes R B (1979) Determinants of compliance: the disease and the mechanics of treatment. In Haynes R B, Taylor D W, Sackett D L (eds) *Compliance in Healthcare*. Baltimore, MD: Johns Hopkins University Press.

Interiano B, Guntupalli K (1993) Metered-dose inhalers: Do health care providers know what to teach? *Archives of Internal Medicine* **153**(1): 81–85.

Kettler L J, Sawyer S M, Winefield H R, Greville H W (2002) Determinants of adherence in adults with cystic fibrosis. *Thorax* **57**: 459–464.

Leventhal H, Deifenbach M, Leventhal E A (1992) Illness cognition: using common sense to understand treatment adherence and affect cognition interactions. *Cognitive Therapy Research* **16**: 143–162.

McGraw C (2004) Multi-compartment medication devices and patient compliance. *British Journal of Community Nursing* **9**(7): 285–290.

Meichenbaum D, Turk D C (1987) Treatment adherence: terminology, incidence and conceptualization. In Meichenbaum D, Turk D C (eds) *Facilitating Treatment Adherence*. New York: Plenum Press.

Mellins R B, Evans D, Zimmerman B, et al. (1992) Patient compliance: are we wasting our time and don't know it? *American Review of Respiratory Disease* **146**: 1376–1377.

Monninkhof E, van der Valk P, van der Palen J, et al. (2003) Effects of a comprehensive self-management programme in patients with chronic obstructive pulmonary disease. *European Respiratory Journal* **22**(5): 815–820.

National Heart, Lung and Blood Institute (1997) *National Asthma Education and Prevention Program. Expert Panel Report II: Guidelines for the Diagnosis and Management of Asthma*. Bethesda, MD: National Institutes of Health.

NCCCC (2004) Chronic obstructive pulmonary disease: National Clinical Guidelines for the management of chronic obstructive pulmonary disease in adults in primary and secondary care. *Thorax* **59** (Suppl 1): 1–232.

Ogren R A, Baldwin J L, Simon R A (1995) How patients determine when to replace their metered dose inhalers. *Annuals of Allergy Asthma Immunology* **75**: 485–489.

Pauwels R, Buist A S, Calverley P M et al. (2001) Global strategy for the diagnosis, management, and prevention of COPD: NHLBI/WHO Global Initiative for Chronic Obstructive Lung Disease (GOLD) workshop summary. *American Journal of Respiratory Critical Care Medicine* **163**: 1256–1276.

Pound P, Britten N, et al. (2005) Resisting medicines; a synthesis of qualitative studies of medicine taking. *Society of Scientific Medicine* **62**: 133–155.

Rand C S, Nides M, Cowles M K, Wise R A, Connett J for the Lung Health Study Research Group (1995) Long term metered dose inhaler adherence in a clinical trial. *American Journal of Respiratory Critical Care Medicine* **152**: 580–588.

Rubin B K, et al. (2004) How do patients determine that their metered dose inhaler is empty? *Chest* **126**: 1134–1137.

Van Mannen J G, Bindels P J, Dekker F W et al. (2002) Risk of depression in patients with COPD and its determinants. *Thorax* **57**: 412–416.

van der Palen J, Klein J J, Kerkoff A H M, van Herwaarden C L A (1995) Evaluation of the effectiveness of four different types of inhalers in patients with COPD. *Thorax* **50**: 1183–1187.

van der Palen J Klein J, van Herwaarden C, et al. (1999) Multiple inhalers confuse asthma patients. *European Respiratory Journal* **14**(5):1034–1037.

3.3 NEBULISED THERAPY AT HOME

British Thoracic Society (1997) Current best practice for nebuliser treatment. *Thorax* **52** (Suppl. 2): S1–S106.

Goldman J M, Teale C, Myers M F (1992) Simplifying the assessment of patients with chronic airflow limitation for home nebuliser therapy. *Respiratory Medicine* **86**(1): 33–38.

Gunawardena K, Smith A, Shankleman J (1986) A comparison of metered dose inhalers with nebulizers from the delivery of ipratropium bromide in domiciliary practice. *British Journal of Diseases and Chest* **80**(2): 170–178.

Jenkins S C, Heaton R W, Fulton T J, Moxham J (1987) Comparison of domiciliary nebulized salbutamol and salbutamol from a metered dose inhaler in stable chronic airflow limitation. *Chest* **91**: 804–807.

Kenderick A H, Smith E C, Wilson R S (1997) Selecting and using nebuliser equipment. *Thorax* **52** (Suppl. 2): S92–S101.

Mestitz H, Copland H M, App B, Mcdonald C F (1989) Comparison of outpatient nebulised treatment V metered dose inhaler terbutaline in chronic airflow obstruction. *Chest* **96**: 1237–1240.

Muers M (1997) Overview of nebuliser treatment. *Thorax* **52** Suppl 2: S25–S30.

O'Driscoll B R (1997) Nebulisers for chronic obstructive pulmonary disease. *Thorax* **52** (Suppl. 2): S49–S52.

O'Driscoll B R, Kay E A, Taylor R J, Berstein A (1990). Home nebulisers; can optimal therapy be predicted by laboratory studies? *Respiratory Medicine* **84**: 471–477.

Pearson M G (2001) Common medical errors and their classification in the investigation and management of COPD. In Wezicha J, Ind P, Miles A (eds) 1st edn. *The Effective Management of Chronic Obstructive Pulmonary Disease.* London: Eculapius Medical Press.

Pounsford J C (1997) Nebulisers for the elderly. *Thorax* **52** (Suppl. 2): S53–S55.

3.4 LONG-TERM OXYGEN THERAPY

British Thoracic Society Working Group on Home Oxygen Services (2005) *Clinical Component for the Home Oxygen Service in England and Wales.*

Calverley P (2000) Supplementary oxygen therapy: is it really useful? *Thorax* **55**: 537–538.

Chaouat A, Weitzenblum E, Kessler R (1999) A randomized trial of nocturnal oxygen therapy in chronic obstructive pulmonary disease patients. *European Respiratory Journal* **14**: 1002–1008.

Cranston J, Crockett A, Moss J, Alpers J, Cranston J (2005) Domiciliary oxygen for chronic obstructive pulmonary disease. Cochrane database of systematic reviews No. 4, p. CD001744 ISSN: 1469–493X.

Earnest M (2002) Explaining adherence to supplementary oxygen therapy. *Journal of General Internal Medicine* **17**: 749–755.

Eaton T, Garrett J, Young P (2002) Ambulatory oxygen improves quality of life in COPD patients: a randomised controlled study. *European Respiratory Journal* **20**: 1192–1193.

Edwards M (2005) Caring for patients with COPD on long-term oxygen therapy. *British Journal of Community Nursing* **10**(9): 404–410.

Gorecka D, Gorzelak K, Sliwinski P (1997) Effect of long-term oxygen therapy on survival in patients with chronic obstructive pulmonary disease with moderate hypoxaemia. *Thorax* **52**: 674–679.

Haidi P, Clement C, Wiese C, Dellweg D, Kohler D (2004) Long term oxygen therapy stops the natural decline of endurance in COPD patients with reversible endurance. *Respiration* **71**: 342–347.

Leach R, Davidson A, Chinn S, Twort C, Cameron I, Bateman N (1992) Portable liquid oxygen and exercise ability in severe respiratory disability. *Thorax* **47**: 781–789.

McDonald C, Blyth C, Lazarus M, Marschner I, Barter C (1995) Exertional oxygen of limited benefit in patients with chronic obstructive pulmonary disease and mild hypoxaemia. *American Journal of Critical Care Medicine* **152**: 1616–1619.

Medical Research Council Working Party (1981) Long term oxygen therapy in chronic hypoxic cor pulmonale complication chronic bronchitis and emphysema. *Lancet* **1**: 681–686.

NCCCC (2004) Chronic obstructive pulmonary disease: National Clinical Guideline for the management of chronic obstructive pulmonary disease in adults in primary and secondary care. *Thorax* **59** (Suppl. 1): 1–232.

Nocturnal Oxygen Therapy Trial Group (1980) Continuous or nocturnal oxygen therapy in hypoxaemic chronic obstructive lung disease: a clinical trial. *Annals of Internal Medicine* **93**: 391–398.

3.5 SURGICAL INTERVENTIONS

Brantigan O C, Mueller E (1957) Surgical treatment of pulmonary emphysema. *Annals of Surgery* **23**: 789–804.

Cooper J D, Trulock E P, Triantafillou A N, Patterson G A, Pohl M S, Deloney P A (1995) Bilateral pneumonectomy (volume reduction) for chronic obstructive pulmonary disease. *Journal of Thoracic Cardiovascular Surgery* **109**: 106–116.

Fishman A, Martinez F, Naunheim K, Piantadosi S, Wise R, Ries A (2003) A randomised trial comparing lung volume reduction surgery with medical therapy for severe emphysema. *New England Journal of Medicine* **348**: 2059–2073.

Gaensler E A, Jederlinie P J, Fitzgerald M X (1986) Patient work-up for bullectomy. *Journal of Thoracic Imaging* **1**: 75–93.

Gaissert H A, Trulock E P, Cooper J D, Sundaresan R S, Patterson G A (1996) Comparison of early functional results after volume reduction or lung transplantation for chronic obstructive pulmonary disease. *Journal of Thoracic Cardiovascular Surgery* **111**: 296–306.

Gross C R, Savik K, Bolman R M, Hertz M I (1995) Long-term health status and quality of life outcomes of lung transplant recipients. *Chest* **108**: 1587–1593.

Hosenpud J D, Bennett L E, Keck B M, Edwards E B, Novick R J (1998) Effect of diagnosis on survival benefit of lung transplantation for end-stage lung disease. *Lancet* **351**: 24–27.

Hosenpud J D, Bennett L E, Keck B M, Fiol B, Boucek M M, Novick R J (1999) The registry of the International Society for Heart and Lung Transplantation: sixteenth official report – 1999. *Journal of Heart Lung Transplant* **18**: 611–626.

Lands L C, Smountas A A, Mesiano G, Brosseau L, Shennib H, Charbonneau M (1999) Maximal exercise capacity and peripheral skeletal muscle function following lung transplantation. *Journal of Heart Lung Transplant* **18**: 113–120.

Lausberg H F, Chino K, Patterson G A, Meyers B F, Toeniskoetter P D, Cooper J D (2003) Bronchial fenestration improves expiratory flow in emphysematous human lungs. *Annals of Thoracic Surgery* **75**: 393–397.

Levine S M, Anzueto A, Peters J I, Cronin T, Sako E Y, Jenkinson S G (1994) Medium term functional results of single-lung transplantation for endstage obstructive lung disease. *American Journal of Respiratory Critical Care Medicine* **150**: 398–402.

Mehran R J, Deslauriers J (1995) Indications for surgery and patient work-up for bullectomy. *Chest Surgery Clinics of North America* **5**: 717–734.

National Emphysema Treatment Trial Research Group (1995) Rationale and design of the national emphysema treatment trial: A prospective randomised trial of lung volume reduction surgery. *Chest* **116**: 1750–1761.

National Emphysema Treatment Trial Research Group (2001) Patients at high risk of death after lung volume reduction surgery. *New England Journal of Medicine* **345**: 1075–1083.

Pellegrino R, Rodarte J R, Frost A E, Reid M B (1998) Breathing by double lung recipients during exercise: response to expiratory threshold loading. *American Journal of Respiratory Critical Care Medicine* **157**: 106–110.

Rendina E A, De Giacoma T, Venuta F, Coloni G F, Meyers B F, Patterson G A (2003) Feasibility and safety of the airway bypass procedure for patients with emphysema. *Journal of Thoracic Cardiovascular Surgery* **125**: 1294–1299.

Schulmann L L (2000) Lung transplantation for chronic obstructive pulmonary disease. *Clinical Chest Medicine* **21**: 849–865.

Sunderesan R S, Shiraishi Y, Trulock E P, Manley J, Lynch J, Cooper J D (1996) Single or bilateral lung transplantation for emphysema? *Journal of Thoracic Cardiovascular Surgery* **112**: 1485–1494.

Toma T P, Hopkinson N S, Hiller J, Hansell D M, Morgan C, Goldstraw P C, Geddes D (2003) Bronchoscopic volume reduction with valve implants in patients with severe emphysema. *Lancet* **361**: 931–933.

Venuta F, De Giacomo T, Rendina E A, Ciccone A M, Diso D, Perrone A (2005) Bronchoscopic volume reduction with one-way valves in patients with heterogeneous emphysema. *Annals of Thoracic Surgery* **79**: 411–416.

Wakabayashi A, Brenner M, Kayaleh R A, Berns M W, Barker S J, Rice S J (1991) Thoracoscopic carbon dioxide laser treatment of bullous emphysema. *Lancet* **337**: 881–883.

4 Smoking Cessation

SUNNY KAUL
King's College Hospital, London

INTRODUCTION

Smoking is the single greatest preventable cause of disease, hospital admissions, GP consultations and death in the United Kingdom (Secretary of State for Health 1998).

"It didn't register with me that it would be a downhill slope if I carried on smoking."

SMOKING PATTERNS AND PREVALENCE

Since the 1970s, there has been a steady decline in smoking in the UK. This levelled off during the 1990s, and is currently falling by 0.4 per cent per year (Figure 4.1). In 2003, 26 per cent of the UK adult population smoked cigarettes: approximately 12.5 million people (National Centre for Social Research 2004). Within the UK there is considerable variation in smoking prevalence according to gender, age, socio-economic status and ethnicity.

GENDER

Some 27 per cent of men and 24 per cent of women smoked cigarettes in 2003. Males smoke an average of 14.5 cigarettes a day, compared with 13.3 smoked by women (National Centre for Social Research 2004) (Figure 4.2).

AGE

Levels of smoking are highest among young people and decline with advancing age. Among 16–24 year olds, 33 per cent of men and 31 per cent of women smoke. Among 25–34 year olds, 38 per cent of men and 29 per cent of women reported smoking.

Managing Chronic Obstructive Pulmonary Disease. Edited by L. Blackler, C. Jones and C. Mooney
© 2007 John Wiley & Sons Ltd

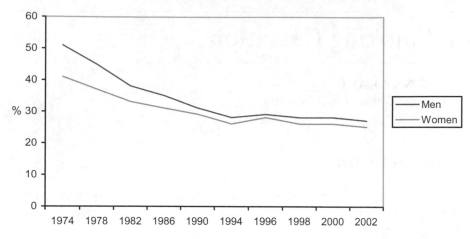

Figure 4.1. Smoking prevalence in the UK, 1974–2002. *Source*: ONS (2004)

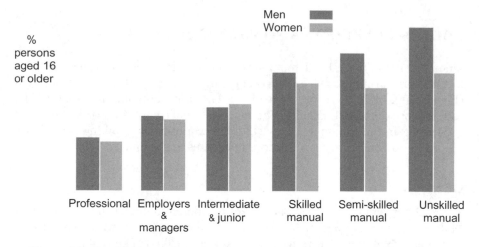

Figure 4.2. Smoking prevalence by occupation and gender. *Source*: ONS (2004)

SOCIO-ECONOMIC STATUS

Smoking behaviour is strongly related to socio-economic status. In relation to occupation, smoking prevalence is lowest in the professional and highest in the semi-skilled manual occupational groups. Among men, 20 per cent of those in managerial and professional households smoke compared with 35 per cent in households with semi-routine and routine occupations. For women, the equivalent figures are 18 per cent and 32 per cent (National Centre for Social Research 2004).

Data on the trend in smoking prevalence within non-manual and manual occupational groups suggest that the difference between these groups has widened in recent years. Smoking cessation rates also show a strong inverse relation with deprivation. Cessation rates have doubled in the most advantaged groups, but have remained almost unchanged over the past two decades in the most disadvantaged sectors of society (Jarvis 1997).

However, other measures of relative poverty or deprivation, including housing tenure, crowding, living in rented accommodation, being divorced or separated, unemployment, low educational achievement, and in women, single parent status, are also independently associated with an increased risk of smoking among adults.

ETHNICITY

There is generally a lower level of cigarette smoking among minority ethnic groups than among the UK population as a whole. But the analysis by gender shows a different picture, and prevalence among younger smokers is higher, reflecting a similar pattern to that for smokers among the UK population as a whole (McEwen & West 1999).

HEALTH RISKS OF SMOKING

About 4,000 chemical compounds have been identified in cigarette smoke, of which over 40 are known to be carcinogenic. Three important components of cigarette smoke include:

- nicotine – the addictive chemical in cigarettes;
- tar – one of the substances produced when tobacco is burnt. It is linked to cancers, lung disease and heart disease;
- carbon monoxide – a gas inhaled by smokers from cigarettes. It is linked to heart disease and has adverse effects in pregnancy.

DEATHS FROM SMOKING

In the UK, cigarette smoking is responsible for approximately 106,000 deaths per year – more than 2,000 per week, 300 per day, 12 per hour (Twigg et al. 2004). On an individual level this means that long-term regular smokers can expect to lose an average of 10 years' life expectancy (Doll et al. 2004). About half to two-thirds of all long-term smokers die prematurely because of their smoking; on average 16 years earlier than if they did not smoke (Doll et al. 2004).

The main causes of death attributable to cigarette smoking are cancers, diseases of the heart and circulation, and lung disease (Table 4.1).

Table 4.1. Deaths attributable to smoking as a percentage of all deaths from that disease, England, 1998–2002

Cause of death	Percentages of deaths attributable to smoking	
	Men	Women
Cancers		
Lung	90	80
Throat and mouth (Callum, 1992)	77	58
Oesophagus	70	72
Bladder	49	23
Kidney	42	7
Stomach	35	12
Pancreas	26	31
Leukaemia	19	12
Heart and circulation		
Ischaemic heart disease	21	12
Aortic aneurysm	64	65
Myocardial degeneration	26	18
Atherosclerosis	22	17
Stroke	10	8
Lung diseases		
Bronchitis and emphysema	87	84
Pneumonia	26	17

Source: Adapted from Twigg et al. (2004)

NICOTINE ADDICTION

Nicotine **addiction** is a recognised disease (WHO 1992). The February 2000 report (Royal College of Physicians 2000) from the Tobacco Advisory Group of the Royal College of Physicians stated that nicotine is a highly addictive psychoactive drug, and regular smokers soon become used to the presence of nicotine in their system.

There are neurobiological theories for the basis of nicotine addiction; some of these involve dopaminergic and **noradrenaline** systems in the brain. The nicotine-addicted brain is neurobiologically different from the non-addicted brain (Leshner 1996).

The power of nicotine addiction is manifest by the fact that 97 per cent of smokers will fail in attempting to quit smoking if they use willpower alone (Hughes et al. 1992; Parrot et al. 1998) and that people who have suffered life-threatening consequences will continue to smoke (Davison & Duffy 1982; Himbury & West 1985).

Nicotine vaporises from smoke particles in the lungs and is rapidly absorbed into the blood and carried to the brain. The nicotine reaches the brain in a 'bolus' with great speed – creating a 'hit' that underpins the addictiveness. The time from inhaling to a rush in the brain is a few seconds. As well as physiological dependence, smoking is sustained by behavioural factors such as movement of the hands and social pressures. The withdrawal syndrome is unpleasant and may start to affect the user within less than one hour of the last cigarette.

The addictive properties of nicotine also mean that simplistic machine measurements of tar and nicotine yields from cigarettes do not reflect real tar and nicotine exposure to smokers. Smokers adjust the way they smoke in order to self-administer a satisfactory dose of nicotine – a process known as 'compensation'. In response to reduced nicotine concentration in smoke, a smoker can adjust nicotine intake back to a satisfactory level by smoking more intensely, holding smoke in the lungs for longer, smoking more of the cigarette, or by blocking ventilation holes in the filter. Cigarette testing machines do not adjust their inhalation profile in response to changes in nicotine. This criticism of cigarette testing is not a minor point; it completely undermines the approach currently used both for regulation of tar and for consumer labelling.

The phenomenon of nicotine 'compensation' has profound implications for the regulation, labelling and branding of cigarettes. The strategy of reducing nominal tar yields has been widely and genuinely assumed by governments and the European Commission to deliver reduced harm to smokers, since it is these other products of tobacco combustion, rather than nicotine itself, that account for most of the harm caused by smoking. The improved understanding of nicotine-seeking behaviour now suggests that this assumption cannot be sustained. The unfortunate truth is that cigarettes labelled as 'low tar' do not necessarily deliver less tar to the smoker. As a result, the official labelling of cigarettes with tar yields expressed as milligrams of tar per cigarette can mislead consumers, and in the case of 'low tar' cigarettes greatly understate the health risks compared to higher tar cigarettes. In the long term, this practice may be more harmful because it may help to perpetuate smoking in people who would otherwise give up completely for health reasons. The problem is further compounded by the use of branding terms such as 'light', 'mild', and 'ultra', which has now changed to colours (e.g. purple, gold). Though based on the government-sanctioned tar yields, such branding makes an implied health claim for low-tar cigarettes that cannot be justified in practice.

ATTITUDES TO SMOKING

In one study 70 per cent of smokers said they wished to stop smoking (Bridgwood et al. 2000) but only 30 per cent actively try to stop each year (West 1997). Cessation rates increase with age: smokers in their twenties and thirties have a quit rate of 2 per cent per year (Stapleton 1998) and this rises to 4 per cent per year among smokers in their forties and fifties. The overall quit rate is around 3 per cent per year (Ginsberg 2005), with many smokers requiring multiple attempts before they are successful (Rose 1996; Ginsberg 2005). Amazingly, smokers who have suffered life-threatening complications still continue to smoke, e.g. almost 50 per cent of lung cancer patients return to smoking within 12 months of surgery (Davison and Duffy 1982) and 38 per cent of smokers who have suffered a myocardial infarction will resume smoking while still in hospital (Himbury & West 1985).

The primary reason that many smokers find it difficult to stop is their dependence on nicotine. Stopping smoking usually brings on a withdrawal syndrome comprising a range of symptoms (Box 4.1). These symptoms, especially urges to smoke, can lead to relapse early in a quit attempt (West et al. 1989b). Most withdrawal symptoms last no longer than two to four weeks (Hughes 1992; West et al. 1989a) so assisting smokers through the first four weeks is important. Tobacco withdrawal symptoms are quite varied and are listed in Box 4.1 (West et al. 1989a, 1989b; Hughes 1992; Hajek et al. 2003; Ussher et al. 2003).

STRATEGIES AVAILABLE

Strategies that can be used, support available and the role of the health-care provider include the following. The evidence and best practice guidelines for smoking cessation practice are set out in guidelines for health professionals published in the journal *Thorax*:

Raw M, McNeill A, West R (1998) Smoking cessation guidelines for health professionals: A guide to effective smoking cessation interventions for the health care system. Health Education Authority. *Thorax* 53 Suppl 5 Pt 1: S1–S19.

Box 4.1. Tobacco withdrawal symptoms

Symptom	Average duration
Depressed mood	<4 weeks
Sleep disturbance	<2 weeks
Irritability	<4 weeks
Difficulty concentrating	<2 weeks
Restlessness	<4 weeks
Increased appetite and increased weight	>10 weeks
Constipation	>4 weeks
Mouth ulcers	>4 weeks
Light-headedness	<2 days
Urges to smoke	>10 weeks

Sources: West et al. (1989a, 1989b); Hughes (1992); Hajek et al. (2003); Ussher et al. (2003); McRobbie et al. (2004)

This is backed up by cost-effectiveness data for commissioners:

Parrott S, Godfrey C, Raw M, West R, McNeill A (1998) Guidance for commissioners on the cost effectiveness of smoking cessation interventions. Health Educational Authority. *Thorax* 53 Suppl 5 Pt 2: S1–38.

An update was published in 2000:

West R, McNeill A, Raw M (2000) Smoking cessation guidelines for health professionals: an update. Health Education Authority. *Thorax* 55: 987–999.

Over two-thirds of smokers say they would like to quit and about one-third try to quit in any year, yet only about 2 per cent succeed. Many smokers will make repeated attempts, with a period of abstinence followed by relapse.

There are two main complementary forms of intervention to assist smoking cessation:

1 Motivation, support and advice.
2 Pharmacological products such as nicotine replacement therapy (NRT) and bupropion.

The first is designed to increase smokers' commitment to stopping, the second to help attenuate cravings and withdrawal. For both, there are approaches with proven efficacy and attractive cost-effectiveness. The benefits of smoking cessation are substantial: immediate improved health, longer life, improved welfare and finances, and reduced passive smoking exposure to family, friends and working colleagues.

COUNSELLING

This is the cornerstone of smoking cessation management. There are three levels of counselling support:

1 *Brief intervention*: ask about smoking status and give brief advice. Many health-care professionals should be able to provide this level of intervention; this should be integrated into a standard consultation process.
2 *Intermediate intervention*: give in-depth advice, assist in stopping smoking and arrange follow-up appointments.
3 *Specialist services*: provide expert advice (identify their cues to smoke and progressively break the link between the cues and smoking), give ongoing assistance (once they quit they learn to prevent relapse) and arrange regular follow-up.

There is evidence for a dose–response relationship between intensity of support (both increased frequency and duration of sessions) and cessation rates (Fiore et al. 1996).

This is a highly cost-effective intervention (Parrott et al. 1998; Prathiba et al. 1998); brief smoking cessation advice (this is just 3 minutes' advice from a doctor with the offer of support only) results in an incremental cost per life-year saved of £174.

There are several strategies available to the health-care provider that will be outlined below.

BRIEF OPPORTUNISTIC ADVICE TO STOP FROM A HEALTH-CARE PROFESSIONAL

This consists of brief advice from health professionals (such as dentists and the dental team, GPs, health visitors, midwives, pharmacists, physiotherapists, practice nurses) delivered opportunistically during routine consultations to smokers whether or not they are seeking help with stopping.

Brief opportunistic advice typically involves asking patients about their current smoking, advising them to stop, offering assistance by way of a referral to a specialist service, advice or a prescription for NRT or bupropion, and arranging follow-up where appropriate.

This advice leads to 1–3 out of 100 smokers receiving it to stop smoking for at least six months (Silagy 2000). This is in addition to the number who would have stopped smoking anyway. It is estimated that approximately 40 per cent of smokers make some form of attempt to quit in response to advice from a GP (Russell et al. 1979; Kreuter et al. 2000). This advice appears to have its effect primarily by triggering a quit attempt, rather than by increasing the chances of success of quit attempts (Russell et al. 1979).

There is correlational evidence that the more time is spent with smokers, the greater the effect in aiding cessation. Direct comparisons between more intensive and less intensive interventions have not been adequate to enable conclusions to be drawn but comparisons across studies suggest that more intensive interventions in terms of frequency of contact and/or duration of contact achieve higher success rates (USDHHS 2000).

There is some evidence that smokers are happier to receive advice to stop when GPs link the advice to their reason for visiting the surgery (Coleman & Wilson 1999; Butler et al. 1998). The BTS offers advice to GPs on helping smokers to quit, and this is summarised in Box 4.2.

FACE-TO-FACE BEHAVIOURAL SUPPORT

This category includes a range of methods of support from focused counselling and advice, through coping skills training to group support. In fact, most programmes tested have been diverse, involving many different components. This support is provided to smokers who are planning to make an attempt to quit and would like help with doing so.

Little is known about the active ingredients of behavioural support so it is difficult to provide evidence-based recommendations regarding the content of behavioural support programmes. It has been proposed that teaching problem-solving skills and social support are useful (USDHHS 2000). There is preliminary evidence that pairing smokers together to make the quit attempt can

---

Box 4.2. BTS advice to GPs

ASK all patients about their smoking history.
ADVISE all patients to quit using personalised but non-judgemental
  language.
ASSESS motivation to quit.

'How do you feel about your smoking?'
'Are you ready to give up?'

ASSIST motivated smokers by giving further advice and prescribing NRT
  or medication.
ARRANGE support follow-up with the local smoking cessation service

---

improve success rates (May & West 2000) and that, with women smokers at
least, a physical activity programme can improve success rates (Ussher et al.
2000).

SELF-HELP MATERIALS

Written self-help materials can be effective in aiding cessation attempts.
Approximately one in 100 smokers using generic self-help materials and
receiving no other form of assistance stop for at least six months who would
not otherwise have done so (Lancaster & Stead 2000). It is unclear how far
adding self-help materials to other forms of intervention, such as brief advice
to stop, is effective (Lancaster & Stead 2000).

Materials that are tailored to the characteristics of a particular smoker can
be more effective than generic materials. There is limited research comparing
generic and tailored materials and in those studies varying approaches to tailoring have been adopted. However, such research as there is suggests that
tailoring in some form may be helpful (Lancaster & Stead 2000).

TELEPHONE COUNSELLING

Proactive, frequent telephone counselling can be effective as an aid to smoking
cessation. There is limited evidence from controlled trials but such evidence
as exists suggests an effect (Lichtenstein et al. 1996; Zhu et al. 1996).

Reactive telephone counselling may be effective as an aid to smoking cessation but is difficult to evaluate in randomised trials. There are no adequate
randomised controlled trials published to date (Lichtenstein et al. 1996) but a
follow-up study (a reactive telephone counselling service) found high self-
reported sustained abstinence rates (Owen 2000). Without control groups, it

is not possible to assess whether these are higher than would have been the case without counselling.

HEALTH BENEFITS FROM SMOKING CESSATION IN COPD

People who manage to stop smoking live longer and healthier lives than those who continue to smoke (Schwartz 1992). The benefits, while greatest for younger smokers, also extend to those who stop at older ages. They apply to people with and without smoking-related diseases (benefits such as improvements in fitness, general health status, teeth, skin, nails, etc.) (Samet 1992). The risk of morbidity and death continues to drop as the abstinence period lengthens (Samet 1992).

As Figure 4.3 illustrates, smoking cessation retards progression of COPD, slowing the age-related decline in lung function to that of a non-smoker within a few months (Fletcher & Peto 1997). Ten years after stopping, an ex-smoker's risk of lung cancer is reduced to become a third to a half of that for a continuing smoker. The risk continues to decline with abstinence (US Dept 1990; American Thoracic Society 1996).

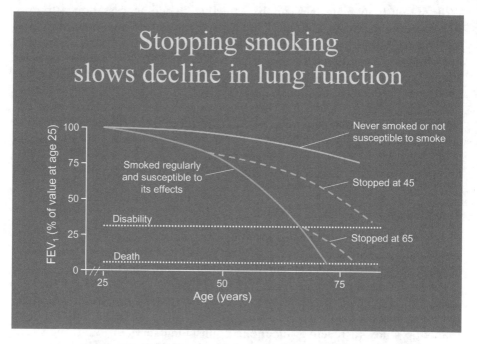

Figure 4.3. Smoking cessation and decline in lung function

The risk of coronary heart disease declines rapidly after smoking cessation. After just one year, the risk of coronary heart disease is halved compared with someone who continues to smoke. The risk continues to decline over time – after 10–15 years it is similar to that for a person who has never smoked (US Dept 1990; American Thoracic Society 1996).

Figure 4.3 illustrates the risks of smoking on lung function: differences between the lines represent effects that smoking, and stopping smoking, can have on the FEV_1 of a man who is liable to develop COPD if he smokes.

FEV_1 declines continuously and smoothly over an individual's life but in most non-smokers and some smokers, clinically significant airflow obstruction never develops (Fletcher & Peto 1997). In susceptible people, however, smoking causes irreversible obstructive changes in the lungs (Fletcher & Peto 1997). Although the damage caused to the lungs by years of smoking is permanent, quitting smoking prevents it from worsening. Consequently, the accelerated decline in lung function in smokers is halted when they stop, returning to the slower rates of decline that occur naturally with ageing (Fletcher & Peto 1997).

In smokers with established COPD, stopping smoking can improve lung function by about 5 per cent within a few months (Fletcher & Peto 1997). Smoking cessation in patients with COPD has also been found to reduce respiratory symptoms such as cough, phlegm, wheezing and dyspnoea (Kanner et al. 1999).

PHARMACOTHERAPIES

NICOTINE REPLACEMENT THERAPY (NRT)

The rationale for NRT is to prevent the withdrawal symptoms by providing nicotine in an alternative form. Nicotine replacement therapy is effective in aiding smoking cessation. It reduces the urges to smoke and other withdrawal symptoms following cessation (Silagy et al. 1998). NRT approximately doubles abstinence rates in smokers who are not already patients irrespective of the intensity of counselling support (Kanner et al. 1999) and is most effective when accompanied by counselling (Fiore et al. 2000a, 2000b).

There are several types of NRT available; these include transdermal patch, gum, nasal spray, inhalator, sub-lingual tablet and lozenges. All six products deliver nicotine to the user's bloodstream but differ in the pattern of nicotine delivery. Few trials have directly compared these drugs with each other and so it is difficult to ascertain if any one is more effective than the other. All are appropriate first-line agents.

The transdermal nicotine patch is the easiest to use. It is put on each morning on a dry, non-hairy part of the skin; it provides a relatively constant dose over 16–24 hours but has the slowest onset of action:

- It comes in strengths of 5, 10 and 15 mg to be worn for 16 hours or 7, 14 and 21 mg to be worn over 24 hours.
- For a >10 a day smoker, a typical course would be 21 mg for 4 weeks, followed by 14 mg for 2 weeks and then 7 mg for 2 weeks.

Nicotine in the gum is absorbed through the **buccal mucosa**; it is important to chew it slowly and not to swallow it (this is wasted nicotine). It comes in 2 mg and 4 mg doses and traditional and mint flavours. Peak blood levels are reached in 20 mins. The nicotine nasal spray acts fastest with blood levels reaching a peak 5–10 mins after administration. Each spray contains 500 mcg and a maximum of 32 sprays per 16 hours to each nostril is permitted. This may be particularly useful in smokers who experience cravings while on other forms of NRT. It does, however, take a little getting used to as it can cause nasal irritation.

The nicotine inhalator consists of a plastic mouthpiece and nicotine cartridges that fit on the end of it. It addresses the hand-to-mouth ritual and users draw on it like a cigarette. The nicotine, however, is absorbed through the buccal mucosa and not the lungs. Each cartridge contains 10 mg of nicotine and the maximum dosage is 12 cartridges per 24 hours. The peak blood nicotine level is reached in 20 mins. Meta-analyses of studies (Lam et al. 1987; Fiore et al. 1994; Agency for Health Care Policy and Research 1996; Hajek et al. 1999) looking at the efficacy of NRT have concluded that the patch at least doubles cessation rates; gum increases the cessation rate by 50 per cent. There have been relatively fewer trials with the inhalator (Tonnenson et al. 1993; Schneider et al. 1996) and nasal spray (Schnider et al. 1990; Sutherland et al. 1992) but those that have been done suggest they approximately double the cessation rates too.

One randomised trial directly compared the efficacy and acceptability of the first four NRT products (Lam et al. 1987); efficacy did not differ among the products, however there was a difference in compliance. Patients were most compliant with the patch and least compliant with the spray.

NRT products can be safely used in combination. Certain combinations have shown greater efficacy than single products (Kornitzer et al. 1995; Blondal et al. 1999). The addition of the nicotine nasal spray to the patch increased the quit rate at 1 year from 11 per cent to 27 per cent. When gum was added to the patch there was an increase in the 6-month quit rate from 15 to 27 per cent but at 1 year the cessation rates (13 per cent v 18 per cent) were not statistically different.

SAFETY OF NRT

NRT is safe in patients with stable cardiovascular disease (Joseph et al. 1996; Benowitz and Gourlay 1997); in acute cardiovascular disease several guidelines recommend against the use of NRT despite the fact NRT has not been studied in this group of patients and despite the fact that the dose of nicotine would be less than that of a cigarette.

Considering administration of NRT during pregnancy, it is unclear how far NRT would carry a risk to the foetus when used in pregnancy but it is almost certainly safer than smoking. Small studies on the effects of NRT on the foetus have not revealed significant problems (Lindblad et al. 1988; Lambers & Clark 1996). Evidence from smokeless tobacco users in India suggests that nicotine may be to some extent implicated in low birth weight (Krishnamurthy & Joshi 1993). However, NRT does not contain the large number of other toxins contained in tobacco smoke and therefore would be expected to be considerably safer than smoking.

The use of NRT while breastfeeding is associated with very few risks to the child. Nicotine does accumulate in breast milk but relatively little is absorbed from the infant's gut, and this then undergoes first pass metabolism resulting in a low plasma concentration (Dempsey & Benowitz, 2001). Any small risk to the child from this low level of nicotine is preferable to the risk of the pregnant woman continuing to smoke.

In its 2002 publication, *Guidance on the Use of Nicotine Replacement Therapy (NRT) and Bupropion for Smoking Cessation*, NICE made it clear that, when considering the use of NRT in smokers with certain conditions (including smokers who are pregnant or breastfeeding and those with cardiovascular disease), the health-care professional should 'take into account the significant harm associated with continuing to smoke and that it can be expected that NRT will deliver less nicotine (and none of the other potentially disease-causing agents) that would be obtained from cigarettes' (NICE 2002).

OVERALL USE

Approximately 25 per cent of quit attempts involve the use of NRT with the transdermal patch being the most popular formulation with smokers. (The majority of smokers attempt to quit using willpower alone, which is the least effective method.) In a number of settings (including OTC sales, smokers' clinics, and hospital inpatients), the nicotine patches were preferred by smokers given the choice (Cummings et al. 1997; Shaw et al. 1998; West et al. 2000).

Most GPs report believing that NRT is effective, and are recommending patients to use it. A recent survey of GPs found that most report accepting the effectiveness of NRT and recommending it or prescribing it, usually on a private prescription (McEwen & West 2000).

BUPROPION (ZYBAN)

Zyban is a sustained-release formulation of bupropion hydrochloride; it is an oral medication for use in helping smokers who are motivated to stop and is the first (and at present only) non-nicotine pharmacotherapy licensed for smoking cessation.

It has a number of actions that are thought to contribute to its ability to help smokers quit:

- The precise mechanism by which bupropion HCl SR enhances the ability of patients to abstain from smoking is not established. However, it does *not* involve substituting one form of nicotine delivery for another.
- Bupropion HCl SR is a relatively weak but selective inhibitor of the neuronal reuptake of dopamine and noradrenaline, with very minimal effect on **serotonin** and does not inhibit monoamine oxidase (Richmond & Zwar 2003).
- As an aid to smoking cessation, bupropion HCl SR is believed to work directly on two pathways in the brain that are important in the addiction process through its dopaminergic and **noradrenergic** properties.
- The dopaminergic activity of bupropion is thought to affect the area of the brain implicated in the positive reinforcing properties of addictive drugs and the development of dependence (Ferry 1999; Covey et al. 2000).
- Its noradrenergic effects in the *locus coeruleus* are thought to play a role in withdrawal from nicotine (Covey et al. 2000; Richmond & Zwar 2003).

Bupropion helps smokers by reducing the severity of withdrawal symptoms, including urges to smoke, making the quit attempt easier and success more likely.

There are now over 20 randomised controlled trials looking at the efficacy of bupropion in a large number of smokers of various ages, ethnic backgrounds and states of health. Combining the results of these studies shows that compared with a placebo, bupropion approximately doubles the chances of remaining abstinent for a year (Hughes et al. 2004). Currently there is not enough evidence to suggest that combining bupropion with NRT is better than using bupropion alone.

When trying to quit, the smoker needs to start bupropion about a week before quitting to allow time for a steady-state concentration to be reached. During this time the client smokes as normal. Bupropion has some common side effects that include a dry mouth, insomnia and sometimes a rash. In common with other antidepressants, there is a rare risk of seizure (1 in 1,000). Contra-indications include: history of seizures, eating disorders, bipolar disease, pregnancy and breastfeeding.

VARIENICLINE

At the time of writing, a new oral drug has been licensed for smoking cessation – Varienicline (Champix). It is a selective nicotinic acetylcholine receptor partial agonist and is designed to bind to the same receptor sites as nicotine.

It alleviates withdrawal symptoms related to quitting smoking, but the drug also blocks the rewarding effects of nicotine (Bender 2005). One study indicates that there is a higher quit rate when compare to bupropion or a placebo at 12 weeks (Gonzales et al. 2006).

REFERENCES

Agency for Health Care Policy and Research (1996) Smoking cessation clinical practice guideline. *JAMA* **275**: 1270–1280.

American Thoracic Society (1996) Cigarette smoking and health. *American Journal of Respiratory Critical Care Medicine* **153**: 861–865.

Bender E (2005) Experimental drug shows promise for smoking cessation. *Psychiatric News* **40**(24): 8.

Benowitz M, Gourlay S (1997) Cardiovascular toxicity of nicotine: implications for NRT. *Journal of American College of Cardiology* **337**: 1195–1202.

Blondal A, Gudmundsson L J, Olafsdottir L, Westin A (1999) Nicotine nasal spray with nicotine patch for smoking cessation: randomised controlled trial with 6 year follow-up. *British Medical Journal* **318**: 285–288.

Bridgwood A, Lilly R, Thomas M, et al. (2000) *Living in Britain: Results from 1998 General Household Survey*. London: The Stationery Office.

Butler C C, Pill R, Stott N C (1998) Qualitative study of patients' perceptions of doctors' advice to quit smoking: implications for opportunistic health promotion. *British Medical Journal* **316**: 1878–1881.

Callum C (1992) UK deaths from smoking. *Lancet* **339**(8807): 1484.

Coleman T, Wilson A (1999) Factors associated with the provision of anti-smoking advice by General Practitioners. *British Journal of General Practice* **49**: 557–558.

Covey L S, Sullivan M A, Johnston J A, et al. (2000) Advances in non-nicotine pharmacotherapies for smoking cessation. *Drugs* **59**(1): 17–31.

Cummings K M, Hyland A, Ockene J K, et al. (1997) Use of the nicotine skin patch by smokers in 20 communities in the United States, 1992–1993. *Tobacco Control* **6**(Suppl. 2): S63–S70.

Davison G, Duffy M (1982) Smoking habits of long-term survivors of surgery for lung cancer. *Thorax* **37**: 331–333.

Dempsey D, Benowitz N (2001) Risks and benefits of nicotine to aid smoking cessation in pregnancy. *Drug Safety* **24**(4): 277–322.

Doll R, Peto R, Boreham J, Sutherland I (2004) Mortality in relation to smoking: 50 years' observations on male British doctors. *British Medical Journal* **328**: 1519–1528.

Ferry L H (1999) Non-nicotine pharmacotherapy for smoking cessation. *Primary Care Clinics in Office Practice* **26**(3): 653–669.

Fiore M C, Bailey W C, Cohen S J, et al. (1996) *Smoking Cessation: Clinical Practice Guideline No 18*. Rockville, MD: Agency for Health Care Policy and Research, US Dept of Health and Human Services, Publication No. 96-0692.

Fiore M C, Bailey W C, Cohen S J, et al. (2000a) For the tobacco use and dependence: Clinical Practice Guideline Panel, Staff and Consortium Representatives. A clinical practice guideline for treating tobacco use and dependence: a US Public Health Service Report. *JAMA* **283**: 3244–3254.

Fiore M C, Bailey W C, Cohen S J, et al. (2000b) *Treating Tobacco Use and Dependence: Clinical Practice Guideline*. Rockville, MD: Public Health Service, US Dept of Health and Human Services. AHRQ Publication No. 00–00032.

Fiore M C, Smith S S, Jorenby D E, Baker T B (1994) The effectiveness of the nicotine patch for smoking cessation: a meta-analysis. *JAMA* **271**: 1940–1947.

Fletcher C, Peto R (1997) The natural history of chronic airflow obstruction. *British Medical Journal* **1**: 1645–1648.

Ginsberg D (2005) Duloxetine for smoking cessation. *Psychopharmacology Reviews*. Available at: www.primarypsychiatry.com/aspx/articledetail.aspx?articleid=129 (accessed 5 Mar. 2006).

Gonzales D, Rennard S I, Nides M, Oncken C, Azoloulay S, Billling C, Watsky E, Gong J, Williams K, Reeves K R (2006) Varieniclin, and alpha4bet 2 nicotinic acetylcholine receptor partial agonist, vs sustained-release bupropion and placebo for smoking cessation: A randomized controlled trial. *JAMA* **296**: 56–63.

Hajek P, Gillison F, McRobbie H (2003) Stopping smoking can cause constipation. *Addiction* **98**(11): 1563–1567.

Hajek P, West R, Nilsson F, et al. (1999) Randomised comparative trial of nicotine polacrilex, a transdermal patch, nasal spray and inhaler. *Archives of Internal Medicine* **159**: 2033–2038.

Himbury S, West R (1985) Smoking habits after laryngectomy. *British Medical Journal* **291**: 514–515.

Hughes J, Stead L, Lancaster T (2004) Antidepressants for smoking cessation. Cochrane Database Systematic Review Oct 18(4): CD000031 Review.

Hughes J R (1992) Tobacco withdrawal in self-quitters. *Journal of Consultant Clinical Psychologists* **60**(5): 689–697.

Hughes J R, Gyulliver S B, Fenwick J W, et al. (1992) Smoking cessation among self-quitters. *Health Psychology* **11**(5): 331–334.

Jarvis M J (1997) Patterns and predictors of smoking cessation in the general population. In Bolliger C T, Fagerström K O (eds) *The Tobacco Epidemic*. Basel: Karger.

Joseph A, Norman S M, Ferry L H, et al. (1996) The safety of transdermal nicotine as an aid to smoking cessation in patients with cardiac disease. *New England Journal of Medicine* **335**: 1790–1798.

Kanner R E, Connett J E, Williams D E, Buist A S (1999) For the Lung Study Research Group. *American Journal of Medicine* **106**: 410–415.

Kornitzer M, Boutsen M, Dramaix M, Thijs J, Gustavsson G (1995) Combined use of nicotine patch and gum in smoking cessation. *Preventive Medicine* **24**: 41–47.

Kreuter M W, Chheda S G, Bull F C (2000) How does physician advice influence patient behaviour? Evidence for a priming effect. *Archives of Family Medicine* **9**: 426–433.

Krishnamurthy S, Joshi S (1993) Gender differences and low birth weight with maternal smokeless tobacco use in pregnancy. *Journal of Tropical Paediatrics* **39**: 253–254.

Lam W, Sacks H S, Sze P, et al. (1987) Meta-analysis of randomised controlled trials of nicotine chewing gum. *Lancet* **2**: 27–30.

Lambers D S, Clark K E (1996) The maternal and foetal physiologic effects of nicotine. *Seminar of Perinatologists* **20**: 115–126.

Lancaster T, Stead L F (2000) Self-help interventions for smoking cessation. Cochrane Database Systematic Review 2: CD001118.

Leshner A L (1996) Understanding drug addiction: implications for treatment. *Hospital Practice* **15**(31): 47–59.

Lichtenstein E, Glasgow R E, Lando H A, et al. (1996) Telephone counselling for smoking cessation: rationales and meta-analytic review of evidence. *Health Education Research* **11**: 243–257.

Lindblad A, Marsal K, Andersson K E (1988) Effect of nicotine on human foetal blood flow. *Obstetrics and Gynaecology* **72**(3 Pt 1): 371–382.

May S, West R (2000) Do social support interventions ('buddy systems') aid smoking cessation? A review. *Tobacco Control* **9**(4): 415–422.

McEwen A, West R (1999) Tobacco use amongst black and minority ethnic groups in England. In *Black and Minority Ethnic Groups and Tobacco Use in England: A Practical Resource for Health Professionals*. London: Health Education Agency.

McEwen A, West R (2000) *GPs' Views on Medications for Treating Tobacco Dependence*. London: Health Education Agency.

McRobbie H, Hajek P, Gillison F (2004) The relationship between smoking cessation and mouth ulcers. *Nicotine Tobacco Research* **6**(4): 655–659.

National Centre for Social Research (2004) *Health Survey for England 2003: Latest Trends*. London: National Centre for Social Research.

NICE (2002) Guidance on the use of nicotine replacement therapy (NRT) and bupropion for smoking cessation. www.nice.org.uk (accessed 12 Feb. 2007).

Office of National Statistics (2004) *Living in Britain: The 2002 General Household Survey*. London: Office of National Statistics.

Owen L (2000) Impact of a telephone helpline for smokers who called during a mass media campaign. *Tobacco Control* **9**: 148–154.

Parrott S, Godfrey C, Raw M, West R, McNeill A (1998) Guidance for commissioners on the cost effectiveness of smoking cessation interventions. Health Educational Authority. *Thorax* **53** Suppl 5 Pt 2: S1–S38.

Prathiba B V, Tjeder S, Phillips C, Campbell I A (1998) A smoking cessation counsellor: should every hospital have one? *Journal of Royal Society for Health* **118**(6): 356–359.

Raw M, McNeill A, West R (1998) Smoking cessation guidelines for health professionals: A guide to effective smoking cessation interventions for the health care system. Health Education Authority. *Thorax* **53** Suppl 5 Pt 1: S1–S19.

Richmond R, Zwar N (2003) Review of bupropion for smoking cessation. *Drug and Alcohol Review* June **22**(2): 203–220.

Rose J E (1996) Nicotine addiction and treatment. *Annual Review of Medicine* **47**: 493–507.

Royal College of Physicians of London (2000) *Nicotine Addiction in Britain: A Report of the Tobacco Advisory Group of the Royal College of Physicians*. London: Royal College of Physicians.

Russell M A, Wilson C, Taylor C, et al. (1979) Effect of general practitioners' advice against smoking. *British Medical Journal* **2**: 231–235.

Samet J M (1992) The health benefits of smoking cessation. *Medical Clinics of North America* **76**: 399–414.

Schneider N G, Olmstead R, Nilsson F, et al. (1990) Efficacy of a nicotine nasal spray in smoking cessation: A placebo controlled double-blind trial. *Addiction* 1671–1682.

Schneider N G, Olmstead R, Nilsson F, et al. (1996) Efficacy of a nicotine inhaler in smoking cessation: A double blind, placebo-controlled trial. *Addiction* **91**(9): 1293–1306.

Schwartz J L (1992) Methods of smoking cessation. *Medical Clinics of North America* **76**(2): 451–477.

Secretary of State for Health and Secretaries of State for Scotland, Wales, Northern Ireland (1998) *Smoking Kills: A White Paper on Tobacco.* London: The Stationery Office.

Shaw J P, Ferry D G, Pethica D, et al. (1998) Usage patterns of transdermal nicotine when purchased as a non-prescription medicine from pharmacies. *Tobacco Control* **7**: 161–167.

Silagy C (2000) Physician advice for smoking cessation. Cochrane Database Systematic Review. 2: CD000165.

Silagy C, Mant D, Fowler G, et al. (1998) Nicotine Replacement Therapy for smoking cessation (Cochrane Review). In The Cochrane Library Issue 2. Oxford: Update Software. Updated Quarterly.

Stapleton J (1998) Cigarette smoking prevalence, cessation and relapse. *Statistical Methods of Medical Research* **7**(2): 187–203.

Sutherland G, Stapleton J, Russell M A, et al. (1992) Randomised controlled trial of nicotine nasal spray in smoking cessation. *Lancet* **340**: 324–329.

Tonnenson P, Norregaard J, Mikkelson K, Jorgenson S, Nilsson F (1993) A double-blind trial of a nicotine inhaler for smoking cessation. *JAMA* **269**: 1268–1271.

Twigg L, Moon G, Walker S (2004) *The Smoking Epidemic in England.* London: Health Development Agency.

US Department of Health and Human Services (1990) *The Health Benefits of Smoking Cessation: A Report of the Surgeon General.* Rockville, MD: US Department of Health and Human Services, Public Health Service, Centers of Disease Control, Center for Chronic Disease Prevention and Health Promotion, Office for Smoking and Health.

US Department of Health and Human Services (2000) *Treating Tobacco Use and Dependence.* Rockville, MD: Agency for Healthcare Research Quality.

Ussher M H, Taylor A H, West R, et al. (2000) Does exercise aid smoking cessation? A systematic review. *Addiction* **95**: 199–208.

Ussher M H, West R, Steptoe A, McEwen A (2003) Increase in common cold symptoms and mouth ulcers following smoking cessation. *Tobacco Control* **12**(1): 86–88.

West R (1997) Getting serious about stopping smoking: A review of products, services and techniques. A report for No Smoking Day. Available at: www.nosmokingday.org.uk/corporate/publications.htm (accessed 5 Mar 2006).

West R, Hajek P, Belcher M (1989a) Time course of cigarette withdrawal symptoms while using nicotine gum. *Psychopharmacology* (Berl) **99**(1): 143–145.

West R J, Hajek P, Belcher M (1989b) Severity of withdrawal symptoms as a predictor of outcome of an attempt to quit smoking. *Psychological Medicine* **19**(4): 981–985.

West R, Hajek P, Nilsson F, et al. (2000) Individual differences in preference for and responses to four nicotine replacement products. *Psychopharmacology* **153**(2): 225–230.

West R, McNeill A, Raw M (2000) Smoking cessation guidelines for health professionals: an update. Health Education Authority. *Thorax* **55**: 987–999.

World Health Organisation (1992) *International Statistical Classification of Diseases and Related Health Problems* (10th rev. vol. 1 ICD-10). Geneva: World Health Organisation.

Zhu S H, Stretch V, Balabanis M, et al. (1996) Telephone counselling for smoking cessation: effects of single-session and multiple-session interventions. *Journal of Consultant Clinical Psychologists* **64**: 202–211.

5 Pulmonary Rehabilitation

AMY GRANT
*Physiotherapist, Lambeth and Southwark Pulmonary Rehabilitation Team,
London*

LAUREN MOORE
*Physiotherapist, Lambeth and Southwark Pulmonary Rehabilitation Team,
London*

Pulmonary rehabilitation (PR) aims to improve the exercise ability, quality of life and functional independence of people with COPD. It consists of a programme of exercise and education, the primary aim being to equip the patients with the appropriate skills to self-manage their chronic lung disease to the best of their ability.

> **"I thought, I can't walk from one chair to another without gasping for breath, how am I going to exercise?"**

The National Institute of Health (NIH) commissioned a PR working party, and in 1994 they published a definition of PR:

> Pulmonary rehabilitation is a multidisciplinary continuum of services directed to persons with pulmonary disease and their families, usually by an interdisciplinary team of specialists, with the goal of achieving and maintaining the individual's maximum level of independence and functioning in the community.
>
> (Cole and Fishman 1994)

BACKGROUND

Charles Dennison first introduced physical exercise for patients with lung disease in 1895 in *Exercise for Pulmonary Invalids* (Garrod 2004). Research into the effects of exercise in COPD, however, did not start until the 1970s. Despite initial scepticism (Belman & Kendregan 1981), the benefits of PR were presented in a review article by Make in 1986. Since then, PR has gained credibility across the world. At least three meta-analyses and several randomised controlled trials have shown that PR leads to clinically significant improvements in exercise capacity and health-related quality of life (Lacasse et al. 1996, 2001; Griffiths et al. 2000; Salman et al. 2003). In 2001, the British Thoracic Society (BTS) published a statement advocating PR in the management of COPD, highlighting its ability to reduce symptoms, improve functional

Managing Chronic Obstructive Pulmonary Disease. Edited by L. Blackler, C. Jones and C. Mooney
© 2007 John Wiley & Sons Ltd

independence and hence quality of life. This recommendation was further strengthened by various national and international guidelines (Troosters et al. 2005), including NICE (2004).

PR is also thought to have the potential to decrease the health-care burden of COPD on the NHS. Griffiths et al. (2001) produced a review article considering the cost effectiveness of PR and concluded that it 'is likely to result in financial benefits to the health service'. Although most of the evidence has examined the effect of PR on COPD patients, there is some suggestion that it is also beneficial for patients with other chronic lung diseases such as **fibrosing alveolitis**, asthma and cystic fibrosis (Foster & Thomas 1990; Kyprianou & Russo 2005). Additionally, it is widely accepted that the benefits of PR are of a greater magnitude than any pharmacotherapy used in COPD with regard to breathlessness, quality of life and exercise capacity.

>   **"Pulmonary rehab has given us a life; we didn't have a life before it."**

>   **"But going to the pulmonary rehab, you're not the only one like this."**

EXERCISE PHYSIOLOGY IN COPD

Patients with COPD are often anxious about becoming breathless and avoid activities that exacerbate these feelings, leading to the adoption of an inactive lifestyle (Casaburi 1993). Chronic inactivity deconditions ambulatory muscles in particular, namely the quadriceps muscle (Man et al. 2003). Lean muscle mass can be reduced by 20–40 per cent in patients with COPD (Schols et al. 1993) causing muscle weakness, increased muscle fatigability and reduced endurance (American Thoracic Society and European Respiratory Society 1999; Debigare et al. 2001). The muscles have a low capacity for **aerobic respiration** due to decreased aerobic enzyme concentrations, capillarity and **mitochondrial** density (Casaburi et al. 1997; Ortega et al. 2002). This results in an early onset of **lactic acidosis** and muscle fatigue during exercise (Casaburi et al. 2001). Additionally, the oxygen requirements of muscle escalate dramatically during exercise. In COPD patients, however, the rate at which oxygen is extracted from circulating blood and used by the working tissues (VO_2) is significantly reduced (Casaburi et al. 1997), resulting in an oxygen deficit. All these factors, along with the progressive nature of COPD, contribute to the patient becoming locked in a downward spiral of increased breathlessness, worsening inactivity and further deconditioning (Figure 5.1).

As outlined above, disuse **atrophy** is certainly a contributory factor to loss of muscle mass in COPD, but the specific process by which quadriceps muscle dysfunction arises is unclear and is likely to be complex and multifactorial. Patients with severe COPD tend to have the greatest degree of quadriceps muscle dysfunction (Bernard et al. 1998). There is also further loss of quadriceps strength during a hospital admission for an exacerbation of COPD (Spruit

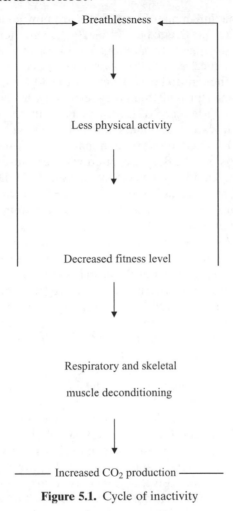

Figure 5.1. Cycle of inactivity

et al. 2003). This obviously has significant implications for those patients frequently admitted to hospital with exacerbations. Reduced peripheral muscle force in COPD has also been shown to correlate with a high consumption of medical resources (Decramer et al. 1994). These two factors combined could precipitate a downward spiral, with patients losing muscle strength during hospitalisation, in turn leading to increased healthcare usage, e.g. re-admission.

Generally, muscle wasting occurs when the rate of muscle protein breakdown (**catabolism**) is greater than the rate of muscle protein synthesis (**anabolism**). Chronic inflammatory processes are now considered to have an important role in COPD (Creutzberg et al. 2000; Dentener et al. 2001). Since inflammatory mediators activate catabolic pathways, this may lead to an anabolic/catabolic imbalance, especially given the reduced circulating levels of anabolic hormones thought to be associated with COPD. Circulating levels of **inflammatory factors** ('pro-inflammatory **cytokines**'), e.g. tumour necrosis factor-α (TNF-α), interleukin-8 (IL-8), are particularly evident in COPD patients with a lower lean muscle mass and higher resting energy expenditure (Schols et al. 1996). Levels of pro-inflammatory cytokines increase further during exacerbations, and IL-8 is associated with leg muscle weakness developing in hospitalised COPD patients (Spruit et al. 2003). Damage to proteins and lipids via increased **oxidative stress** may also contribute to the loss of muscle mass in COPD (Couillard & Prefaut 2005), as might a prolonged use of steroids (Decramer et al. 1994).

A patient with COPD becomes breathless on exertion predominantly due to ventilatory limitation. At rest, the loss of elastic recoil combined with increased resistance to expiratory airflow can lead to lung hyperinflation (static hyperinflation). On exertion, hyperinflation can progressively worsen (dynamic hyperinflation) resulting in a reduced inspiratory capacity that is insufficient in meeting the ventilation requirement of the exercise. Further increases in ventilation are thus achieved by increasing the respiratory rate. A patient with COPD, therefore, experiences breathlessness sooner than a subject without ventilatory limitation at a given level of exercise.

Dynamic hyperinflation also changes the operating characteristics of the lung and chest wall resulting in decreased compliance, increased work of breathing and inspiratory muscle weakness. The capacity of the patient with severe COPD to achieve appropriate inspiratory volumes is diminished further as dynamic hyperinflation increases. The imbalance between the increased load on the respiratory system and reduced ventilatory capacity results in increased central respiratory drive. This increase is disproportionately greater than the increase in ventilation during exercise in COPD patients ('neuromechanical uncoupling') (Sinderby et al. 2001), leading to increased breathlessness. Gas exchange is often impaired also, contributing further to the ventilatory limitation (Casaburi 1993). Finally, a genetic predisposition may underlie the variable nature of disability observed in this disease.

WHY EXERCISE?

Exercise is the cornerstone of a PR programme in patients with COPD, which has been shown to do the following:

- Reduce dyspnoea on exertion (Gigliotti et al. 2003).
- Increase muscle strength (Simpson et al. 1992; Clark et al. 2000).

- Reduce sensation of breathlessness (Fernal and Daniels 1984).
- Increase muscle endurance (Clark et al. 2000).
- Increase exercise tolerance (Guell et al. 2000).
- Improve health-related quality of life (Wedzicha et al. 1998; Griffiths et al. 2000).

There is, however, no evidence to suggest that exercise reduces airways obstruction on lung function testing or improves the ventilatory limitation in patients with COPD (Ortega et al. 2002). Exercise, however, is critical in breaking the cycle of chronic inactivity experienced by these patients. The deconditioning process may be halted, if not reversed, through regular exercise.

Randomised controlled trials investigating the efficacy of PR have reported significant improvements in maximal exercise capacity, walking distance and endurance capacity after PR. The exact way in which these improvements occur is not entirely clear but it is thought they are due to the reversal of a number of the above-mentioned physiological changes that occur in patients with COPD.

Porszasz et al. (2005) showed that exercise training in patients with severe COPD could reduce dynamic hyperinflation. This reduces breathlessness at a given level of exercise by increasing inspiratory capacity which, in turn, leads to improvements in submaximal exercise endurance. Endurance training increases aerobic enzyme concentration and capillary density within the quadriceps muscle (Maltais et al. 1996) as well as lowering blood lactate levels and increasing VO_2 kinetics (Casaburi et al. 1997). The physiological benefits of strength training are only just starting to emerge within the realm of COPD. The healthy elderly population has shown improvements in strength, mobility and muscle mass following strength training (Charette et al. 1991). These effects may well be applicable to the COPD population as Simpson et al. (1992) demonstrated a 30 per cent increase in strength with an 8-week weight-lifting regime with COPD patients.

In addition, exercise training combined with breathlessness management (including positioning, **breathing control**, pursed-lip breathing and pacing) can reduce patients' perception of breathlessness as measured on a modified Borg scale (see Box 5.1) (Hochstetter et al. 2005). Exposure to breathlessness within the safety of the PR setting enables patients to reduce their fear of becoming short of breath and gives them the confidence to become more active in their day-to-day life.

REFERRAL TO PULMONARY REHABILITATION (PR)

PR should be considered for all COPD patients with an FEV_1 below 80 per cent of the predicted value (GOLD consensus document – Fabbri & Hurd 2003) who experience symptoms of breathlessness. It is vital for the patient to

Box 5.1. Borg Breathlessness Score

0	nothing at all
0.5	very, very slight (just noticeable)
1	very slight
2	slight (light)
3	moderate
4	somewhat severe
5	severe (heavy)
6	
7	very severe
8	
9	very, very severe (almost maximal)
10	maximal

Name, address and telephone number

Date of Birth

Past Medical History (especially details of any cardiac disease)

Drug History

Respiratory Function Tests (RFTs)

MRC score (see Box 5.2)

Figure 5.2. Necessary patient information

be motivated to participate in rehabilitation (Troosters et al. 2005), otherwise compliance is likely to be poor and consequently the patient is unlikely to gain any benefit.

Each hospital/institution will have a different referral process but the whole multidisciplinary team (MDT) needs to be aware of the availability and accessibility of PR in their area. Referrals may be accepted from all MDT members working in both primary and secondary care. It is possible to accept self-referrals, as long as the diagnosis is confirmed by the patient's GP and relevant medical information is obtained prior to assessment and enrolment onto the programme.

It is essential that the following information is provided on referral to enable the PR team to assess the suitability of the patient for pulmonary rehabilitation, see Figure 5.2.

EXCLUSION CRITERIA

Again, these may differ between institutions but will usually include the following:

- unstable angina (BTS 2001)
- aortic stenosis
- aortic valve disease (BTS 2001)
- a serious cardiac event within the past six weeks
- uncontrolled cardiac arrhythmias
- uncontrolled hypertension
- uncompensated left ventricular failure (LVF)
- any medical problems that severely restrict ability to exercise or comply with the programme, e.g. dementia, severe arthritis.

ASSESSMENT OF A PATIENT FOR PULMONARY REHABILITATION

RESPIRATORY FUNCTION TESTS (RFTS)

RFTs are essential for an accurate diagnosis. It is important to confirm that the patient's breathlessness is primarily due to lung disease to ensure appropriate delivery of treatment and advice. Furthermore, effective spirometry ensures that the patient is provided with optimal inhaled therapy for their disease severity (NICE Guidelines 2004). RFTs should be conducted when the patient is stable and not during an exacerbation, when used as part of the diagnostic pathway. They can be carried out in primary as well as secondary care, now that GPs and practice nurses are becoming increasingly confident and competent at carrying out spirometry. It is hoped that the bulk of initial spirometry testing will be done in primary care, so reducing the need for patients to travel to hospital and minimising waiting times.

MEDICATION

Patients should be on the optimal inhaled therapy for their disease severity (NICE Guidelines 2004) ideally before commencing PR, in order to gain the most benefit possible from the exercise. Therapists working in PR should identify on assessment those patients whose respiratory medications are not optimal, referring them to the GP, COPD nurse or chest consultant as appropriate for a review. Patients who need oxygen (long-term oxygen therapy or ambulatory oxygen) may need to bring their own portable cylinders depending on the setting, as most community sites would not be able to provide oxygen.

EXERCISE TESTING

It is essential to employ an exercise tolerance test both pre- and post-rehabilitation to accurately and repeatedly measure exercise ability. A significant amount of research has been done to demonstrate the reliability, validity and sensitivity of a number of simple 'field tests' which are described below. Each is validated for use with COPD patients and any of the tests may be appropriate.

Objective measures such as heart rate, peripheral oxygen saturations (SpO_2) and Borg Symptom Scale rating for dyspnoea and leg fatigue should be taken before, during and after the exercise tests. To ensure reproducible and reliable testing, it is advisable to standardise the degree of encouragement given to the patient during the test and to repeat the test at least once after a sufficient rest (20–30 minutes is advised).

The incremental shuttle walk test (ISWT) is an externally paced exercise test that exercises the patient to a symptom-limited maximum (Singh et al. 1992). Pre-recorded instructions ensure that the description of the test given to the patient is standardised. It is easily repeatable as the walking speed is set by beeps on a tape/CD. The patient walks between two cones set 10 metres apart and is instructed to complete the 10 m distance before the next beep on the tape/CD. The time between the beeps decreases at certain intervals throughout the test, so that the patient needs to walk progressively faster to complete the 10 m course – hence an incremental test. The test continues until the patient is unable to complete the 10 m lap in the allotted time, which may be due to breathlessness or leg fatigue. A practice walk is recommended to familiarise patients with the nature of the test and ensure that patients reach their maximal exercise ability. The ISWT shows a strong correlation with VO_2 max, enabling health-care professionals to prescribe a level of exercise intensity appropriate to each patient (Singh et al. 1994). An increase of 48 m post PR has been shown to be required to deem the improvement as significant (Singh et al. 1992). To date, the minimum clinically important distance for the ISWT has not been established. As the ability of patients can vary so considerably, a standardised percentage improvement would perhaps be the most useful outcome measure in clinical practice.

The endurance shuttle walk test (ESWT) specifically tests endurance ability. It requires an ISWT to be carried out first, making it a fairly lengthy test to administer, especially as patients are required to complete a practice ISWT and ESWT to obtain good reproducibility. The patient is asked to walk for as long as possible at a speed calculated at 85 per cent of the maximal walking speed achieved during the ISWT, the speed being externally set by beeps on a tape or CD (Revill et al. 1999). The ESWT appears to be more sensitive to changes after pulmonary rehabilitation than the ISWT (Revill et al. 1999). It could also be used as a tool for endurance training within the PR class and to form the basis of a home walking programme for patients as they become accustomed to the walking speed.

The six-minute walking distance (6 MWD) is a sub-maximal test (a 3MWD or 12MWD can also be used). The patient walks a 10 m distance as for the ISWT and is instructed to cover as many metres as possible in the scheduled time. The patient should feel they are exercising to their maximum by the end of the test, although they can stop and rest as frequently as needed within the allocated time. It is, therefore, not so easily repeatable and relies heavily on patient motivation. It is recommended that a patient undertakes at least one practice walk to overcome the learning effect (Guyatt et al. 1984). Further repetitions of the test may result in a 3 per cent improvement each time, but as this is not considered significant, one practice test is acceptable. Redelmeier et al. (1997) identified the minimal significant clinical distance for the 6 MWD as an increase of 54 m after an intervention. However, the results of many studies into PR have demonstrated changes smaller than 54 m that still reach statistical significance (Knox et al. 1988; Elpern et al. 2000). Normal reference values are documented (Enright & Sherill 1998) enabling predicted values to be calculated.

AMBULATORY OXYGEN

The BTS 2001 statement indicates that 'supplementary oxygen during training should be provided where clinically important desaturation is documented at the training workload'. This evidence arises from a number of publications that show an improvement in exercise tolerance and relief of dyspnoea with supplemental oxygen in patients who demonstrate arterial desaturation (Somfay et al. 2002). According to the Royal College of Physicians (Wedzicha 1999), a trial of supplementary oxygen should be initiated where clinically significant desaturation is demonstrated (a fall of >4 per cent and below 90 per cent). If there is a clinically relevant improvement in distance (48 m or 35 per cent ISWT and 50 m 6 MWD) or relief of dyspnoea, the patient should be provided with oxygen titrated to maintain saturations of 89 per cent or above during peak workload. In practice, this may require a patient to repeat the ISWT on 2 litres and then 4 litres of oxygen to determine the optimum level.

MUSCLE TESTING

Both **isometric** and **isokinetic** muscle strength have been shown to be significantly reduced in COPD patients compared to healthy subjects (Decramer et al. 1994; Gosselink et al. 1996) with lower limb muscle strength being particularly affected (Bernard et al. 1998; Gosselink et al. 2000). This is of importance because skeletal muscle function is an independent marker of disease severity (Debigare et al. 2003) and COPD patients with significant muscle weakness appear to respond better to PR (Troosters et al. 2001).

Assessment of peripheral muscle strength can assist with optimising exercise prescription within PR, as it enables health-care professionals to target the weaker muscle groups. Muscle strength testing can be measured in a variety of ways, some of which require specific equipment that can prove to be expensive.

The Medical Research Council (1976) Manual Muscle Testing Scale 0–5 (Petty and Moore 1998) is the simplest way of testing peripheral muscle strength. However, this test may have questionable inter-rater and intra-rater reliability and is not always very sensitive when recording differences in muscle strength above grade 3 (active movement against gravity).

One-repetition maximum (1-RM) – weightlifting for **isotonic muscle** force – is a dynamic method for measuring the maximum weight that can be lifted at any one time during a standard weightlifting exercise. Weight increments between 1 kg and 5 kg are used with rests of between 1 and 5 minutes between attempts. This method has been shown to be safe in COPD patients (Kaelin et al. 1999).

Dynamometry is used to measure isometric muscle force. Handgrip dynamometry has been shown to be reliable and normal values are available (Mathiowetz et al. 1984, 1985). Hand-held dynamometry can be used for all muscle groups and has been effectively implemented with COPD patients in various studies (Troosters et al. 1999; Gosselink et al. 2000). Again, normal values are available (Andrews et al. 1996). Computer-assisted dynamometers can measure isokinetic and isometric muscle strength and have the advantage of measuring maximal muscle strength over a wide range of joint positions and velocities, although they require expensive equipment and thus are not available to many practitioners.

HEALTH-RELATED QUALITY OF LIFE (HRQL)

QOL questionnaires aim to measure a person's perception of how their chronic disease affects their life and general well-being. These subjective measures complement the objective measures to give a complete assessment of a patient's level of function. Lacasse et al. (2001) suggest that quality of life should be the primary outcome measure in pulmonary rehabilitation, given that symptomatic control is so crucial to the care of patients with COPD (ATS 1995).

DISEASE-SPECIFIC QUESTIONNAIRES

There are many HRQL questionnaires, which can be generic or disease-specific. The disease-specific questionnaires which have been designed and validated for patients with respiratory disease are:

• the chronic respiratory disease questionnaire – CRDQ (Guyatt et al. 1987);

- the St George's respiratory questionnaire – SGRQ (Jones et al. 1992);
- the breathing problems questionnaire – BPQ (Hyland et al. 1994);
- the quality of life in respiratory illness questionnaire – HRQoLRIQ (Maille et al. 1997).

Any one of these is appropriate to assess health-related quality of life pre- and post-PR. The two most commonly used in clinical practice are the CRDQ and the SGRQ.

ACTIVITIES OF DAILY LIVING (ADLS)

The cycle of inactivity that many COPD patients experience can lead to the elimination of daily activities from the patient's lifestyle. Restrick et al. (1993) showed that 78 per cent of patients with COPD experienced breathlessness when walking around at home and had difficulty performing routine ADLs.

There are three validated disease-specific ADL questionnaires available:

- the pulmonary functional status and dyspnoea questionnaire – PFSDQ (Lareau et al. 1994);
- the Manchester respiratory activities of daily living questionnaire – MRADL (Yohannes et al. 2000);
- the London chest activity of daily living scale – LCADL (Garrod et al. 2000).

ANXIETY AND DEPRESSION

It is well known that people with COPD can become anxious and/or depressed due to a variety of factors related to their chronic disease. These often include breathlessness itself, fear of the future (given the progressive nature of the disease), frustration at not being able to do all they wish to and social isolation. Anxiety in COPD patients has been shown to correlate with the risk of re-hospitalisation after an admission for an exacerbation of COPD (Gudmundsson et al. 2005).

It can, therefore, be valuable to record anxiety and depression scores pre- and post-PR. Anecdotally, PR can reduce anxiety by providing patients with skills to self-manage their disease, thus increasing their confidence. PR can also have an impact on depression by providing patients with a means of regular exercise and a social support network.

In light of the strong correlation between COPD, anxiety and depression, a PR programme can benefit from close links with psychology and counselling teams as part of the education programme, and for individual assessment and treatment where appropriate.

DYSPNOEA

The Borg Scale of Perceived Dyspnoea (Box 5.1) is a 10-point scale (Modified Borg) on which the patient is asked to rate how breathless they feel (Borg 1982). It has been validated for use with COPD patients (Kendrick et al. 2000) and shows a high level of sensitivity, but is an entirely subjective measure and can be interpreted differently by each patient. Its reliability, therefore, is questionable. Despite its shortcomings, the BORG Scale is widely used clinically to evaluate how breathless patients become during exercise testing and during the class itself. Patients can also use it themselves to monitor their own breathlessness when exercising. It is generally accepted that patients need to exercise until they are moderately to somewhat severely out of breath (a score of 3–4 on the BORG scale) in order to achieve a training effect.

An alternative way of evaluating how breathless a patient becomes during a PR class and to ensure they are working at a sufficient level, is to use their ability to speak a sentence (e.g. 'this exercise programme is going to do me good'). They should be able to say the sentence slowly with a few stops. Again, patients can use this method to monitor their own level of breathlessness when walking or exercising independently.

The MRC Dyspnoea Scale (Box 5.2) is a self-administered, valid and reliable 5-point scale, which describes a patient's degree of breathlessness related to activities (Bestall et al. 1999). Its use is recommended in the NICE Guidelines (2004) and it can be used to stratify patients according to ability.

The NICE Guidelines (2004) recommend that patients with an MRC score of 3–5 should be offered PR. There has been some concern that patients with an MRC grade of 5 may not benefit from PR. Heatley et al. (1999) reviewed PR outcomes when patients are categorised into MRC scale grades 3, 4 and 5 and demonstrated that the outcome measures (ISWT and CRDQ) improved

---

Box 5.2. The MRC Dyspnoea Scale

Grade 1 – I only get breathless with strenuous exercise.

Grade 2 – I get short of breath when hurrying on the level or walking up a slight hill.

Grade 3 – I walk slower than people of the same age on the level because of breathlessness or have to stop for breath when walking at my own pace on the level.

Grade 4 – I stop for breath after walking 100 yards or after a few minutes on the level.

Grade 5 – I am too breathless to leave the house, or breathless on dressing or undressing.

less in the MRC grade 5 group. Participation in PR, however, still resulted in clinically significant improvements in health status in patients with an MRC scale grade of 5.

Anecdotal evidence shows that patients with an MRC of 1 or 2 can achieve significant improvements in exercise capacity and quality of life from attending PR, but may only require shorter supervised programmes to introduce them to regular exercise. It may then be more appropriate for them to join an 'exercise referral' scheme. These are run nationwide and comprise community-based exercise sessions for people with a variety of medical problems, supervised by fitness instructors. These patients, however, can still benefit from the education component of PR and so it may in fact be appropriate for them to complete the whole PR course.

There is no evidence at present to suggest whether or not patients with an MRC of 1 benefit from PR, or whether 'exercise on referral' may be more appropriate. However, it is fair to suggest that some of these patients may still require certain components of the education programme. On the whole, therefore, patients with MRC scores between 2 and 5 should be considered for PR, although it may still be worthwhile to assess patients with an MRC of 1 to clinically decide the best treatment option. It should also be taken into consideration that breathlessness, and hence MRC score, is not necessarily linked to disease severity, again emphasising the importance of assessing each person's individual needs.

THE PULMONARY REHABILITATION PROGRAMME

EXERCISE COMPONENT

Exercise is the primary component of a successful pulmonary rehabilitation programme. The overall object of the exercise regime is to stimulate the cardiovascular system and skeletal muscle, leading to physiological adaptations, which reverse the deconditioning process and increase cardio-respiratory fitness. Until there is evidence to prove otherwise, it is generally accepted that the specific parameters of exercise programmes for healthy, inactive individuals can also be applied to patients with chronic disease, details of which will be discussed later in this section. The exercise regime needs to accommodate each patient's respiratory limitation, tailoring the programme to address individual functional problems. Specific goals should be set with the patient, focusing on activities that they find particularly difficult due to breathlessness. Choosing a goal based on a task or activity pertinent to the individual may increase motivation to exercise. The exercise regime may also need to be adapted to take account of other musculoskeletal and cardiovascular limitations.

Despite the weight of evidence in favour of exercise for the COPD population, the optimal duration, frequency, length, and intensity of training sessions are not well defined at present (BTS 2001), nor is the ideal type of training – endurance versus strength. Current guidelines, however, provide a consensus regarding each parameter of the exercise regime. Further research would help to confirm the ideal training programme for patients with COPD, to ensure they are gaining the most benefit possible.

DURATION

Programmes lasting between 4 and 12 weeks have been shown to be effective (Lake et al. 1990; Bendstrup et al. 1997) with the general consensus being that longer programmes result in a greater improvement. There is, however, a paucity of research directly comparing length of programme. One study demonstrated that a seven-week, twice weekly programme was more effective than a four-week programme (Green et al. 2001). Furthermore, six months of rehabilitation have been shown to yield more significant results than three months (Troosters et al. 2002). It is important to consider that shorter programmes are less expensive per patient and will enable more patients to access pulmonary rehabilitation (Troosters et al. 2005). On the other hand, longer programmes may be needed to change a person's behaviour, i.e. permanently adopt a more active lifestyle (Sneed & Paul 2003). The general recommendation currently is 6–8 weeks (BTS Guidelines 2002).

FREQUENCY

The current exercise guidelines for healthy subjects are 3–5 times per week for 20–30 minutes (American College of Sports Medicine 1998). It is generally accepted that these parameters are transferable to the COPD population, as no evidence exists to the contrary. The BTS advocates at least three exercise sessions per week, two of which should be supervised. General practice reflects these recommendations, with most PR programmes running twice weekly classes but encouraging patients to do at least one other exercise session at home per week.

It is important to encourage and enable the patients to exercise at home in addition to attending the classes regularly in order the gain the most benefit from the programme. Tools such as home exercise diaries, home walking programmes and PR exercise videos should therefore be considered, in order to maximise patients' compliance. It is also advisable, where possible, to make some of the exercises in the class transferable to the home environment, again to facilitate home exercising.

ENDURANCE VS STRENGTH

In clinical practice, PR programmes either comprise solely endurance exercise or a combination of strength and endurance exercise to help patients achieve their individual goal. To date, there has been no consensus in the field of PR on the role of strength training in PR exercise programmes (Puhan et al. 2005).

When comparing endurance-only, strength-only and combination regimes, significant improvements in exercise ability (measured by ISWT or 6MWD) have been found in all types of protocols (Ries et al. 1988; Sivori et al. 1998; Bernard et al. 1999; Wurtemberger & Bastian 2001; Normandin et al. 2002; Ortega et al. 2002; Spruit et al. 2002; Mador et al. 2004). One can expect to find a greater increase in exercise capacity with endurance-only exercises, as opposed to the combination approach, but this is in fact not borne out in the literature. As expected, combination regimes resulted in a larger increase in muscle strength when compared to endurance-only regimes, but this did not translate into significant benefits in terms of HRQL or exercise capacity (Bernard et al. 1999; Ortega et al. 2002; Mador et al. 2004). Despite this, however, the bulk of evidence on this subject does suggest that strength exercise tends to improve HRQL more than endurance alone. Hence, one of the conclusions made from a recent systematic review of exercise modalities is that strength training should be routinely included in the exercise component of a PR programme (Puhan et al. 2005).

Translating this into clinical practice, perhaps the emphasis should once again be brought back to the individual patient, as some may benefit from concentrating more on one exercise modality, depending on the specific limitation of each patient.

CONTINUOUS VS INTERVAL

Historically PR has tended to use interval training, whereas cardiac rehabilitation tends to use a continuous exercise programme in the form of a circuit class. There is evidence to show significant improvements in HRQL, maximum exercise capacity and peak oxygen uptake using both exercise regimes with no significant difference between them. However, studies demonstrate that interval training elicits fewer symptoms (Coppoolse et al. 1999; Vogiatzis et al. 2002).

This may be explained by the postulation that interval training elicits less dynamic hyperinflation when compared with continuous exercise, and so may be more appropriate for patients with more severe hyperinflation (Vogiatzis et al. 2002). Many COPD patients would find continuous exercise impossible and certainly very unpleasant due to severe breathlessness, needing a specific time for recovery between exercises.

As patients are diagnosed sooner and referred to PR earlier in the course of their disease, the patient group accessing PR will hopefully become less severe and so continuous exercise programmes may well become an option within PR. There are many aspects to bear in mind when considering this option. For example, the range of disease severities within one group and so whether continuous exercise is appropriate for all, the transferability of a circuit class to the home setting for independent home exercises and whether it allows for a truly individual, goal-based exercise programme.

FUNCTIONAL EXERCISE

Sewell et al. (2005) compared the use of patient-specific functional exercises to a general programme of strengthening exercises. No significant differences were seen in exercise testing, HRQL or ADL-specific questionnaires. This would infer that there is no benefit in designing programmes to specifically include functional exercises such as hoovering and bed making, rather that general upper limb and lower limb exercises are sufficient.

INTENSITY

In healthy subjects, aerobic or fitness training is usually targeted at 60–90 per cent of the predicted maximal heart rate or 50–80 per cent of the maximal oxygen uptake (ACSM 1998). This would be considered high-intensity exercise. It was initially suggested that due to their ventilatory limitation, patients with severe COPD may not be able to achieve a high enough training level to produce a physiological training effect (Belman et al. 1981). However, the interval approach to exercise appears to provide a way for COPD patients to sustain a sufficiently high intensity to result in a training effect, seen clinically as an improvement in exercise ability.

The evidence favouring high-intensity over low-intensity exercise has methodological flaws (Puhan et al. 2005) and so is of limited use in determining the optimal exercise intensity for the COPD population. It remains of interest, however, that exercising patients with moderate COPD at 80 per cent of the peak work rate resulted in a greater significant physiological response than when exercised at 40 per cent peak work rate (Casaburi et al. 1991). Functionally, high-intensity endurance exercise programmes have also been shown to improve exercise tolerance and muscle function in the severe COPD population (Casaburi et al. 1997) but in slight contrast, Maltais et al. (1997) showed that training at 60 per cent of the peak work achieved in a maximal incremental exercise test resulted in a significantly improved exercise tolerance. This may suggest, therefore, that exercising patients at moderate intensities may be sufficient to improve functional performance.

RECOMMENDATIONS FOR EXERCISE PRESCRIPTION

As outlined above, evidence for precise exercise prescription is not convincing and further research is warranted. It would appear beneficial to include both endurance and strength exercises and adopt an interval-based training strategy. Endurance training at a moderate or high intensity would seem necessary to improve the aerobic capacity of skeletal muscle, although there is also some suggestion that strength training is linked with increased oxidative capacity in healthy subjects (Frontera et al. 1990). Strength training in the healthy elderly has been shown to improve mobility and decrease the incidence of falls (ACSM 1998), and it would seem reasonable to assume this is also applicable to the elderly COPD population. A generalised upper and lower limb strengthening programme combined with endurance training is popular in clinical practice and has yielded effective improvements in walking distance and functional ability. As COPD patients have particularly weak ambulatory muscles, however, it may be more important to focus on these muscle groups with, for example, cycling, walking and step-ups combined with specific strengthening exercises.

EDUCATION COMPONENT

The PR programme should benefit from a multidisciplinary approach to the education component with input from specialities such as psychology, dietetics, occupational therapy, physiotherapy, palliative care, nursing and medicine (see Box 5.3).

The efficacy of education specifically within pulmonary rehab is yet to be established convincingly but the aim is to improve patients' self-management skills. One study by Bourbeau et al. (2003) in Canada showed a reduction in health-care utilisation after a disease-specific self-management intervention. Trained health professionals randomised patients to receive either a two-month comprehensive patient education programme consisting of weekly visits, or the usual care. Results showed significant reductions in hospital admissions (39.8 per cent) and accident and emergency visits (41 per cent) in

---

Box 5.3. Example of education sessions

- What is COPD?
- Managing breathlessness
- Secretion clearance
- Energy saving
- Nutrition
- Why exercise?
- Medication
- Stress and relaxation
- Living with a chronic disease
- Managing infections
- Palliative care
- How should we breathe?
- Oxygen
- NIV and advances in COPD management

the intervention group. Rea et al. (2004) compared usual care to a disease management programme including a COPD management guideline, a patient-specific care plan and pulmonary rehabilitation. Hospital admission data was compared for 12 months prior to and during the trial. Results showed a reduction in mean hospital bed days from 2.8 to 1.1 in the intervention group whereas those for the group receiving usual care increased from 3.5 to 4.0.

HEALTH RESOURCE UTILISATION AND HEALTH ECONOMICS

Hospital admissions for COPD currently place a huge burden on the NHS (Man et al. 2004). The potential of PR to reduce this burden is only just becoming apparent through recent research into this field. In comparison to the effect of PR on exercise capacity and health status, there is little data available from randomised controlled trials regarding the effect on health-care utilisation and health economics, not helped by the fact that these are relatively difficult parameters to measure. It has, however, been demonstrated by several *non-randomised* and *observational* studies that there is a trend towards a decrease in the length of hospitalisation in the year following a PR programme compared to the year preceding rehabilitation (Guell et al. 2000; Hui & Hewitt 2003).

There are few randomised controlled trials that have used health resource usage as an outcome measure. Griffiths et al. (2001) showed no difference between the rehabilitation and control groups in the number of hospital admissions. However, the number of days spent in hospital was significantly less in the rehabilitation group (mean 10.4 days versus 21.0 days) as was the number of GP home visits. Ries et al. (1995), however, found that duration of hospital stay between the two groups was not significant. In a recent small study, Man et al. (2004) showed that commencing PR two weeks after a hospital admission for an exacerbation resulted in fewer GP visits, hospital admissions and bed days. Again, recently, PR has been shown to be effective in reducing health-care resources over the 18 months following PR (California Pulmonary Rehabilitation Collaborative Group 2004). The data, however, were collected by self-reported questionnaire – possibly a less reliable method than objective measures used in other studies. Bourbeau et al. (2003) also showed a reduction in hospital admissions following a disease-specific self-management programme, comprising education sessions only.

Programme costs depend on location, class capacity, staffing levels and transport provision. In the UK, the cost of PR per patient has been estimated to be between £400 and £725 based on six to seven weeks' rehabilitation (White et al. 1997; Singh et al. 1998; Griffiths et al. 2001). Given the fact that *one* bed day on a medical ward has been estimated to cost in the region of £300, PR clearly has cost-saving potential if future research continues to demonstrate its ability to reduce length of stay and even keep patients out of hospital altogether.

THE FUTURE OF PULMONARY REHABILITATION

The evidence to prove that pulmonary rehabilitation improves the lives of patients with COPD is conclusive; thus PR is now recognised as an essential part of the management of patients with COPD. In 2002, however, it was found that only 1.7 per cent of the COPD population had access to a PR programme (BTS and BLF Pulmonary Rehabilitation Survey 2002). PR services have certainly expanded since, but this expansion needs to continue if the shortfall between demand and capacity is to be met.

COMMUNITY-BASED PULMONARY REHABILITATION PROGRAMMES

Traditionally PR programmes have always been hospital-based. This, along with the fact that the services are relatively sparse throughout the UK, may mean that patients have to travel significant distances to access the programmes. There is also often a significant waiting list for hospital-based programmes. Community-based PR is a comparatively recent development in the UK but may offer a solution to the current demand and capacity imbalance. PR can be run in many locations, e.g. local leisure centres, community halls or church halls. Community programmes make PR much more accessible for patients, which, in turn, may help to optimise compliance with completing the course. Setting up PR in the community is likely to enable more classes to be run, as hospital physiotherapy gyms can be in high demand.

Community-based programmes, however, will not be appropriate for all patients. Some patients with severe COPD or with multiple pathologies may be reliant on hospital transport to access a PR programme or may need to exercise in an acute hospital setting from a safety aspect, at least initially.

With sufficient supervision from health-care professionals and an appropriate risk assessment of the facilities, the community environment provides a very viable option for expanding pulmonary rehabilitation across the country.

LONG-TERM BENEFITS OF PR AND MAINTENANCE PROGRAMMES

As shown throughout this chapter, PR is a highly evidence-based intervention. It is much less clear, however, how long these benefits last. A review of the research in 1999 indicated that significant improvements in exercise capacity could be sustained for up to nine months after rehabilitation (Cambach et al. 1999). This presents a problem to those in the field of pulmonary rehabilitation, as if over time, patients lose the benefits gained from PR and return to their previous level of function, they are likely to be frequently re-referred, placing an ever-increasing demand on PR services. Hence, maintenance classes run in the community have been proposed as being one way of enabling patients to continue with regular exercise, in an attempt to maintain the benefits.

There is currently, however, little evidence to support the use of maintenance programmes. Research into this area is particularly challenging because COPD patients will naturally decline in function as their disease progresses. Furthermore, they will fluctuate day to day, with the weather or exacerbations affecting their ability to commit to regular exercise. For example, Griffiths et al. (2000) found that only 25 per cent of patients attended the majority of weekly maintenance sessions.

If maintenance programmes are thought to have the potential to sustain improvements after PR, then how often do patients need to attend to achieve this goal? This question is yet to be answered. Monthly exercise follow-up, in the main, has been shown to be ineffective in maintaining all improvements a year after PR (Ries et al. 1995; Brooks et al. 2002; Bestall et al. 2003). Interestingly, however, the control groups in all the studies actually deteriorated further, which would suggest that monthly exercise may at least have a role in slowing down the decline of this chronic progressive illness. In support of maintenance, weekly classes have been shown to reduce length of hospital stay and GP home visits (Griffiths et al. 2000). Additionally, an 8-week maintenance class post PR led to further improvements in walking distance and dyspnoea (Johnson et al. 2001), although the ability of weekly classes to maintain the physical and psychological benefits of PR in the long term is yet to be investigated.

Motivating and enabling any patient group to exercise for life are challenges, especially those with a chronic progressive disease. Ideally, patients should continue exercising at home, at least three times a week, but this relies on considerable self-motivation. Maintenance programmes, therefore, have the potential to keep patients motivated to exercise and anecdotally, this is most certainly the case. The social support that can be provided between patients at a maintenance group is also highly valuable. In fact, patients report feeling better equipped to deal with their illness from this one factor alone. Gym or studio classes are not to everyone's liking and it is widely accepted that adherence to any exercise programme will be significantly better if the activity is enjoyable for the individual. The ultimate goal therefore, must to be to provide choice for patients, for example, swimming, walking or dancing groups. Walking groups especially are growing nationwide, as the importance of exercise for patients with chronic disease becomes increasingly recognised. Maintenance classes can also become over-subscribed and with limited resources, other avenues need to be investigated to allow all patients with COPD to exercise as they choose.

CONCLUSION

Pulmonary rehabilitation is now recognised as being crucial to the management of patients with COPD. Its benefits are manifold, improving both physical function and quality of life, as well as having the potential to reduce the financial burden of COPD on the NHS.

What is most striking about PR in its clinical context is the magnitude of the improvements seen and how patients feel their life has changed for the better so dramatically. PR helps patients to regain control of their lives by increasing their understanding of their disease and enabling them to help themselves. This alone can be immensely powerful. Subsequently, it can be a very rewarding area of clinical practice in which to work.

Unfortunately, PR is not yet widely available across the UK, although the number of programmes is continually on the increase. In order to provide PR for all COPD patients who are limited by their breathlessness, which ultimately is our aim, services will need to expand into the community. This way, PR can become more accessible and thus more attractive to patients, as well as being able to provide a larger capacity to meet the ever-increasing demand on the service. The community setting may also be more effective at encouraging and empowering patients to exercise for life. This change in lifestyle is key, if patients are to maintain the benefits of PR and delay the progressive nature of this chronic disease.

REFERENCES

American College of Sports Medicine Position Stand (1998) The recommended quantity of exercise for developing and maintaining cardiorespiratory and muscular fitness, and flexibility in healthy adults. *Medical Science Sports* Exercise **30**: 975–991.

American Thoracic Society (1995) Standards for the diagnosis and care of patients with COPD. *American Journal of Respiratory Critical Care Medicine* **152**: S77–S120.

American Thoracic Society (1999) Skeletal muscle dysfunction in chronic obstructive pulmonary disease: a statement of the American Thoracic Society and European Respiratory Society. *American Journal of Respiratory Critical Care Medicine* **159**(4): 2S–40.

Andrews A W, Thomas M W, Bohannon R W (1996) Normative values for isometric muscle force measurements obtained with hand-held dynamometers. *Physical Therapy* **76**: 248–259.

Belman M J, Kendregan B A (1981) Exercise training fails to increase skeletal muscle enzymes in patients with chronic obstructive pulmonary disease. *American Review of Respiratory Disease* **123**: 256–261.

Bendstrup K E, Ingermann J J, Holm S, Bengtsson B (1997) Outpatient rehabilitation improves activities of daily living, quality of life and exercise tolerance in COPD. *European Respiratory Journal* **10**: 2801–2806.

Bernard S, Leblanc P, Whittom F, et al. (1998) Peripheral muscle weakness in patients with COPD. *American Journal of Respiratory Critical Care Medicine* **158**: 629–634.

Bernard S, Whitton F, LeBlanc P, et al. (1999) Aerobic and strength training in patients with COPD. *American Journal of Respiratory Critical Care Medicine* **159**: 896–901.

Bestall J C, Paul E A, Garrod R, Garnham R, Jones P W (2003) Longitudinal trends in exercise capacity and health status after pulmonary rehabilitation in patients with COPD. *Respiratory Medicine* **97**: 173–180.

Bestall J C, Paul E A, Garrod R, Garnham R, Jones P W, Wedzicha J A (1999) Usefulness of the MRC dyspnoea scale as a measure of disability in patients with COPD. *Thorax* **54**: 581–586.

Borg C (1982) Psychophysical basis of perceived exertion. *Medical Science Sports Exercise* **14**: 377–381.

Bourbeau J, Julien M, Maltais F, Rouleau M, Beaupre A, Begin R, Renzi P, Nault D, Borycki E, Schwartzman K (2003) Reduction of hospital utilisation in patients with chronic obstructive pulmonary disease: a disease-specific self-management intervention. *Archives of Internal Medicine* **163**: 585–591.

British Thoracic Society (2001) Society Standards of Care statement on pulmonary rehabilitation. *Thorax* **56**: 827–834.

British Thoracic Society and British Lung Foundation (2002) Pulmonary rehabilitation survey. Available at: http:// www.brit-thoracic.org.uk (accessed January 2006).

Brooks D, Krip B, Mangovski-Alzamora S, Goldstein R S (2002) The effect of post-rehabilitation programmes among individuals with COPD. *European Respiratory Journal* **20**: 20–29.

California Pulmonary Rehabilitation Collaborative Group (2004) Effects of pulmonary rehabilitation on dyspnea, quality of life and healthcare costs in California. *Journal of Cardiopulmonary Rehabilitation* **24**(1): 52–62.

Cambach W, Wagenaar R C, Koelman T W, Ton van Keimpema A R J, Kemper H C G (1999) The long-term effects of pulmonary rehabilitation in patients with asthma and COPD: a research synthesis. *Archives of Physical Medicine Rehabilitation* **80**: 103–111.

Casaburi R (1993) Exercise training in chronic obstructive lung disease. In Casaburi R, Petty T L (eds) *Principles and Practice of Pulmonary Rehabilitation*. Philadelphia, PA: WB Saunders Company.

Casaburi R, Patessio A, Loli F, et al. (1991) Reduction in exercise lactic acidosis and ventilation as a result of exercise training in patients with obstructive lung disease. *American Review of Respiratory Diseases* **143**: 9–18.

Casaburi R, Porszasz J, Burns M R, Carithers R, Chang R S Y, Cooper C B (1997) Physiological benefits of exercise training in rehabilitation of patients with severe COPD. *American Review of Respiratory Diseases* **155**: 1541–1551.

Charette S L, McEvoy L, Pyka G, et al. (1991) Muscle hypertrophy response to resistance training in older women. *Journal of Applied Physiology* **70**: 1912–1916.

Clark C J, Cochrane L M, Mackay E, et al. (2000) Skeletal muscle strength and endurance in patients with mild COPD and the effects of weight training. *European Respiratory Journal* **15**: 92–97.

Cole T M, Fishman A P (1994) Workshop on pulmonary rehabilitation research: a commentary. *American Journal of Physical Medicine and Rehabilitation* **73**: 132–133.

Coppoolse R, Scols A M, Baarends E M, et al. (1999) Interval versus continuous training in patients with severe COPD: a randomised controlled trial. *European Respiratory Journal* **14**: 258–263.

Couillard A, Prefaut C (2005) From muscle disuse to myopathy in COPD: potential contribution of oxidative stress. *European Respiratory Journal* **26**: 703–719.

Creutzberg E C, Schols A M, Weling-Scheepers C A, Buurman W A, Wouters E F M (2000) Characterization of non-response to high caloric oral nutritional therapy in depleted patients with chronic obstructive pulmonary disease. *American Journal of Respiratory Critical Care Medicine* **161**: 745–752.

Debigare R, Cote C H, Maltais F (2001) Peripheral muscle wasting in chronic obstructive pulmonary disease: clinical relevance and mechanisms. *American Journal of Respiratory Critical Care Medicine* **164**: 1712–1717.

Debigare R, Marquis K, Cote C, et al. (2003) Catabolic/anabolic balance and muscle wasting in patients with COPD. *Chest* **124**(1): 83–89.

Decramer M, Lacquet L M, Fagard R, Rogiers P (1994) Corticosteroids contribute to muscle weakness in chronic airflow obstruction. *American Journal of Respiratory Critical Care Medicine* **150**: 11–16.

Dentener M A, Creutzberg E C, Schols A M, Mantovani A, van t Veer C, Buurman W A, Wouters E F M (2001) Systemic anti-inflammatory mediators in COPD: increase in soluble interleukin 1 receptor II during treatment of exacerbations. *Thorax* **56**: 721–726.

Elpern E H, Stevens D, Kesten S (2000) Variability in performance of timed walk tests in pulmonary rehabilitation programmes. *Chest* **158**: 1384–1387.

Enright P L, Sherill D L (1998) Reference equations for the six-minute walk in healthy adults. *American Journal of Respiratory Critical Care Medicine* **58**: 1384–1387.

Fabbri L M, Hurd S S (2003) Global strategy for the diagnosis, management and prevention of COPD: 2003 update. *European Respiratory Journal* **22**: 1–2.

Fernal B, Daniels F S (1984) Electroencephalographic changes after a prolonged running period: evidence for a relaxation response. *Medicine and Science in Sports and Exercise* **16**: 181.

Foster S, Thomas H M (1990) Pulmonary rehabilitation in lung disease other than COPD. *American Review of Respiratory Disease* **141**: 601–604.

Frontera W R, Meredith C N, O'Reilly K P, Evans W J (1990) Strength training and determinants of VO2 max in older men. *Journal of Applied Physiology* **68**: 329–333.

Garrod R (2004) Disability and handicap in COPD. In Garrod R (ed.) *Pulmonary Rehabilitation: An Interdisciplinary Approach*. London: Whurr Publishers Ltd.

Garrod R, Bestall J C, Paul E A, Wedzicha J A, Jones P W (2000) Development and validation of a standardised measure of activity of daily living in patients with severe COPD: the London Chest Activity of Daily Living Scale (LCADL). *Respiratory Medicine* **94**: 589–596.

Gigliotti F, Coli C, Bianchi R, Romagnoli I, Lanini B, Binazzi B, Scano G (2003) Exercise training improves exertional dyspnoea in patients with COPD: evidence of the role of mechanical factors. *Chest* **123**: 1794–1802.

Gosselink R, Troosters T, Decramer M (1996) Peripheral muscle weakness contributes to exercise limitation in COPD. *American Journal of Respiratory Critical Care Medicine* **153**: 976–980.

Gosselink R, Troosters T, Decramer M (2000) Distribution of respiratory and peripheral muscle weakness in patients with stable COPD. *Journal of Cardiopulmonary Rehabilitation* **20**: 353–358.

Green R H, Singh S J, Williams J, Morgan M D (2001) A randomised controlled trial of four weeks versus seven weeks of pulmonary rehabilitation in COPD. *Thorax* **56**: 143–145.

Griffiths T L, Burr M L, Campbell I A, et al. (2000) Results at 1 year of outpatient multi-disciplinary pulmonary rehabilitation: a randomised controlled trial. *Lancet* **355**: 362–368.

Griffiths T L, Phillips C J, Davies S, et al. (2001) Cost effectiveness of an outpatient multidisciplinary pulmonary rehabilitation programme. *Thorax* **56**: 779–784.

Gudmundsson G, Gislason T, Janson C, Lindberg E, Hallin R, Ulrik C S, Brondum E, Nieminen M M, Aine T, Bakke P (2005) Risk factors for rehospitalisation in COPD: role of health status, anxiety and depression. *European Respiratory Journal* **26**: 414–419.

Guell R, Casan P, Belda J, Sangenis M, Morante F, Guyatt G H, Sanchis J (2000) Long term effects of outpatient rehabilitation of COPD: a randomised controlled trial. *Chest* **117**: 976–983.

Guyatt G H, Berman L B, Townsend M, Pugsley S O, Chambers L W (1987) A measure of quality of life for clinical trials in chronic lung disease. *Thorax* **42**: 773–778.

Guyatt G H, Pugsley S O, Sullivan M J, et al. (1984) Effect of encouragement on walking test performance. *Thorax* **39**: 818–822.

Heatley M, Foster S, Dogan S, Jefferson D, Price D C, Afolabi O A, Peel E T (1999) Outcomes of post pulmonary rehabilitation when COPD patients are categorised into MRC dyspnoea scales 3, 4 and 5. *Thorax* **54**: 60.

Hochstetter J K, Lewis J, Soares-Smith L (2005) An investigation into the immediate impact of breathlessness management on the breathless patient: randomised controlled trial. *Physiotherapy* **91**: 178–185.

Hui K P, Hewitt A B (2003) A simple pulmonary rehabilitation program improves health outcomes and reduces hospital utilisation in patients with COPD. *Chest* **124**: 94–97.

Hyland M E, Bott J, Singh S J, et al. (1994) Domains, constructs and the development of the breathing problems questionnaire. *Quality of Life Research* **3**: 245–256.

Johnson L C, Backley J, Gray B, Moxham J (2001) A controlled pilot study of a community based maintenance class for patients with severe COPD following pulmonary rehabilitation. *Thorax* **56**: Supplement III, iii37.

Jones P W, Quirk F H, Baveystock C M, Littlejohns P (1992) A self-complete measure of health status for chronic airflow limitation: The St George's Respiratory Questionnaire. *American Review of Respiratory Disease* **145**: 1321–1327.

Kaelin M E, Swank A M, Adams K J, et al. (1999) Cardiopulmonary responses, muscle soreness, and injury during the one repetition maximum assessment in pulmonary rehabilitation patients. *Journal of Cardiopulmonary Rehabilitation* **19**: 366–372.

Kendrick K, Baxi S, Smith R (2000) Usefulness of the modified 0–10 Borg scale in assessing the degree of dyspnea in patients with COPD and asthma. *Journal of Emergency Nursing* **26**(3): 216–222.

Knox A J, Morrison J F, Muers M F (1988) Reproducibility of walking test results in COPD. *Thorax* **43**: 388–392.

Kyprianou A, Russo R (2005) Defining the role of pulmonary rehabilitation in non-COPD lung disease. *Journal of Respiratory Disease* **26**: 105–114.

Lacasse Y, Brosseau L, Milne S, Martin S, Wong E, Guyatt G H, Goldstein R S (2001) Pulmonary rehabilitation for chronic obstructive pulmonary disease. Cochrane database *System Review* 3: CD003793.

Lacasse Y, Wong E, Guyatt G H, et al. (1996) Meta-analysis of respiratory rehabilitation in Chronic Obstructive Pulmonary Disease. *Lancet* **348**(9035): 1115–1119.

Lake F R, Henderson K, Briffa T, Openshaw J, Musk A W (1990) Upper-limb and lower-limb exercise training in patients with chronic airflow obstruction. *Chest* **97**: 1077–1082.

Larcau S C, Meek P M, Roos P J (1994) Development and testing of the Pulmonary Functional Status and Dyspnoea Questionnaire (PFSDQ). *Heart and Lung: Journal of Acute and Critical Care* **23**: 242–250.

Mador M J, Bozkanat E, Aggarwal A, et al. (2004) Endurance and strength training in patients with COPD. *Chest* **125**: 2036–2045.

Maille A R, Koning C J, Zwinderman A H, et al. (1997) The development of the quality of life for respiratory illness questionnaire (QOL-RIQ): a disease specific questionnaire for patients with mild to moderate chronic non-specific lung disease. *Respiratory Medicine* **91**: 297–309.

Make B J (1986) Pulmonary rehabilitation: myth or reality? *Clinical Chest Medicine* **7**(4): 519–540.

Maltais F, LeBlanc P, Jobin J, et al. (1997) Intensity of training and physiologic adaptation in patients with COPD. *American Journal of Respiratory Critical Care Medicine* **155**: 555–561.

Maltais F, LeBlanc P, Simard C, et al. (1996) Skeletal muscle adaptation to endurance training in patients with COPD. *American Journal of Respiratory Critical Care Medicine* **154**: 442–447.

Man W D-C, Polkey M I, Donaldson N, Gray B, Moxham J (2004) Community pulmonary rehabilitation after hospitalisation for acute exacerbations of COPD: randomised controlled trial. *British Medical Journal* **329**: 1209.

Man W D-C, Soliman M G, Nikoletou D, Harris M L, Rafferty G F, Mustfa N, Polkey M I, Moxham J (2003) Non-volitional assessment of skeletal muscle strength in Chronic Obstructive Pulmonary Disease. *Thorax* **58**: 665–669.

Mathiowetz V, Dove M, Kashman N, et al. (1985) Grip and pinch strength: normative data for adults. *Archives of Physical Medicine Rehabilitation* **66**: 69–72.

Mathiowetz V, Weber K, Volland G, et al. (1984) Reliability and validity of grip and pinch strength evaluations. *Journal of Hand Surgery* **9**: 222–226.

NICE Guidelines (2004) *Chronic Obstructive Pulmonary Disease: Management of Chronic Obstructive Pulmonary Disease in Adults in Primary and Secondary Care. Clinical Guideline.* London: HMSO.

Normandin E A, McCusker C, Connors M, et al. (2002) An evaluation of two approaches to exercise conditioning in pulmonary rehabilitation. *Chest* **121**: 1085–1091.

Ortega F, Toral J, Cejudo P, et al. (2002) Comparison of effects of strength and endurance training in patients with COPD. *American Journal of Critical Care Medicine* **166**: 669–674.

Petty N, Moore A (1998) *Neuromusculoskeletal Examination and Assessment: A Handbook for Therapists.* London: Churchill Livingstone.

Porszasz J, Emtner M, Goto S, Somfay A, Whipp B, Casaburi R (2005) Exercise training decreases ventilatory requirements and exercise induced hyperinflation at submaximal intensities in patients with COPD. *Chest* **128**: 2025–2034.

Puhan M A, Schunemann H J, Frey M, Scharplatz M, Bachmann L M (2005) How should COPD patients exercise during respiratory rehabilitation? Comparison of exercise modalities and intensities to treat skeletal muscle dysfunction. *Thorax* **60**: 367–375.

Rea H, McAuley S, Stewart A, Lamont C, Roseman P, Didsbury P (2004) A chronic disease management programme can reduce days in hospital for patients with COPD. *Internal Medicine Journal* **34**(11): 608–614.

Redelmeier D A, Bayoumi A M, Goldstein R S, Guyatt G H (1997) Interpreting small differences in functional status: the six-minute walk test in chronic lung disease patients. *American Journal of Respiratory Critical Care Medicine* **155**: 1278–1282.

Restrick L J, Paul E A, Braid G M, Cullinan P, Moore-Gillon J, Wedzicha J A (1993) Survey of activities of daily living in patients with COPD. *Thorax* **48**: 936–946.

Revill S M, Morgan M D L, Singh S J, et al. (1999) The endurance shuttle walk test: a new field test for the assessment of endurance capacity in chronic obstructive disease. *Thorax* **54**: 231–232.

Ries A L, Ellis B, Hawkins R W (1988) Upper extremity exercise training in COPD. *Chest* **93**: 688–692.

Ries A L, Kaplan R M, Limberg T M, et al. (1995) Effects of pulmonary rehabilitation on physiologic and psychosocial outcomes in patients with chronic obstructive pulmonary disease. *Annals of Internal Medicine* **122**: 823–832.

Salman G F, Mosier M C, Beasley B W, et al. (2003) Rehabilitation for patients with Chronic Obstructive Pulmonary Disease: meta-analysis of randomised controlled trials. *Journal of General Internal Medicine* **18**(3): 213–221.

Schols A M, et al. (1993) Prevalence and characteristics of nutritional depletion in patients with stable COPD eligible for pulmonary rehabilitation. *American Review of Respiratory Disease* **147**(5): 1151–1156.

Schols A M, et al. (1996) Evidence for a relation between metabolic derangements and increased levels of inflammatory mediators in a subgroup of patients with chronic obstructive pulmonary disease. *Thorax* **51**: 819–824.

Sewell L, Singh S J, Williams J E, Collier R, Morgan M D (2005) Can individualized rehabilitation improve functional independence in elderly patients with COPD? *Chest* **128**: 1194–1200.

Simpson K, Killian K, McCartney N, et al. (1992) Randomised controlled trial of weightlifting exercise in patients with chronic airflow limitation. *Thorax* **47**: 70–75.

Sinderby C, et al. (2001) Diaphragm activation during exercise in chronic obstructive pulmonary disease. *American Journal of Respiratory Critical Care Medicine* **163**(7): 1637–1641.

Singh S J, Morgan M D L, Hardman A E, et al. (1994) Comparison of oxygen uptake during conventional treadmill and the shuttle walking test in chronic airflow limitation. *European Respiratory Journal* **7**: 2016–2020.

Singh S, Morgan M, Scott S, et al. (1992) Development of a shuttle walking test of disability in patients with chronic airways obstruction. *Thorax* **47**(12): 1019–1024.

Singh S J, Smith D L, Hyland M E, et al. (1998) A short outpatient Pulmonary Rehabilitation programme: Immediate and longer-term effects on exercise performance and quality of life. *Respiratory Medicine* **92**(9): 1046–1054.

Sivori M, Rhodius E, Kaplan P, et al. (1998) Exercise training in COPD: Comparative study of aerobic training of lower limbs vs. combination with upper limbs. *Medicina* **58**: 717–727.

Sneed N V, Paul S C (2003) Readiness for behavioural changes in patients with heart failure. *American Journal of Critical Care* **12**: 444–453.

Somfay A, Porzasz J, Lee S M, Casaburi R (2002) Effect of hypoxia on gas exchange and lactate kinetics following exercise onset in non-hypoxaemic COPD patients. *Chest* **121**: 393–400.

Spruit M A, Gosselink R, Troosters T, et al. (2002) Resistance versus endurance training in patients with COPD and peripheral muscle weakness. *European Respiratory Journal* **19**: 1072–1078.

Spruit M A, et al. (2003) Muscle force during an acute exacerbation in hospitalised patients with COPD and its relationship with CXCL8 and IGF-I. *Thorax* **58**: 752–756.

Troosters T, Casaburi R, Gosselink R, Decramer M (2005) Pulmonary rehabilitation in COPD. *American Journal of Respiratory Critical Care Medicine* **172**: 19–38.

Troosters T, Gosselink R, Decramer M (1999) Reliability of handheld spirometry to measure peripheral muscle strength in COPD. *European Respiratory Journal* **14**: 481.

Troosters T, Gosselink R, Decramer M (2001) Exercise training in COPD: how to distinguish responders from non-responders. *Journal of Cardiopulmonary Rehabilitation* **21**: 10–17.

Troosters T, Gosselink R, Van Hove P, Derom E, et al. (2002) Effects of pulmonary rehabilitation in a clinical setting. *American Journal of Respiratory Critical Care Medicine* **165**: A735.

Vogiatzis I, Nanas S, Roussos C (2002) Interval training as an alternative modality to continuous exercise in patients with COPD. *European Respiratory Journal* **20**: 12–19.

Wedzicha J A (1999) Domiciliary oxygen therapy services: clinical guidelines and advice for prescribers. Summary of a report of the Royal College of Physicians. *Journal of Royal College of Physicians of London* **33**: 445–447.

Wedzicha J A, Bestall J C, Garrod R, et al. (1998) Randomised controlled trial of PR in severe COPD patients, stratified with the MRC dyspnoea scale. *European Respiratory Journal* **30**: 363–369.

White R J, Rudkin S T, Ashley J, et al. (1997) Outpatient Pulmonary Rehabilitation in severe COPD. *Journal of the Royal College of Physicians of London* **31**(5): 541–545.

Wurtemberger G, Bastian K (2001) Functional effects of different training in patients with COPD. *Pneumologie* **55**: 553–562.

Yohannes A M, Roomi J, Winn S, Connolly M J (2000) The Manchester Respiratory Activities of Daily Living questionnaire: development, reliability, validity and responsiveness to pulmonary rehabilitation. *Journal of American Geriatric Society* **48**: 1496–1500.

6 Quality of Life

6.1 FATIGUE MANAGEMENT

TANYA NAVARRO
King's College Hospital, London

Fatigue is one of most debilitating symptoms of COPD. It cannot be cured; however, it can be managed. Fatigue management is a collection of principles/ techniques, that allow someone who is fatigued to better manage their daily life and activities. It is hoped that this section will increase awareness of fatigue and its management, but it is not intended to serve as a sole guide for those planning to run a fatigue management group.

"Things you took for granted, like changing the curtains, using a hoover, getting in and out of the bath, your life will never be the same again."

FATIGUE IN COPD

Despite fatigue being identified as a major problem for COPD patients, little research has been completed on the impact it has on patients' symptoms and activities of daily living (Small & Lamb 1999).

An early study carried out by the First National Health and Nutrition Examination Survey (Chen 1986) showed that the risk of fatigue in pulmonary patients was greater than in patients with rheumatoid arthritis or anaemia. A comprehensive study by Breslin et al. (1998) showed a positive relationship between fatigue and disease severity, exercise tolerance, depression and overall quality of life. This study demonstrated that fatigue was an important symptom requiring evaluation and management, as it actively prevented patients from doing the things they wanted to do. Furthermore, it was hypothesised that the perception of fatigue may serve as a self-protective function, providing a warning that activity needs to be limited. More recently, a large study was carried out (n = 209) using information from those close to or who had cared for recently deceased patients. Fatigue or 'weakness' was rated as the second most common symptom (96 per cent), which was present 'all of the time or sometimes', where breathlessness was the most common symptom (98 per cent) (Elkington et al. 2005): it is clear that fatigue is a major symptom affecting the life of those with COPD.

Managing Chronic Obstructive Pulmonary Disease. Edited by L. Blackler, C. Jones and C. Mooney
© 2007 John Wiley & Sons Ltd

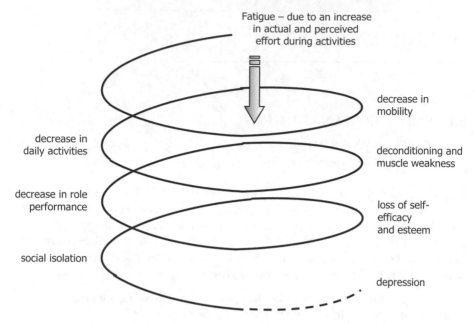

Figure 6.1.1. The impact of fatigue on daily life. *Source*: Adapted from The Disability Spiral (Oliver & Sewell, in Turner et al., 2002)

Figure 6.1.1 shows a hypothetical negative cycle of decline resulting from fatigue in COPD.

FATIGUE

Fatigue can be described as the perception of generalised tiredness, exhaustion, or lack of energy (Tack 1990; Belza et al. 1993). There are two types of fatigue: acute and chronic. Acute fatigue is normal or expected tiredness, has a rapid onset, and is usually of short duration. Chronic fatigue is a prolonged, debilitating fatigue that persists or recurs (CancerMail 2002). Although there is a variety of factors involved in the development of fatigue, only the physiological mechanisms in relation to COPD will be discussed here.

FATIGUE IN CHRONIC DISEASE

Fatigue is common in patients with chronic illness (Swain 2000). Despite this, fatigue is often ignored by medical clinicians, due to its subjective nature and the lack of an effective therapy (Small & Lamb 1999). There has been a significant amount written about fatigue in non-pulmonary diseases. Oncology patients identify severe fatigue as the symptom which interferes most with their normal routines (Lipman & Lawrence 2004). Similarly, palliative care patients report fatigue to be the symptom which has the most profound effect on their quality of life (Lane 2005). The effect of fatigue on quality of life has been studied in a number of chronic diseases, including rheumatoid arthritis (Wolfe et al. 1996; Huyser et al. 1998), multiple sclerosis (Freal et al. 1984; Krupp et al. 1988) and systemic lupus erythematosus (Krupp et al. 1990; Denburg et al. 1997). Patients consistently identify fatigue as one of the most problematic aspects of their disease and one of the key factors leading to a decrease in their quality of life (Swain 2000).

APPROACH TO FATIGUE MANAGEMENT

Fatigue management is a compensatory approach, often undertaken by occupational therapists (Downey 1981, in Pedretti & Early 2001; Oliver & Sewell, in Turner et al. 2002), which can enable people to carry out their daily activities in a more energy-efficient way. This allows people to conserve their energy resources, so that they can complete those activities which are most important to them (Downey 1981, in Pedretti & Early 2001). It can also include relaxation techniques, and an analysis of any difficulties with activities of daily living, as well as the recommendation or provision of equipment or environmental adaptations. Fatigue management is commonly referred to as energy conservation; however, this term can be misleading. Upon asking a COPD patient what this term referred to, she wondered whether it was about using low-energy light bulbs . . .

MECHANISMS FOR CAUSES OF FATIGUE WITHIN COPD

Studies by Baarends et al. (1997), using cycling as exercise, found that energy expended during exercise as well as total daily energy expenditure, was higher in COPD patients compared with healthy subjects. This may be due to the increased amount of energy needed for breathing, possibly due to higher airway resistance. A later study by Velloso et al. (2003) used upper limb exercise as COPD patients often find these activities very tiring. The results showed that moderate to severe COPD patients exhibited a significantly higher VO_2[1] when compared to their own maximum value. This means that compared to healthy controls, patients with moderate to severe disease have a higher oxygen cost for the same task, with the patient having to exert themselves more, in relative terms, than someone without COPD.

Similarly, a study by Steiner et al. (2005) measured biochemical changes within skeletal muscle in COPD patients, and age-matched healthy volunteers. Muscle biopsy samples were taken at rest and following a constant workload cycle test performed at 80 per cent peak workload. The results showed that even though all individuals were working at 80 per cent of their peak capacity, COPD patients achieved far lower speeds than healthy controls, despite their metabolism working at the same rate. They also demonstrated a significant level of metabolic stress during these tasks. A healthy volunteer would have to work at a much harder level to elicit an equivalent response.

This study demonstrates that COPD patients show significant metabolic stress at low absolute workloads, similar to those required for activities of daily living, and therefore find such tasks physically demanding. This means that a COPD patient would have greater fatigue levels carrying out normal everyday tasks. These levels of fatigue are equivalent to tasks categorised as heavy exercise in non-COPD patients. These results may explain why patients with moderate to severe COPD often feel fatigued. Metabolically speaking, their bodies appear to work less efficiently.

TREATMENT FOR FATIGUE

There is no pharmacological treatment for fatigue, but fatigue management principles and techniques can be useful to improve fatigue levels. This is best done in conjunction with pulmonary rehabilitation (PR), in order to build up strength and stamina. There is much evidence for the efficacy of PR; this is discussed in Chapter 5.

RESEARCH INTO FATIGUE MANAGEMENT

Case reports by Branick (2003) using a pulse oximeter and adaptive techniques during activities of daily living found that fatigue management could be beneficial. More research has been carried out with patients with chronic diseases such as cancer, multiple sclerosis and rheumatoid arthritis. Mathiowietz et al. (2001) showed a significant improvement in levels of fatigue, quality of life measures as well as increased use of energy conservation behaviours. Patients attending the fatigue management workshops report finding the sessions very useful; however, further research is needed to look at the efficacy of fatigue management with COPD patients.

TECHNIQUES TO COUNTER FATIGUE

Patients are often expert at managing their own condition and have developed coping mechanisms for many areas but there are also areas where they may be struggling. The main principles behind fatigue management as well as some tips and techniques for common areas of difficulty within each activity area are now presented.

Prioritisation

Establishing what the patient actually does each day, as well as what they really want to do, is a vitally important starting point. This enables them to identify

---

Box 6.1.1. Prioritisation and planning list

What tasks/activities do I do?
What tasks/activities do I do for others, if any?
Beside each activity, mark VIP if it is very important to you that you do
  this activity YOURSELF or No if it is not so important.
What tasks/activities would I like to be able to do but find very difficult/
  impossible?
Consider whether any of these can be made easier/done less often/using
  less energy?
Ask family/friend/carer for their opinion.
Consider those tasks marked with No. Do I really want to use my valuable
  energy for this? Can anyone else do this for me (family/friend/carer)?

---

where their energy and time is being 'spent'. They may only be able to carry
out a few activities that are actually important, which will affect confidence as
well as satisfaction and quality of life. Box 6.1.1 presents a prioritisation and
planning list to help to structure thinking about whether activities are 'important' or 'not important' and prompt solutions to difficult tasks. Activities that
are not important could be left out or considered for delegation to a family
member/friend/social services/private agency.

Planning

Once this has been done, the tasks that are important but difficult can be
broken down, to check if there may be an easier way of doing them. They
could be done less frequently (e.g. shopping/hoovering only once per week),
or reducing the energy load of the task by using a wheeled trolley instead of
bags/hoovering only one room at a time.

The most important activities should be carried out first, while the patient
is feeling more energetic. It is vital to organise time for a rest before and after,
or even during the activity if it is very tiring. For example, Mrs D spends an
hour most days standing in the kitchen, ironing. She considered this important,
but difficult.

After analysis of this task, the difficult elements are standing and lifting her
arms above waist height (often difficult for people with COPD). This could be
made easier by shortening the task – only 15 minutes per day, or doing the
task sitting on a high stool, and having the ironing board adjusted to a lower
position, so her arms are not so high. Mrs D chose to sit and adjusted the
ironing board lower than usual – she found sitting odd at first but reports less
fatigue after completing the task.

Pacing

Many patients with moderate to severe COPD find that they have good and bad days. On a good day, they may feel as if they have more energy than usual. So they complete many activities until they are exhausted. The following days are characterised by a slump in energy levels and an inability to carry out anything but the most basic personal care tasks, see Figure 6.1.2. Note that there are more 'bad days' than 'good days'.

The key to successful pacing involves including regular rest periods through-out the day and planning to carry out only moderate amounts of activity, whether it is a 'good' or 'bad' day. In this way, the body will not become over-tired and will have time to recover between activities. Thus the patient will be able to maintain a reasonable level of activities every day, rather than only every few days. See Figure 6.1.3 for an illustration of this.

TIPS AND TECHNIQUES

The following tips for fatigue management are a combination of suggestions from patients and the website http://cc.ucsf.edu/crc/hm_conserving_energy. html (2001) adapted from 'Suggested Strategies for Energy Conservation' by the Oncology Nursing Society 2001.

Washing and dressing

• Plan ahead and allow plenty of time and rest breaks to avoid rushing.
• Sit on a shower board when showering. Use long-handled sponges and brushes.

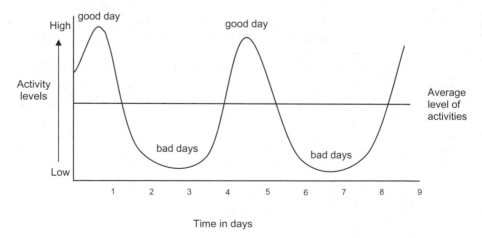

Figure 6.1.2. Activity levels over good and bad days

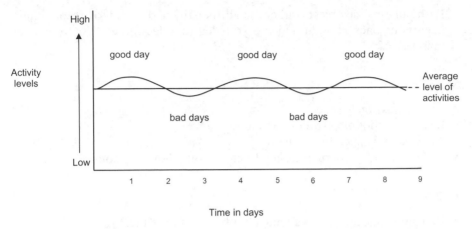

Figure 6.1.3. Improved activity levels due to pacing

- Use a towelled dressing gown instead of drying off.
- Lay out all clothes and toiletries before dressing.
- Minimise leaning over to put on clothes and shoes. Lift foot to the opposite knee to put on socks and shoes. Fasten bra at front, then turn to back.
- Install grab rails next to the toilet or a raised toilet seat if the toilet is low.
- Apply to social services/occupational therapists for a bath lift, if having difficulty getting in/out of bath.

Meal preparation

- Use ready-made foods/chilled frozen meals.
- Arrange the kitchen to allow easy access to frequently used items.
- Prepare food sitting down on a high stool.
- Soak dishes in water before washing and let them dry.
- Prepare larger portions and freeze the leftovers.
- Consider having hot meals delivered.

Housework

- Plan weekly household tasks to prevent over-activity on one day.
- Stop working *before* becoming overly tired.
- Sit when ironing and take rest periods, or leave out ironing altogether.
- Do housework sitting down, where possible. Use long-handled dusters, etc.
- If heavy housework is something you would rather not do, delegate if possible.

- Push/pull or slide objects rather than lifting. If you do need to lift something, keep your back straight and use your leg muscles rather than your back muscles.

Shopping

- Shop at less busy times.
- Lean on a shopping trolley for support.
- Request assistance in getting to the car.
- Use a wheeled shopping trolley to carry your shopping home.

Childcare

- Delegate childcare to give yourself a break, if possible.
- Plan activities that can be done sitting down (e.g., drawing pictures, playing games, reading, and computer games) rather than being lifted.

Paid work

- Plan workload to take advantage of peak energy times. Alternate physically demanding tasks with less demanding tasks.
- Arrange work environment for easy access to commonly used equipment and supplies.

Hobbies/leisure

- Select activities that match your energy level.
- Try and sit down, if possible.

Balance activity and rest – to prevent getting over-tired.

NOTE

1 VO_2 is defined as oxygen uptake, i.e. how much oxygen is used by the body during any activity.

6.2   NUTRITION AND HEALTHY EATING

RICHARD C. WILSON
King's College Hospital, London

In evolutionary terms the human body is the same as it was 5,000 years ago. By contrast our diet has changed beyond all recognition even in the past 50 years. We are putting twenty-first-century food into Stone Age bodies and many of the chronic diseases we suffer are a direct consequence of this. There is a worldwide pandemic of obesity, diabetes and heart disease, directly related to the nutritive environment we inhabit. Patients suffering from COPD are likely to have these co-morbidities. In severe disease and during acute exacerbations, poor nutrition and unintentional, often debilitating, weight loss are common.

A healthy diet for an individual with COPD will vary depending upon their condition. If the patient is relatively fit and well, then a healthy diet is necessary to maintain that healthy situation. When the patient is unwell, then a healthy diet has the aim of maintaining weight, strength and function.

WHAT IS A HEALTHY DIET?

We have known for some time now what a healthy diet is. Essentially it is the type of diet our bodies are designed for, the type of diet our hunter-gatherer ancestors would have eaten. A healthy diet is:

- *high in fibre* – lots of roots, nuts, seeds, berries and fruit. The human colon is perfectly designed for a high fibre intake and it is colonised with bacteria, which aid digestion and produce many useful nutrients for us. If the colon is supplied with insufficient fibre then normal motility is affected and constipation, **diverticular disease** and haemorrhoids ensue.
- *low in salt* – the diet of our ancestors was low in salt. Salt was so scarce that it was used as currency by the Romans and is the root of the word 'salary'. In modern times salt has become more readily available and prior to refrigeration it was widely used to preserve food. We have become accustomed to a high salt diet, and this is a strong contributory factor to hypertension, heart disease and stroke.
- *low in fat* – our ancestors did not have domestic animals. If they wanted to eat meat or drink milk, then they would have to chase after and capture or kill an animal. This was a risky and difficult exercise and meat would not have been a common ingredient of diet. The meat that was eaten would have been from wild animals – leaner and containing a lot less saturated fat than modern domestic animals.
- *low in sugar* – sucrose (common table sugar) is not common in the plant world. Only sugar beet and cane are cultivated to produce it. The diet of our ancestors would have contained very little sugar. Wild honey would have been a rare treat acquired only after the great discomfort of many stings.
- *high in fruits, seeds, nuts, berries and antioxidant vitamins* – fruits, nuts and berries in season along with leaves, roots and seeds would have been the staple fare. These foods are rich in fibre and the antioxidant vitamins A, C and E.

WHAT ARE THE DIETARY ISSUES FOR PATIENTS WITH COPD?

Patients with COPD should be weighed regularly. A patient of normal and stable weight should maintain their health by eating a healthy diet. The two main health issues affecting diet for this group of patients are obesity and unintentional weight loss, problems of energy balance. There are 3500 kcal (15 MJ) in 0.5 kg of human flesh. Maintaining a healthy and stable weight is dependent upon energy balance:

- If energy in (i.e. calories from food and drink) is *equal to* energy out (i.e. energy expended in the activities of daily living), then weight will remain stable.
- If energy in is *more* than energy out, the body can do nothing with the excess energy other than store it. Accumulated excess energy in will lead to weight increase – 0.5 kg for every 3,500 kcal (15 MJ) accumulated.
- If energy in is *less* than energy out, the body's stores will diminish and weight loss will ensue – 0.5 kg loss for every 3,500 kcal (15 MJ) of deficit.

This whole process is cumulative – minute after minute, day after day, month after month and year after year. A relatively small imbalance can lead to dramatic weight change. An excess of just 35 kcal (about half the calorie content of an apple) would build up to 3500 kcal in 100 days, 0.5 kg gained; 14,000 kcal in a year, 2 kg gained; 140,000 kcal in ten years, 20 kg gained!!! Weight loss can be just as insidious, a negative energy balance of just 35 kcal leading to 20 kg weight loss in ten years.

MANAGEMENT OF OBESITY

Many patients with COPD are obese (i.e. body mass index greater than 30 kg/m^2). They are ill equipped to carry this extra weight and should be encouraged to lose it. Most obese patients would benefit by losing 10 per cent of their initial weight, regardless of the starting point: for a patient weighing 90 kg that would be 9 kg. It is often motivating to ask the patient how they would manage carrying a 9 kg bag of potatoes! How much easier their life would be without that 9 kg!

Changing diet and lifestyle to achieve permanent weight loss is very difficult and requires a great deal of motivation and help and support from carers and professionals. The following points are worth bearing in mind:

- The patient must be in control. Imprisonment and forced labour are not permitted in the modern NHS! All decisions about lifestyle change need to be made by the patient with appropriate guidance and support.
- Aim for sensible weight loss of about 0.5 kg per week. More rapid weight loss is undesirable and unsustainable – lean tissue will be lost and it will be hard to recover.

- Maintain maximum levels of activity in order to maximise energy output and maintain muscle strength and fitness.

Weight loss is all about achieving negative energy balance. There are an infinite number of ways to achieve this and the health-care professional's role is to assist and support the patient in finding the solution that suits them and can be sustained.

PHARMACEUTICAL SUPPORT FOR WEIGHT LOSS

At the time of writing, there are two medicines licensed for prescription on the NHS to aid weight loss. They are an aid to weight loss and not a substitute for diet and lifestyle change. Orlistat (trade name Xenical) and sibutramine (trade name Reductil) work in quite different ways. Orlistat blocks the activity of the enzyme lipase and dramatically reduces fat absorption. When taking orlistat, patients must severely restrict fat intake (i.e. calorie intake), otherwise the unabsorbed fat will cause severe diarrhoea. Sibutramine affects the appetite centres in the hypothalamus and increases the feeling of satiety: patients feel fuller on less food (i.e. fewer calories). Patients will need to consult their medical team in order to discuss the usefulness and the side effects of these drugs in relation to their other treatments.

MANAGEMENT OF UNDERNUTRITION

Severe, unintentional weight loss can compromise patients with COPD quite severely. Unintentional weight loss of more than 10 per cent over a 3–6-month period is severe. It is important that this is recognised early. Patients who are obese need to lose weight in a controlled fashion and weight loss needs to be combined with optimised or increased activity to maintain lean body mass. Weight loss resulting from poor appetite and a failure to eat a healthy, balanced diet will be indiscriminate and result in a disproportionate loss of lean tissue – including respiratory muscle. Unintentional and unmanaged weight loss will make COPD worse and should be identified quickly and treated. Patients should have their weight recorded regularly and any unintentional losses should be investigated and acted upon accordingly.

The aim of treatment in this situation is to improve energy balance in order to stabilise body weight. The recovery of weight lost needs to be carefully managed, patients need full rehabilitation including the optimisation of or an increase in activity if the energy supplied in the diet is to be used effectively for the production of lean tissue. Excess energy that is not being used to replace and repair lean body mass will be stored as fat and will also increase the respiratory load.

A full medical history should be taken when investigating unintentional weight loss. Underlying conditions such as chest infections, depression, constipation or dehydration can adversely affect appetite and they should be treated. Patients with poor appetite should be encouraged to do the following:

- Take small frequent meals and snacks. They should always be nibbling, chewing sweets or taking nourishing drinks.
- Take nourishing drinks, e.g. full fat milk, sugary drinks but fizzy drinks are probably best avoided.
- Avoid drinking immediately before a meal as this may fill them up and reduce appetite.
- Fortify food with butter, cream, sugar, etc. The aim is to get as many calories into every mouthful as possible.
- Eat biscuits, cakes, bread and butter, sweets, toffees and chocolate as snacks.

A consultation with a dietician might be useful to develop a diet plan and consider the use of prescribable supplements, which may help. When using these supplements it is important to monitor the patient and make sure that the supplements are indeed supplementary to food and they are not being used as a substitute for food. When appetite is poor, it is also worth considering advising the patient to take a multi-vitamin supplement. Every patient is different and treatment for unintentional weight loss needs to be individually tailored.

CONCLUSION

Patients with COPD are nutritionally at risk and it is important to ensure that their nutrition is optimal. Weight should be monitored and recorded regularly. Overweight patients should be encouraged to lose weight. Unintentional weight loss should be detected early and treated quickly.

6.3 CONTINENCE

SUE FOXLEY
King's College Hospital, London

INTRODUCTION

This section aims to provide an overview of continence promotion and management of incontinence in people with COPD.

The NHS Plan, published in 2000, set out an ambitious programme of change and modernisation for the National Health Service (NHS). It requires investment in technology, capacity and capability to deliver patient access, choice, consistency and quality of care. To achieve this, the government has committed to increasing overall expenditure on health and remains focused on ensuring that the NHS gains the very best value for money in all areas of expenditure.

Incontinence has a great impact on the nation's health and the provision of many health-associated services, but possibly the level of continence care varies across the country (Foxley 2005). Norton (1995) suggests that the provision, quality and quantity of continence products are at the discretion of each primary and secondary care trust.

Continence is a human skill, basic to living in a complex social environment. Helping people to achieve continence or manage incontinence is a core nursing activity that is used on a daily basis (Norton 2001).

Patients experiencing the symptoms of COPD, cough, breathlessness which is possibly worse at night (Fehrenbach 2002), heart failure and its associated problems, those needing assisted ventilation, help with mobility and dexterity, this all can impact upon the patient's ability to remain continent. Plus the added fear that they are not able to get to the toilet on time.

There are many demands on the time of health-care professionals; a need is required to prioritise workloads. A continence assessment may be a low priority among other pressing needs, yet incontinence has a high priority with patients and their carers. Often there is no quick fix answer to the management of incontinence; however, new approaches are emerging that improve patients' quality of life.

DEFINITIONS AND PREVALENCE

The International Continence Society states, 'Urinary Incontinence is a condition while voluntary loss of urine is a social and hygienic problem and is objectively demonstrable' (Abrams 2002). Table 6.3.1 presents the medical definitions to describe incontinence.

Fehrenbach (2002) states that about 1 per cent of the UK population (600,000 people) has a diagnosis of COPD, while, on the other hand, over six million people in the UK have a bladder problem: that is more than the number of people who have asthma and diabetes put together (Incontact 2003). Box 6.3.1 shows the prevalence of urinary incontinence.

THE CAUSES OF URINARY AND FAECAL INCONTINENCE

Incontinence does not 'just happen': there should always be a reason. Until the cause or causes have been correctly identified for each individual, by the health-care professional completing a continence assessment, any attempt at treatment or management is futile. The causes may be many and complex, but can be broadly divided into two main categories:

1 Bladder and bowel problems.
2 Factors making the patient unable to cope with normal function, which will precipitate incontinence.

Table 6.3.1. Medical definitions of incontinence

Void	Term used to pass urine
Urgency	A strong desire to pass urine
Urge incontinence	Urgency is severe; patient is not able to reach the toilet on time
Stress incontinence	Leak of urine upon physical exertion
Nocturia	Waking at night to void
Passive incontinence	Voiding without knowledge
Functional incontinence	The patient requires assistance to achieve continence

---

Box 6.3.1. Prevalence of urinary incontinence

For people living at home

- Between 1 in 20 and 1 in 14 women aged 15–44.
- Between 1 in 13 and 1 in 7 women aged 45–64.
- Between 1 in 10 and 1 in 5 women aged 65 and over.
- Over 1 in 33 men aged 15–64.
- Between 1 in 14 and 1 in 10 men aged 65 and over.

For people (both sexes) living in institutions

- 1 in 3 in residential homes.
- Nearly 2 in every 3 in care homes with nursing.
- 1 in 2 to 2 in 3 in wards for the elderly and elderly mentally infirm.

Source: DOH (2000a)

The causes of urinary incontinence

Table 6.3.2 shows the causes of urinary incontinence.

NEW DRUG THERAPY FOR URINARY INCONTINENCE

A drug had recently been licensed specifically for the treatment of moderate to severe stress incontinence.

Duloxetine is a selective serotonin and noradrenaline re-uptake inhibitor that enhances pudendal nerve activity and contraction of the urethral sphincter, used in combination with pelvic floor exercises. Main side effects include fatigue and insomnia.

Drug therapy for the overactive bladder includes the **antimuscarinics**, these act by trying to reduce bladder contractions and to increase bladder capacity. They work on the smooth bladder muscle, targeting the M receptor cells.

Table 6.3.2. Causes of urinary incontinence

Type of incontinence	Symptoms	Probable cause in patients with COPD	Treatment options
Stress	Urine leakage on mild to severe cough On a laugh, or strain in any way Due to an incompetent urethral sphincter Atrophic changes in post-menopausal women	Pelvic floor laxity Multiple childbirth Obstetric trauma Obesity Atrophic vaginitis Post-prostatectomy Breathlessness Chronic cough	• Pelvic floor exercises • Dietary advice • Surgery • Medication review • Lifestyle changes • Drugs
Urge	Urgency to void Frequency Wetting on the way to the toilet Nocturia Wetting the bed at night	Associated neurological disease Diuretic drug therapy Stress and anxiety Poor mobility Assisted ventilation Excessive fluid intake Urinary tract infection Gynaecological problems	• Lifestyle changes • Medication review • Effective nurse care planning • Toileting programme • Pelvic floor exercises • Medication • Bladder retraining • Product assessment
Overflow	Bladder does not empty properly = residual urine Poor flow Hesitancy Straining Dribbling Urinary tract infections	Obstruction Prostatic enlargement Fibroids Uterine prolapse Constipation Stricture Atonic Neurological problems Diabetes	• Effective bowel care • Instruction re voiding techniques • Medication review • Surgery • Catheterisation • Product assessment
Passive and Functional	Incontinence without warning – day and night Reduced patient awareness Mental impairment Confusion Dementia Anxiety/stress/fear	Poor mobility Breathlessness Chronic cough Poor dexterity Being attached to Oxygen therapy No one around to assist safe mobility Disorientation Poor motivation Carers unaware of patients needs	• Holistic toileting programme • Reality orientation • Gaining coping strategies • Lifestyle review • Medication review • Provision of suitable products • Effective care planning with regular review

Detrusitol and oxybutynin are two of the most commonly used. Oxybutynin is currently available in patch format.

BOWEL PROBLEMS

Frequency of bowel emptying varies between individuals, as does the perception of when problems occur (Colley 2000). Defecation is a private and seldom mentioned bodily function, which people prefer to take for granted and seldom consider.

Adults who are unable to control their bowel function are faced with coping not only with physical symptoms, but also with the embarrassment, shame, social isolation and stigma, should others become aware of their problem. Prevalence of this problem is shown in Box 6.3.2. Table 6.3.3 shows the causes of bowel problems.

INABILITY OF THE PATIENT WITH COPD TO COPE WITH BLADDER AND BOWEL PROBLEMS

Many different problems can affect the patient's ability to cope with normal elimination needs, thus predicting incontinence, and a comprehensive continence assessment will highlight these; some of the commonest include:

1 *Immobility* – If mobility is limited or poor, ability to reach the toilet may be impaired, especially if the patient also has a strong desire to void. Good footwear, suitable mobility aids or provision of assistance or a urinal/commode may help.
2 *Dexterity and vision* – The patient with poor manual dexterity may be unable to remove clothing or position themselves onto the toilet. Good eyesight is also important; in order to see where you are going, plus avoid any obstacles.
3 *Mental ability* – The confused or disorientated patient may lose touch with social conventions, or be unable to find the correct place to pass urine. In patients with severe dementia, the concept of the meaning of continence may be lost.

Box 6.3.2. Prevalence of faecal incontinence

Faecal incontinence affects:

- 1% of adults living at home
- 17% of the elderly.
- 25% of people living in institutional care.

Source: DOH *Good Practice in Continence Services* (2000a)

Table 6.3.3. Causes of bowel problems

Type of problem	Causes linked with COPD	Symptoms	Treatment options
Constipation	Psychological factors Psychiatric problem – depression Neurological problem Metabolic Gastrointestinal Lack of exercise Breathlessness Poor diet Drug therapy Laxative abuse Anxiety Worry/stress Poor mobility	Infrequent passage of a hard stool General malaise Loss of appetite Nausea and vomiting Urinary incontinence Abdominal bloating Rectal discomfort Faecal incontinence	Identify cause • Lifestyle changes • Diet/fluid advice • Medication review • Drug therapy • General advice • Occupational therapy and physiotherapy input
Faecal incontinence	Anal sphincter damage Pelvic floor damage Neurological disease Impaction with overflow Lifestyle Environment Idiopathic Stool consistency Poor mobility Poor dexterity Breathlessness	Uncontrolled passage of a formed/liquid faeces Poor control of flatus Soiling of underwear	Identify cause – continence assessment • Treat constipation • General advice • Lifestyle advice • Diet and fluid care • OT and physio

4 *Environment* – Distance to the toilet, presence of oxygen cylinders, sign-posting and lighting problems can influence the patient's ability to reach the toilet. Products which facilitate independence can make continence achievable.

5 *Drugs* – Several drugs can affect bladder function: those which can cause urinary incontinence include salbutamol and atrovent (Table 6.3.4).

6 *Emotions* – Anxiety often affects bladder function aggravating frequency and urgency to void. The patient worried about incontinence may get into a vicious circle of increasing anxiety and incontinence.

7 *Constipation* – Severe problems will aggravate urinary incontinence, avoidance is best.

Table 6.3.4. Effect of drugs on continence problems

Drug	Main uses	Action upon urinary tract	Possible effect on continence
Salbutamol	Bronchospasm of asthma or COPD	Increases smooth muscle tone in outflow tract	Voiding difficulties and retention. May relieve stress incontinence
Atrovent	Antimuscarinic bronchodilator	Increases smooth muscle tone in outflow tract	Voiding difficulties and retention. May relieve stress incontinence

8 *Urinary tract infection* – From a poor fluid intake or possibly poor personal hygiene, this can lead to a variety of symptoms and serious consequences.

9 *Nurses* – Nursing attitude and the planning of care appropriate to the elimination needs of each patient can make a difference between continence and incontinence.

10 *Fluid intake* – Many patients with continence problems will often, as a coping mechanism, restrict their fluid intake hoping that they will produce less urine. A daily intake of 1.5 litres (eight cups or six mugs) of fluid a day is recommended (Getcliffe & Dolman 2003).

Bladder and bowel incontinence may be frequent occurrences for those patients suffering from chronic disease. Improvements in quality of life, which has an impact on nursing care and the financial consequences, may be provided by knowledge of the nature of the bladder and bowel problem. A careful evaluation of the problem is often all that is necessary to provide the improvements sought.

6.4   SLEEP

LAURA BLACKLER

Guy's and St Thomas' Hospital, London

Sleep takes up nearly one-third of our lives, and its quality and quantity have a huge impact on the time we are awake. Sleep is defined as a state where the perception of, and response to, the external environment is reduced or absent (George and Bayliff 2003).

Sleep is divided into two states: **rapid eye movement (REM)** and **non-rapid eye movement (NREM)**. NREM sleep has four stages; stage 1 is the deepest level of sleep and stage 4 the lightest. During NREM sleep, there is a reduction in the alveolar ventilation from being awake to NREM and an increase in

Table 6.4.1. Factors influencing sleep

External factors	Internal factors
Room temperature	Age
Drugs	Underlying medical condition
Noise	Less sleep = greater need for sleep
Comfort	Circadian rhythm

arterial CO_2; this decrease in ventilation is due to the small reductions in tidal breathing volume with little or no change in breathing (Mohsenin 2005). Respiration is irregular and the mean respiratory frequency is increased in NREM. REM is a state of paralysis where only eyes, respiratory muscles and the diaphragm move, and is where most of the dreaming occurs. There is a significant reduction in ventilation during REM despite an increase in the respiratory rate and the CO_2 response is further decreased.

Sleep normally progresses though a cycle with REM sleep alternating with NREM approximately every 90 minutes. The pattern, rate and effectiveness of breathing are linked to the sleep state, and the ventilatory responses to hypoxaemia and hypercapnia will differ from REM to NREM (Douglas 2000). In healthy adults, breathing is affected by sleep because there is increased airway resistance as a result in changes in airway calibre due to mild nocturnal **bronchoconstriction** and a relaxation of the upper respiratory muscles (Carlson & Mascarella 2003).

The timing and type of sleep depend on the time of day it occurs, and there are a number of external and internal factors that also influence sleep (Table 6.4.1).

THE EFFECTS OF COPD ON SLEEP

Sleep disturbance is common in COPD, and may contribute to depression, cognitive dysfunction, and lessened quality of life in this disease (Croxton et al. 2003). In a study carried out by Klink and Quan (1987) more than 50 per cent of the patients with COPD had difficulties in falling asleep and/or remaining asleep, and 25 per cent complained of excessive day-time sleepiness.

It is well recognised that sleep-related hypoxaemia and hypercapnia, particularly during REM sleep, occurs in those with COPD (McNicholas 2000). When the individual with COPD enters the REM period, they will have a loss of functional residual capacity because of a combination of intercostal muscle **hypotonia** and an ineffective, flattened diaphragm (O'Donohue & Bowman 2000). Participants in the Sleep Heart Health Study (Saunders et al. 2003), with an FEV_1/FEC ratio of less than 65 per cent, had an increased risk of oxygen desaturation. Even patients with mild hypoxaemia, when awake, can develop significant nocturnal oxygen desaturation according to Fletcher et al. (1989). Recurrent episodes of hypoxaemia and hypercapnia occur due to an increase in airway resistance and reduction in the minute ventilation during sleep (McNicholas 2000). This is supported by a study undertaken by O'Donoghue et al. (2004); they looked at whether the respiratory drive was altered during sleep and found that the minute volume fell by approximately 25 per cent between wakefulness and NREM sleep in a hypercapnic COPD group.

Disrupted sleep in individuals with COPD has been attributed to a number of factors (Calverley et al. 1982; Goldstein et al. 1984; Cormick et al. 1986; Klink and Quan 1987; Brand et al. 1991):

- respiratory symptoms – cough, wheezing, sputum production
- nocturnal oxygen desaturation
- hypercapnia
- **circadian rhythm** changes in airway calibre and resistance.

NOCTURNAL OXYGEN DESATURATION (NOD)

Nocturnal oxygen desaturation (NOD) occurs occasionally in many healthy individuals but the frequency, severity and length of time are increased in those with COPD (O'Donohue & Bowman 2000). NOD was divided into two types by Wynne et al. (1978):

1 Type 1 – short episodes lasting from a few seconds to a few minutes, associated with alterations in breathing, e.g. hypopnoea, apnoea.
2 Type 2 – longer periods lasting from several minutes to more than 30 minutes with no specific alterations in the breathing pattern. The longer periods normally occur during REM and are linked to elevations in pulmonary artery pressure.

Alveolar **hypoventilation** is the prime cause of oxyhaemoglobin desaturation and, according to Lewis (2001), there are a number of factors that contribute to this which have been observed in patients with COPD:

- increase in upper airway resistance;
- reduced responsiveness to carbon dioxide during sleep;
- lower arterial PO_2 when awake;
- reduced tidal volume in individuals with elevated ventilatory dead space;
- hypotonia of voluntary skeletal muscles occurs during REM sleep, leading to hypoventilation in those with hyperinflation who rely on accessory muscles to generate their tidal volume.

Desaturation is also linked to the alteration in the ventilation–perfusion ratio during REM sleep because oxygen uptake is increased and there is a disassociation between diaphragmatic and intercostal muscle activity (Fleetham 2003).

SLEEP APNOEA

Approximately 10–15 per cent of individuals with COPD have **obstructive sleep apnoea**, according to Chaouat et al. (1995). These individuals are more likely to develop severe hypoxaemia during sleep and are therefore more prone to developing complications such as cor pulmonale and polycythaemia (McNicholas 2000). Where these two conditions occur, the individual will have greater oxygen desaturation and sleep disruption than someone with only one condition.

INVESTIGATIONS INTO SLEEP DISTURBANCES

There is no universal agreement about when and how COPD patients should be checked to determine whether they have developed nocturnal hypoxaemia because of the controversy about when treatment should be implemented, according to Gay (2004). However, sleep studies are not generally indicated in patients with COPD because the PaO_2 level when awake is the best predictor of the likelihood of nocturnal oxygen desaturation.

ASSESSMENT OF SLEEP PATTERN

It is important that an assessment should include asking about sleep patterns because this can give vital information about the patient's physical and psychological health. It is also important, with the patient's permission, that you speak to their bed partner as they may have noticed if the patient stops breathing, suddenly wakes or is restless during the night. Sleep disturbance can affect the partner, as well as the individual with COPD, causing them to have interrupted sleep and may have caused them to sleep separately.

Questions that should be asked, adapted from Carlson and Mascarella (2003):

- What is their usual bedtime routine?
- How long does it usually take to fall asleep?
- How often do they wake up during the night?
- Do they wake up coughing, wheezing, feeling breathless, gasping?
- What time of night are they most likely to wake up?
- How long does it take to fall asleep again?
- Do they have a nap during the day?
- Do they feel sleepy during the day?
- What interventions have they tried to improve their sleep?

Maladaptive behaviour towards sleep can develop because sleep disturbances occur over a long time, therefore it is important to identify these through your assessment.

MANAGEMENT OF SLEEP DISRUPTION

The first thing to do is to ensure that the individual is on optimal therapy and review their medication because some drugs can interfere with sleep. These are:

- corticosteroids;
- B-agonists – may produce sufficient adrenergic stimulation to interfere with initiating and maintaining sleep;
- stimulants – nicotine, caffeine;
- some antidepressants – monamine oxidase inhibitors, certain selective serotonin reuptake inhibitors.

Review behavioural approaches to sleep as these have been shown to be as effective in dealing with late-life insomnia as sedatives in both the short term and the long term in a study carried out by Morin et al. (1999). Advice that can be given to help this problem, adapted from George and Bayliff (2003), is:

- Go to bed when sleepy.
- Use the bed for sleeping or sex only.
- Get up at the same time *every day* – this leads to regular bed time.
- Exercise.
- Environment – insulate against sound and light, maintain temperature cool enough to sleep.
- Do not go to bed hungry or very full.
- Avoid excessive fluid intake in the evening.
- Avoid caffeine drinks in the evening.
- Avoid alcohol in the late evening.
- Avoid sleeping during the day-time.
- Do not try to fall asleep – this leads to increased frustration and makes it harder to fall asleep.
- Remove clocks from the bedside – this takes away the pressure of not being asleep by a certain time.

CONCLUSION

The reasons for sleep disturbances are many and varied and it is important that this aspect of life is addressed and optimised because of its impact on an individual's quality of life. It also has a significant impact on the life of their partner and their relationship; therefore, it is an area health-care professionals must consider when looking at the issues affecting the patient's life.

6.5   TRAVEL AND HOLIDAYS

CAROLINE MOONEY
Papworth Hospital, Cambridge

Going on holiday requires a great deal of planning and organisation for all of us. However, for those people with COPD, extra considerations need to be taken into account and planned.

WHERE TO GO?

Air quality

The environment in which we live, or travel to, can contribute to the worsening of respiratory symptoms. A number of studies have demonstrated the association between the prevalence of respiratory diseases and air pollution (Dockery et al. 1989). Exposure to high levels of air pollution has been related to a higher risk of COPD admission (Anderson et al. 1997); particularly particles and ozone are related to emergency hospital admissions for people with respiratory conditions (Dockery & Pope 1994).

Fusco et al.'s (2001) study found that CO (carbon monoxide), NO_2 (nitrogen dioxide) and O_3 (ozone) are important contributors to respiratory hospitalisation. In particular, CO plays a major role for admissions among adults. The effects of air pollutants, at least that of CO, seems to be stronger during the warm season. Sunyer et al. (1991) found a positive association between admissions for COPD and black smoke, SO_2 (sulphur dioxide) and CO.

Temperature

It is suggested that temperature may contribute to exacerbations (MacNee 2002). Patients with COPD often experience a greater sensation of dyspnoea when they are exposed to low temperatures. Cooling of the facial skin causes a reflex reaction of increasing respiratory rate and an immediate fall in FEV_1 (Kosela et al. 1996): this often results in a decreased exercise capacity (Kosela et al. 1998). Cold weather is associated with an increased risk of exacerbation caused by viral infections. Donaldson et al. (1999) found that exacerbations are significantly related to outdoor temperature. At the other extreme, very hot weather has also been associated with increased admissions for people with COPD (MET Office 2005).

A forecast model has been developed by the MET Office (2005) to predict the risk of COPD exacerbations, in order to improve patients' quality of life and help plan services.

When considering temperature, it is also important that patients check their medication, as some may be affected by extreme temperature (British Thoracic Society 2002).

High altitude

Lower oxygen levels at high altitude can make breathing worse. For this reason it is recommended that patients should check to see if their destination is at a high altitude. The BTS recommendations state that patients who require in-flight oxygen should also receive oxygen when visiting high altitude destinations (British Thoracic Society 2002).

What type of accommodation do you require?

It is essential for people to think about their needs. There are many questions that people need to have answered before they book their holidays. Examples include:

• Will their accommodation suit their requirements?
• Is there wheelchair access?
• Is there air conditioning available?
• How will I get around when I get there?

HOW TO GET THERE?

There are many ways for people to travel: by coach, train, car, boat and air. Whenever people are arranging their journey, it requires careful planning to avoid unnecessary complications that could interfere with their safety and comfort. There are several leaflets produced by travel companies that address disabled people's needs. The main consideration for the health of COPD sufferers concerns air travel.

Air travel

Breathing air at 2483 m (8000 ft) is equivalent to breathing 15.1 per cent oxygen at sea level. When healthy individuals fly, their PaO_2 will be influenced by their age and minute ventilation, but their PaO_2 is likely to fall to 7.0–8.5 kPa (53–64 mm Hg, SpO_2 85–95 per cent) (Nunn 1987). However, in healthy people this is thought not to cause any difficulties.

The effect of acute hypoxaemia in patients with stable COPD is not well studied and, subjectively, many patients appear to tolerate hypoxaemia well (Gong 1991). Patients with COPD can exhibit falls in PaO_2 that average 3.3 kPa (Christensen et al. 2000).

To enhance the safety for respiratory patients travelling by air and to improve recognition among health-care professionals, the British Thoracic Society (2002) has produced guidelines for managing passengers with lung disease planning air travel. The guidelines highlight the fact that clinical assessment may be required for people with respiratory disease prior to travelling by air.

For people with COPD, a pre-flight assessment is recommended that includes:

- history and physical examination;
- previous flying experience;
- spirometry;
- arterial blood gases/SpO_2; arterial blood gases are preferred if hypercapnia is known or suspected.

RESULTS OF SCREENING ASSESSMENT

The results of screening assessments are shown in Table 6.5.1.
Additional risk factors include

- hypercapnia
- FEV_1 < 50 per cent predicted
- lung cancer
- restrictive lung disease
- ventilator support
- cerebrovascular or cardiac disease
- within 6 weeks of an exacerbation of chronic lung or cardiac disease (BTS 2002).

Following this screening process, patients will further be assessed about their suitability to fly.

There are currently three procedures used to assess whether patients are fit to fly:

1 *The 50 metre walk*: Traditionally, this has been favoured by airlines because of its simplicity. People who are unable to complete the task (either distance or within time period), or those who record moderate or severe distress on a breathlessness score will alert the doctor and patient to the possible need for in-flight oxygen.

Table 6.5.1. Screening assessments and recommendations

Screening results at sea level	Recommendation
SpO_2 > 95%	No oxygen required
SpO_2 92–95% and no risk factor	No oxygen required
SpO_2 92–95% and additional risk factor	Oxygen may be required (further assessment is required with a hypoxic challenge test)
SpO_2 < 92%	In-flight oxygen required
Uses long-term oxygen	May need increased flow while at cruising altitude

Table 6.5.2. Results of the hypoxic challenge

Hypoxic challenge result	Recommendation
PaO$_2$ > 7.4 kPa (>55 mmHg)	Oxygen not required
PaO$_2$ 6.6–7.4 kPa (50–55 mmHg)	Borderline; a walk test may be useful
PaO$_2$ < 6.6 kPa (<50 mmHg)	In-flight oxygen (2 l/min)

2 *Predicting hypoxaemia from equations*: Some centres use equations to predict PaO$_2$ or SpO$_2$, from measurements at sea level (BTS 2002).
3 *The hypoxic challenge test*: This test is the ideal test. Cabin altitude of 2483 metres (8000 ft) can be simulated at sea level with a gas mixture containing 15 per cent oxygen in nitrogen. People undergoing the test are usually asked to breathe the hypoxic gas mixture for 20 minutes. During the procedure, saturation is monitored throughout and arterial blood gases are measured before and on completion.

The results of the hypoxic challenge test (15 per cent FiO$_2$ for 20 minutes) with AHCPR testing are shown in Table 6.5.2.

However, some researchers have expressed concern that simulated hypoxia under resting conditions does not adequately reproduce the stresses of flight, and has led them to include a modest exercise stress to simulate cabin movement (Naughton et al. 1995; Seccombe et al. 2004). Advice regarding using/arranging in-flight oxygen by those who already use LTOT is given in Box 6.5.1.

RISK OF PNEUMOTHORAX

COPD patients with large bullae are theoretically at increased risk of pneumothorax during air travel. This is because of volume expansion at reduced cabin pressures (BTS 2002). The BTS states that there is 'no data to state with any confidence what the maximum volume of a bulla should be before it reaches an unacceptable level of rupture leading to tension pneumothorax, pneumomediastinum or air embolism'. Therefore, there is no evidence that pressure changes during air travel will precipitate a pneumothorax (Johnson 2003).

There are restrictions for COPD patients who have previously had a pneumothorax. Airlines recommend that a pneumothorax should have settled completely before air travel and that flying should be avoided for at least six weeks. However, there appears to be no evidence to support this six-week recommendation, as it does not take into account the type of treatment that may have been given (Johnson 2003).

For this reason, the BTS (2002: 292) states that 'although reoccurrence is unlikely during the flight, the consequences at altitude may be significant given

---

Box 6.5.1. Advice for patients who require in-flight supplemental oxygen

If screening indicates the need for in-flight supplemental oxygen, patients should seek advice from the flight companies before booking their flights, as not all airlines will provide oxygen and others have restrictions (Johnson 2003). Patients should also consider the cost of supplemental oxygen when comparing air ticket prices, as considerable variation exists (BTS 2002).

If the airline is able to accommodate the needs of patients who require supplementary oxygen, the airline medical department will issue a medical form. This form is required to be completed by both the patient and the GP or hospital specialist. It details the patient's diagnosis, the reason for supplementary oxygen, and the duration of oxygen therapy (intermittent or continuous) with a further section for information on the patient's mobility and need for special boarding or seating arrangements. The airline's Medical Officer will then evaluate the patient's needs. Most airlines have a medical department that may be helpful, although getting through can be time-consuming (Stoller et al. 1999).

Other advice for people who are travelling using oxygen:

- A direct flight is recommended. If connecting flights are unavoidable, separate arrangements must be made for oxygen while on the ground.
- If the patient requires humidification, they should inform the airline.
- Airlines do not provide oxygen for use at the airport. Some airports restrict oxygen use in the airport because of the risk of explosions, so it is advisable to check with your booking agent.
- In-flight oxygen flow is usually limited to 2 l/min or 4 l/min.
- Patients cannot use their own cylinder and concentrator but may be able to take them as baggage if empty. They should check with the airlines first, as some have restrictions and others may charge for this service.
- The main oxygen distributors have their own international distribution network and can supply oxygen at intended destinations.
- Patients normally using long-term oxygen therapy (LTOT) should ensure that they have LTOT throughout their stay.
- Those who require oxygen should carry a copy of their medical form and must be accompanied.
- Arrangements should be made for the return as well as the outward journey.

---

the absence of prompt medical care'. This is particularly true for those with co-existing lung disease. Passengers may wish to consider alternative forms of transport within one year of the event.

General considerations for travelling by air for all patients with COPD are listed in Box 6.5.2.

Box 6.5.2. General considerations for COPD sufferers

- Individuals who do not use supplementary oxygen should remain mobile during the flight, in light of the recent recommendations regarding the incidence of venous thrombosis and pulmonary embolism.
- Portable nebuliser machines may be used at the discretion of the cabin crew. Patients should check with the carrier when booking.
- Many airports can provide wheelchairs for transport to and from the aircraft.
- Passengers should carry all their necessary medication in their hand luggage and may need to carry a prescription with them.
- A letter confirming the medical necessity of any electrical equipment such as nebuliser machines, CPAP/NIPPV machines or oxygen concentrators is essential with current tight airline security (Johnson 2003).

CONCLUSION

The main consideration for people with COPD when going on holiday is to plan all aspects of their stay. It is imperative that health-care professionals provide consistent and correct information to assist people to go on holiday. People with COPD have enough limitations placed on their lives, without additional ones being placed on them when they travel.

6.6 VACCINATIONS

CAROLINE MOONEY
Papworth Hospital, Cambridge

Vaccinations play an important part in reducing infectious diseases and mortality. The aim of vaccination is to provide protective immunity by inducing lasting immune memory in response to an infectious microorganism, using a non-toxic antigen preparation (Lydyard & Whelan 2000). For COPD patients, the NICE Guidelines (2004) recommend that patients have influenza and pneumococcal vaccines. These diseases, vaccines and evidence of use in relation to COPD patients will be discussed. Box 6.6.1 gives definitions of relevance to vaccinations.

INFLUENZA

What is it?

Influenza is an acute viral infection of the respiratory tract. There are three types of influenza virus: A, B and C. Influenza A and influenza B are the most

---

Box 6.6.1. Definitions of relevance to vaccinations

What is an epidemic?
An epidemic is the occurrence in a community or region of cases of an
illness in excess of what might be normally expected.
What is a pandemic?
A pandemic is an epidemic occurring over a very wide area and usually
affecting a large portion of the population (HPA 2005a).
How are vaccines administered?
Pneumococcal and influenza vaccines can be administered at the same
time. The vaccines should be given at separate sites, preferably in different limbs. Vaccines are routinely given into the upper arm or antero-
lateral thigh. However, for individuals with bleeding disorders, vaccines
should be given by deep subcutaneous injection to reduce the risk of
bleeding.

---

important types as they are responsible for most clinical illness. Influenza is
highly infectious with an incubation period of one to three days. The infectious
period varies but an infected person can probably pass on the disease the day
before their symptoms appear and remain potentially infectious for 3–5 days
(Health Protection Agency 2005a).

Symptoms

The disease is characterised by the sudden onset of fever, chills, headache,
myalgia and extreme fatigue. Other common symptoms include a dry cough,
sore throat and stuffy nose.

Who is affected?

For the majority of people, influenza is not life-threatening. Those deemed
most at risk of serious illness and mortality from influenza are neonates, older
people and those with underlying chronic respiratory and cardiac disease, and
those who are immunosuppressed (Dept of Health 2005a).

How is it spread?

Influenza infections are spread by respiratory droplets produced by coughing
or sneezing. Spread can also occur through fine aerosols and by hand to
mucous membrane contact. Influenza spreads rapidly especially among closed
communities. Most cases in the UK tend to occur during a 6–8-week period
during the winter, although technically influenza is not bound by seasons, and
can occur all year round in tropical climates (Health Protection Agency 2005a).

A possible explanation for the high influenza activity in winter is the fact that people congregate indoors during winter, facilitating the transmission of the virus, and this is confounded by the fact that humid air indoors may prolong the survival of the virus (Health Protection Agency 2005a).

Seasonal influenza varies in timing, extent and severity. Influenza A viruses cause outbreaks most years and these viruses usually cause epidemics. Influenza B tends to cause less severe disease and smaller outbreaks, although in children the severity of illness may be similar to that associated with influenza A.

The influenza virus is unstable and new strains and variants are always emerging. Changes in the principal surface antigens of influenza A – haemagglutinin (H) and neuraminidase (N) – make these viruses antigenically liable. Minor changes (**antigenic drift**) to the amino acid sequence of the haemagglutinin molecules occur progressively from season to season. Major changes (**antigenic shift**) occur periodically, resulting in the emergence of a new sub-type with a different haemagglutinin (Dept of Health 2005a). As this is different to previous viruses, it can lead to major epidemics or pandemics as populations have little or no immunity to the new strain. Three influenza pandemics occurred in the last century. Influenza B viruses are subject to antigenic drift but with less frequent changes.

Influenza immunisation has been recommended in the UK since the late 1960s with the aim of directly protecting those at a higher risk of serious morbidity and mortality. In 2000, the policy was extended to include all people aged 65 years and over. It also extends to those who are a main carer for an elderly or disabled person.

The World Health Organisation (WHO) monitors influenza viruses throughout the world. Each year the WHO makes recommendations about the strains to be included in vaccines. To provide continuing protection, annual immunisation is necessary with vaccines against the current prevalent strains.

Influenza vaccines are prepared using virus strains in line with WHO recommendations. Current vaccines are trivalent, containing two subtypes of influenza A and one type of B virus. The viruses are grown in embryonated hens' eggs, they are then chemically inactivated, further treated and purified.

Three types of influenza vaccine are currently available (Dept of Health 2005a):

1 'Split virion, inactivated' or 'disrupted virus' vaccines containing virus components prepared by treating whole viruses with organic solvents or detergents;
2 'Surface antigen, inactivated' vaccines contain highly purified haemagglutinin and neuraminidase antigens prepared from disrupted virus particles;
3 'Surface antigen, inactivated, virosome' vaccines containing highly purified haemagglutinin and neuraminidase antigens prepared from disrupted virus particles reconstituted into virosomes with phospholipids.

The vaccines are equivalent in efficiency and adverse reactions. As the vaccines are inactivated, they do not contain live organisms and therefore cannot cause the disease. The current available influenza vaccines give 70–80 per cent protection against infection from the influenza virus strains well matched with those in the vaccine (Fleming et al. 1995).

After immunisation, antibody levels may take up to 10–14 days to reach protection. While influenza activity is not usually significant before the middle of November, the influenza season can start early, and therefore the ideal time for immunisation is between September and early November.

Patients should be advised that many other organisms cause respiratory infections similar to influenza during the influenza season, e.g. the common cold or respiratory syncytial virus (RSV). The influenza vaccine will not protect against these diseases (Wongsurakiat et al. 2004).

There are very few individuals who cannot receive influenza vaccine. However, the vaccines should not be given to those who have had:

- a confirmed anaphylactic reaction to a previous dose of the vaccine or to any component of the vaccine;
- a confirmed anaphylactic response to egg products.

Patients with chronic underlying illnesses such as COPD have an increased risk of respiratory illness-related hospitalisations during influenza outbreaks (Advisory Committee on Immunization Practices 1993). The administration of the flu vaccine has been shown to reduce serious morbidity and mortality in COPD patients by 50 per cent (Nichol et al. 1994).

Miller (2005) reports that the influenza vaccination is highly effective in preventing influenza-related acute respiratory illness in patients with COPD, regardless of the severity of their COPD. A Cochrane review (Poole et al. 2005) found that inactivated vaccine might reduce exacerbations in COPD patients. They found that in the elderly, there was an early increase in adverse effects with vaccination, but these are usually mild and transient. The influenza vaccine has been shown to reduce the risk of admission into hospital (Nichol et al. 1999). However, the EFRAM study (Garcia-Aymerich et al. 2001) found that the vaccine was associated with a higher risk of admission.

Despite the evidence of the effectiveness of the influenza vaccination, rates of uptake are not optimal (Nguyen-Van Tam & Nicholson 1993). It has been identified that there is patient and physician concern that vaccination may induce acute exacerbations in those with COPD (Rothbarth et al. 1995). However, routine influenza vaccination in the general UK population of older individuals with COPD does not increase the short-term incidence of adverse respiratory outcomes or the need for oral corticosteroid prescriptions (Tata et al. 2003).

In order to improve vaccination rates, further promotion should occur. Primary health-care workers and public education are key to this aim (Nguyen-Van-Tam & Nicholson 1993).

What happens if, despite vaccination, people develop influenza? There are antiviral drugs available that can be used under certain circumstances to either prevent influenza or treat it. The National Institute for Clinical Excellence (2003) issued guidance on the treatment and prevention of influenza with antiviral drugs.

Osetamivir® and Amantadine® are licensed drugs for the prevention of influenza, and Zanamivir®, Osetamivir® and Amantadine® are licensed for the treatment of influenza. However, NICE does not recommend Amantadine® for the treatment of influenza. Zanamivir® and OsetamivirA are neuramini-dase inhibitors, and have been shown to be effective in treatment of influenza A and B; Amantadine® is an M2 inhibitor, active against influenza A only. Zanamivir® should be used with caution in people with asthma or COPD because there is a risk of bronchospasm. These drugs are an important tool in the management of influenza, but are not substitutes for immunisation (Dept of Health 2005a).

PNEUMOCOCCAL VACCINATIONS

Pneumococcal disease is the term used to describe infections caused by the bacterium Streptococcus pneumoniae (pneumococcus) (Dept of Health 2005b). Streptococcus pneumoniae (S. pneumoniae) is a Gram positive encap-sulated bacterium that usually gains entry into the human host by colonising the nasopharyngeal mucosal epithelium. Over 90 different pneumococcal serotypes have been identified. S. pneumoniae is a major cause of bacterial meningitis, invasive pneumococcal disease (IPD) and community acquired pneumonia (CAP) and is therefore a major cause of morbidity and mortality (Health Protection Agency 2005b).

Pneumococcal disease particularly affects neonates, the elderly, those with an absent or non-functioning spleen, and those with other causes of impaired immunity (Dept of Health 2005b). Pneumococcal disease is a major public health problem all over the world. It is a public health priority due to many factors: the increased risk of pneumococcal disease with advancing age, the costs associated with infection, and the rising rates of drug resistance (US Dept of Health and Human Services 2000).

Two types of pneumococcal vaccine are available:

1 Pneumococcal polysaccharide vaccine contains 25 mcg of purified capsular polysaccharide for each of 23 capsular types of pneumococcus. These 23 types account for about 96 per cent of the pneumococcal isolates causing serious infection in Britain (George & Melegaro 2000). This vaccine is the one given to adults who are deemed to be at risk of developing pneumococ-cal disease.

2 Pneumococcal conjugate vaccine contains polysaccharide from seven common capsular types. It is estimated that the seven capsular types in the

vaccine would provide cover for 66 per cent of isolates from invasive infections in England and Wales (George & Melegaro 2000). This type is administered to children under the age of 5.

Following the administration of the vaccine, most people develop a good antibody response within three weeks. The length of protection is not known and may vary between capsular types. Although there is evidence of a decline in protection with time (Shaprio et al. 1991), there are no studies showing additional protection from further immunisation, which is therefore not recommended (Dept of Health 2005b). The vaccines are inactivated and do not contain live organisms. This means that they cannot cause the diseases against which they protect.

It is difficult to reach firm conclusions about the effectiveness of the polysaccharide vaccine, but overall efficacy in preventing pneumococcal bacterium is probably 50–75 per cent (Melegaro & Edmunds 2004). They are inexpensive, effective and safe (Nichol et al. 1999).

The vaccines should not be given to those who have had a confirmed anaphylactic reaction to a previous dose or any component of the vaccines. Confirmed anaphylaxis is rare. Other allergic conditions, such as rashes, may occur more commonly but are not contraindications to further immunisation if it is deemed necessary.

Driver (2002) states that it is preferable not to vaccinate someone who has an acute infection (febrile or obviously unwell), but mild infections or antibiotics do not interfere with efficiency. De Roux et al. (2004) found that systemic steroids did not influence the antibody response.

The rate of pneumococcal disease is high among patients with COPD (Lipsky et al. 1986), and is probably due to their defective clearance mechanisms (Alfageme et al. 2005). In these patients, community acquired pneumonia (CAP) is an infectious illness that frequently leads to hospital admission and increased risk of mortality. Streptococcus pneumoniae is felt to be the causative organism in up to 43 per cent of cases (Torres et al. 1996). Pneumococcal vaccine has been shown to reduce the risk of pneumococcal pneumonia (Fine et al. 1994).

Alfageme et al. (2005) found that the pneumococcal polysaccharide vaccine should be given to COPD patients younger than 65 years of age, especially if they have severe airflow obstruction.

CONCLUSION

Vaccinations are an important component of preventing morbidity and mortality in patients with COPD. Pre-existing lung disease has the highest predicted odds for patients requiring hospitalisation for influenza and pneumonia (Foster et al. 1992). This section has provided evidence of the benefits of having vaccinations for this group of patients. Hedlund et al. (2003) showed that hospital mortality rates were lower for pneumonia, COPD and cardiac failure following vaccinations.

Health-care professionals who administer vaccinations must understand both the vaccines they administer as well as the disease, as nothing is more counterproductive to public confidence than conflicting advice (Driver 2002). It is a challenge to all involved to ensure that patients are encouraged and well informed about having vaccinations. Their effects on health status should be promoted.

6.7   SEXUALITY

CHRISTINE JONES
King's College Hospital, London

Sex and sexuality are often used interchangeably by society. Sexuality is not just about the physical act, and it affects the whole person, influencing every aspect of their life (Webb 1994). Sexuality is a highly complex phenomenon 'relating to gender, self-expression, race and culture, sexual orientation, sexual intercourse, relationship to others, love, emotions and feelings' (Gamlin 1999).

"You could let yourself go and not bother about your appearance."

"I'm so determined to look my best each day."

Sexuality is an important aspect of an individual's life and therefore should be considered when planning care with clients of all ages, making a medical diagnosis and within a variety of different settings (Poorman 1988). However, lack of knowledge about sexuality, traditional attitudes and anxiety among health-care professionals are common and can prevent an open discussion (Wilson & Williams 1988).

Patients diagnosed with chronic obstructive pulmonary disease (COPD) are often over the age of 65, and may be in the palliative stages of their disease. Ageist assumptions deem that the elderly are non-sexual adults, according to Agronin (2001), or people for whom a relationship, if any is besieged by dysfunction and lack of sexual stimulation and fulfilment (Starr & Weiner 1981).

Health professionals managing the care of the COPD patient may reinforce ageist stereotypes, giving the impression that sexuality and body image are not priority issues (White 2003) particularly when one is faced with a life-threatening illness or is dyspnoeic.

BARRIERS TO SEXUAL DISCUSSION

There are a number of barriers which can prevent individuals from discussing their sexuality, including culture and perceptions about what is acceptable within society. One of the main barriers that has been identified by a number of authors that prevents patients from discussing sexuality is the embarrassment of the health-care professional.

"I think they would be too embarrassed."

"They are so young and we're older, they may think we are not at it."

SPECIFIC ISSUES THAT CAN AFFECT A PATIENT WITH COPD

Specific issues that can affect a patient with COPD are:

- *Hypoxia*: COPD patients who suffer from hypoxia have lower levels of testosterone, which can cause erectile dysfunction. It has been suggested that hypoxaemia suppresses the hypothalamic–pituitary–testicular axis (Semple et al. 1984).
- *Breathlessness*: this can contribute to avoidance of any activities that could worsen the degree of breathlessness (Mooradian & Greiff 1990). The partner may fear inducing breathlessness and therefore avoid any sexual activities (Sexton & Munro 1985), and this could cause miscommunication between the couple. Avoidance may be interpreted as rejection and no longer finding the person attractive.

"What I don't like is that I am now on my own, and I know if I met someone, huffing and puffing is not very romantic."

- *Fatigue*: many patients experience fatigue and lethargy, and this can affect how they feel as a person and the way they relate to others.
- *Depression*: this can diminish levels of adrenal hormones (Gift & McCrone 1993) and 90 per cent of patients with COPD suffer from clinical depression/anxiety according to Gore et al. (2000).
- *Low self-esteem and poor body image*: psychological distress that accompanies chronic illness can make people feel asexual. The loss of role, changes in physical condition e.g. weight loss/gain, excessive sputum production, coughing are all factors that can make patients feel asexual.

"I split up with my ex-husband, I was too tired to be bothered."

- *Changes in relationships*: partners can become carers and pre-existing relationship problems can be exacerbated by the stress of a chronic illness (McInnes 2003). If a partner becomes the carer, this can alter the relationship, and may interfere with sexual feelings and emotions of both parties.
- *Communication*: very few couples discuss their sexual lives; therefore, this can cause significant problems when difficulties arise (Finger & Quillen 2006).

MEDICATIONS THAT AFFECT LIBIDO

Common therapies such as bronchodilators can exacerbate existing problems by causing nervousness and anxieties. Steroids can cause many side effects such as weight gain, mood swings and depression which in turn affect libido as well as sense of self (Haggerty 2004). Kochar et al. (1999) suggest that as many as 25 per cent of all cases of erectile dysfunction may be attributed to drug therapy.

Drugs that can affect the libido include:

- theophylline
- diuretics
- protein pump inhibitors
- antidepressants
- anxiolytics, e.g. diazepam
- beta blockers
- antihypertensives
- tobacco and alcohol.

This is not an exhaustive list and all medication should be reviewed if a patient expresses any issues regarding sexuality.

GENDER DIFFERENCES

It has been suggested that women have fewer sexual problems than men. Walbroehl (1992) believes that this is due to a number of factors including the fact that erectile dysfunction is more visible than loss of vaginal lubrication, and changes in the dynamics of relationships as traditionally women have taken the more passive role with the sexual side of the relationship.

THE ROLE OF THE HEALTH-CARE PROFESSIONAL

Health-care professionals do not need to be an expert; patients often just need a listening ear and reassurance that having a chronic illness does not mean the end of their sexual needs. Over half of disabled patients questioned stated that they would like to have the opportunity to discuss their sexual function with a health-care professional (Sadoughi et al. 1971) and there is no evidence to suggest that this view has changed. A key role is to encourage communication between the couple which will help them to face potential problems and find solutions acceptable to both.

It is essential that the health-care professional knows their own limitations and refers the patient to the appropriate person, or advises patients where they can go for further information/advice. Practical strategies to encourage sexuality are shown in Box 6.7.1.

CONCLUSION

Patients with a chronic illness can become disinterested or sexually inactive because of misconceptions about safety, their ability to have sex, body image

---

Box 6.7.1. Practical strategies to encourage sexuality

- Plan and ensure adequate rest.
- Do not plan any activities after a heavy meal or with alcohol.
- Use the reliever inhaler before commencement.
- Practise breathing control.
- Maintain maximum physical condition.

Source: Adapted from Hagherty (2004)

---

issues or psychosocial factors (Carter 1990). Depression, fatigue, pain, stress and anxiety can also contribute to further difficulties with sexuality; however, it must be emphasised that touch and physical intimacy are important for any relationship (Schover 2000). To overcome problems, health-care professionals should explore the different ways of expressing affection that do not expend energy. Planning and setting realistic goals can help to resolve these issues.

Sexuality is intrinsic to a person's sense of self and can be an intimate form of communication that helps relieve suffering and lessens the threat to person-hood in the face of a life-limiting illness (Hordern & Currow 2003).

"It's not so much sex, but someone of your own age for company."

Therefore, this aspect of a person's life should not be ignored as it can have a negative effect on quality of life.

REFERENCES

6.1 FATIGUE MANAGEMENT

Baarends E, Scholes A, Mostert R, Wouters E (1997) Peak exercise response in relation to tissue depletion in patients with chronic obstructive pulmonary disease. *European Respiratory Journal* **10**(12): 2807–2813.

Belza B L, Henke C J, Yelin E H, et al. (1993) Correlates of fatigue in older adults with rheumatoid arthritis. *Nursing Research* **42**: 93–99.

Branick L (2003) Integrating the principles of energy conservation during everyday activities. *Caring* **22**(1): 30–31.

Breslin E, van der Schans C, Breukink S, Meek P, Mercer K, Volz W, Louie S (1998) Perception of fatigue and quality of life in patients with COPD. *Chest* **114**: 958–964.

Chen M K (1986) The epidemiology of self-perceived fatigue among adults. *Preventative Medicine* **15**: 74–81.

Denburg S D, Carbotte R M, Denburg J A (1997) Psychological aspects of systemic lupus erythematosus: cognitive function, mood, and self-report. *The Journal of Rheumatology* **24**: 998–1003.

Downey C (1981) Guidelines for analysis and testing of ADL with Cardiac Patients. In Pedretti L W, Early M B (2001) (eds) *Occupational Therapy: Practice Skills for Physical Dysfunction*. St Louis, MO: Mosby.

Elkington H, White P, Addington-Hall J, Higgs R, Edmonds P (2005) The healthcare needs of chronic obstructive pulmonary disease patients in the last year of life. *Palliative Medicine* **19**(6): 485–491.

Freal J G, Kraft G H, Coryell J K (1984) Symptomatic fatigue in multiple sclerosis. *Archives of Physical Medicine and Rehabilitation* **5**: 135–137.

Huyser B A, Parker J C, Thoreson R, Smarr K L, Johnson J C, Hoffman R (1998) Predictors of subjective fatigue among individuals with rheumatoid arthritis. *Arthritis and Rheumatism* **41**: 2230–2237.

Krupp L B, Alvarez L A, LaRocca N G, Scheinberg L C (1988) Fatigue in multiple sclerosis. *Archives of Neurology* **45**: 435–437.

Krupp L B, LaRocca N G, Muir J, Steinberg A D (1990) A study of fatigue in systemic lupus erythematosus. *The Journal of Rheumatology* **17**: 1450–1452.

Lane I (2005) Managing cancer-related fatigue in palliative care. *Nursing Times* **101**(18): 38–41.

Lipman A J, Lawrence D P (2004) The management of fatigue in cancer patients. *Oncology* **18**(12): 1527–1535.

Mathiowietz V, Matuska K, Murphy M (2001) Efficacy of an energy conservation course for persons with multiple sclerosis. *Archives of Physical Medicine and Rehabilitation* **82**(4): 449–446.

Oliver K, Sewell L (2002) Cardiac and respiratory disease. In Turner A, Foster M, Johnson S E (eds) *Occupational Therapy and Physical Dysfunction: Principles, Skills and Practice*. Edinburgh: Churchill Livingstone.

Pedretti L W, Early M B (2001) (eds) *Occupational Therapy: Practice Skills for Physical Dysfunction*. St Louis, MO: Mosby.

Small S, Lamb M (1999) Fatigue in chronic illness: the experience of individuals with chronic obstructive pulmonary disease and with asthma. *Journal of Advanced Nursing* **30**(2): 469–478.

Steiner M, Evans R, Deacon A, et al. (2005) Adenine nucleotide loss in the skeletal muscles during exercise in chronic obstructive pulmonary disease. *Thorax* **60**(11): 932–936.

Swain M (2000) Fatigue in chronic disease. *Clinical Science* **99**: 1–8.

Tack B (1990) Fatigue in rheumatoid arthritis: Conditions, strategies, and consequences. *Arthritis Care Research* **3**(2): 65–70.

Turner A, Foster M, Johnson S E (eds) (2002) *Occupational Therapy and Physical Dysfunction: Principles, Skills and Practice*. Edinburgh: Churchill Livingstone.

Velloso M, Stella S, Cendon S, Silva A, Jardim J (2003) Metabolic and ventilatory parameters of four activities of daily living accomplished with arms in COPD patients. *Chest* **123**(4): 1047–1053.

Wolfe F, Hawley D J, Wilson K (1996) The prevalence and meaning of fatigue in rheumatic disease. *Journal of Rheumatology* **23**: 1407–1417.

WEBSITES

National Cancer Institute, CancerMail. FatigueInformation from PDQ – for Health Professionals (2002) cancernet@cancerweb.org.uk

http://cc.ucsf.edu/crc/hm_conserving_energy.html (2001) adapted from 'Suggested Strategies for Energy Conservation' by the Oncology Nursing Society 2001.

6.2 NUTRITION AND HEALTHY EATING

More information and advice about healthy eating and the management of obesity can be found on the Food Standards Agency – Eatwell website: www. eatwell.gov.uk; referenced February 2006.

More information about eating well with COPD can be found at: www.clevelandclinic. org/health/health-info/docs/2400/2411.asp?index=9451; referenced February 2006.

6.3 CONTINENCE

Abrams P (2002) Report from the standardisation sub-committee of the International Continence Society: The standardisation of terminology in lower urinary tract function. *Neurology and Urodynamics* **21**(2): 167–176.

Colley W (2000) Constipation 1, Causes and assessment. *Nursing Times Practical Procedures for Nurses No. 27*, EMAP Healthcare.

Department of Health (2000a) *Good Practice in Continence Services*. London: HMSO.

Department of Health (2000b) *NHS Plan*. London: HMSO.

Fehrenbach C (2002) Chronic obstructive pulmonary disease. *Nursing Standard* **17**(10): 45–51.

Foxley S (2005) *It's a Risky Business: Product Interventions and Best Practice.* Coloplast UK.

Getcliffe K, Dolman M (2003) *Promoting Continence: A Clinical and Research Resource*. London: Baillière Tindall.

Incontact (2003) www.incontact.demon.co.uk Address: Redbank House, St Chads Street, Cheetham, Manchester, M8, promocon2001@disabledliving.co.uk.

Norton C (1995) Continence: A challenge for us all. *British Journal of Nursing* **4**(6): 307–308.

Norton C (2001) *Nursing for Continence*. Bucks: Beaconsfield Publishers Ltd.

6.4 SLEEP

Brand P L, Postma D S, Kerstjens H A (1991) The Dutch CNSLD study group: relationship of airway hyperresponsiveness to respiratory symptoms and diurnal peak flow variation in patients with obstructive lung disease. *American Review of Respiratory Disease* **143**: 916–921.

Calverley P M, Brezinova V, Douglas N J, Catterall J R, Flenley D C (1982) The effect of oxygenation on sleep quality in chronic bronchitis and emphysema. *American Review of Respiratory Disease* **126**: 206–210.

Carlson B W, Mascarella J J (2003) Changes in sleep patterns in COPD: A new vital sign in the management of people with chronic obstructive pulmonary disease. *American Journal of Nursing* **103**(12): 71–74.

Chaouat J R, Weitzenbum E, Krieger J (1995) Association of chronic obstructive pulmonary disease and sleep apnea syndrome. *American Journal of Respiratory Critical Care Medicine* **151**: 82–86.

Cormick W, Olson L G, Hensley M J (1986) Nocturnal hypoxaemia and quality of sleep in patients with chronic obstructive pulmonary disease. *Thorax* **41**: 846–854.

Croxton T L, Weinmann G G, Senior R M, Wise R A, Crapo J D, Buist A S (2003) Clinical research in chronic obstructive pulmonary disease: needs and opportunities. *American Journal of Respiratory and Critical Care Medicine* **167**(8): 1142–1149.

Douglas N J (2000) Respiratory physiology: control of ventilation. In Kryger M H, Roth T, Dement W C (eds) *Principles and Practice of Sleep Medicine* (3rd edn). Philadelphia, PA: Saunders.

Fleetham J A (2003) Is chronic obstructive pulmonary disease related to sleep apnea–hypopnea syndrome? *American Journal of Respiratory and Critical Care Medicine* **167**: 3–4.

Fletcher E C, Luckett R A, Miller T (1989) Pulmonary vascular haemodynamics in chronic lung disease patients with and without oxyhemoglobin desaturation during sleep. *Chest* **95**: 757–766.

Gay P C (2004) Chronic obstructive pulmonary disease and sleep. *Respiratory Care* **49**(1): 39–51.

George G F, Bayliff C D (2003) Management of insomnia in patients with chronic obstructive pulmonary disease. *Drugs* **63**(4): 379–387.

Goldstein R S, Ramcharan V, Bowes G (1984) Effect of supplemental nocturnal oxygen on gas exchange in patients with severe obstructive lung disease. *New England Journal of Medicine* **310**: 425–429.

Klink M, Quan S F (1987) Prevalence of reported sleep disturbances in a general adult population and their relationship to obstructive airway disease. *Chest* **91**: 540–546.

Lewis D A (2001) Sleep in patients with asthma and chronic obstructive pulmonary disease. *Current Opinion in Pulmonary Medicine* **7**(2): 105–112.

McNicholas W T (2000) Impact of sleep in COPD. *Chest* **117** (Suppl. 2): 48S–53S.

Mohsenin V (2005) Sleep in chronic obstructive pulmonary disease. *Seminars in Respiratory and Critical Care Medicine* **26**(1): 109–116.

Morin C M, Colechi C, Stone J (1999) Behavioural and pharmacological therapies for late-life insomnia: a randomised controlled trial. *JAMA* **281**: 991–999.

O'Donoghue F J, Catcheside P G, Eckert D J, Doug McEvoy R (2004) Changes in respiration in NREM sleep in hypercapnic chronic obstructive pulmonary disease. *Journal of Physiology* **559**(2): 663–673.

O'Donohue W J, Bowman T J (2000) Hypoxemia during sleep in patients with chronic obstructive pulmonary disease: Significance, detection and effects of therapy. *Respiratory Care* **45**(2): 188–191.

Saunders M H, Newman A B, Haggerty C L, Redline S, Lebowitz M, Samet J, O'Connor G T, Punjab N M, Shahar E for Sleep Heart Health Study (2003). Sleep and sleep-disordered breathing in adults with predominantly mild obstructive airway disease. *American Journal of Respiratory and Critical Care Medicine* **167**: 7–14.

Wynne J W, Block A J, Hunt L A, Flick M R (1978) Disordered breathing and oxygen desaturation during daytime naps. *Johns Hopkins Medical Journal* **143**(1): 3–7.

6.5   TRAVEL AND HOLIDAYS

Anderson H R, Spix C, Medina S, Schouten J P, Castellsague J, et al. (1997) Air pollution and daily admissions for chronic obstructive pulmonary disease in 6 European cities: results from the APHEA project. *European Respiratory Journal* **10**: 1064–1071.

British Thoracic Society (2002) Managing patients with respiratory disease planning air travel: British Thoracic Society recommendations. *Thorax* **57**: 289–304.

Christensen C C, Ryg M, Refvem O K, et al. (2000) Development of severe hypoxaemia in chronic obstructive pulmonary disease patients at 2483 m (8000 ft) altitude. *European Respiratory Journal* **15**: 635–639.

Dockery D W, Pope C A III (1994) Acute respiratory effects of particulate air pollution. *Annual Review Public Health* **15**: 107–132.

Dockery D W, Speicer F E, Frank E, et al. (1989) Effects of inhalable particles on respiratory health of children. *American Review of Respiratory Disease* **139**: 587–594.

Donaldson G C, Seemungal T, Jefferies D J, Wedzicha J A (1999) Effect of temperature on lung function and symptoms in chronic obstructive pulmonary disease. *European Respiratory Journal* **13**(4): 844–849.

Fusco D, Forastiere F, Michelozzi P, Spadea T, Ostro B, Arca M, Perucci C A (2001) Air pollution and hospital admissions for respiratory conditions in Rome, Italy. *European Respiratory Journal* **17**: 1143–1150.

Gong H (1991) Air travel and patients with pulmonary and allergic conditions. *Journal of Clinical Immunology* **87**: 879–885.

Johnson A C (2003) Chronic Obstructive Pulmonary Disease 11: Fitness to fly in COPD. *Thorax* **58**: 729–732.

Kosela H, Pihlajamaki J, Pekkarinene H, Tukiainen, H O (1998) Effect of cold air on exercise capacity in COPD: Increase or decrease? *Chest* **113**: 1560–1565.

Kosela H O, Kosela A K, Tukiainen H O (1996) Bronchoconstriction due to cold weather in COPD: The role of direct effects and cutaneous reflex mechanisms. *Chest* **110**: 632–636.

MacNee W (2002) Acute exacerbations of COPD: Consensus Conference on Management of Chronic Obstructive Pulmonary Disease. *Journal of Royal College Physicians, Edinburgh* **32**: 16–26.

MET Office/NHS Winter 2004/05 (2005) *Anticipatory Care for COPD*. London: DHS. Met Office, Fitz Roy Rd, Exeter EX1 3PB, www.metoffice.gov.uk (accessed 6 April 2006).

Naughton M, Rochford P, Pretta J, et al. (1995) Is normbaric simulation of hypobaric hypoxia accurate in chronic airflow limitation? *American Journal of Respiratory Critical Care Medicine* **152**: 1956–1960.

Nunn J F (1987) *Applied Respiratory Physiology* (3rd edn). London: Butterworths.

Seccombe L M, Kelly P T, Wong C K, Rogers P G, Lim S, Peters M J (2004) Effect of simulated commercial flight on oxygenation in patients with interstitial lung disease and chronic obstructive pulmonary disease. *Thorax* **59**: 966–970.

Stoller J K, Hoisington E, Auger G (1999) A comparative analysis of arranging in-flight oxygen aboard commercial air carriers. *Chest* **115**: 991–995.

Sunyer J, Anto J M, Murillo C, Saez M (1991) Effects of urban air pollution on emergency room admissions for chronic obstructive pulmonary disease. *American Journal of Epidemiology* **134**: 277–286.

6.6 VACCINATIONS

Advisory Committee on Immunization Practices (1993) Practices, prevention and control of influenza. *MMWR* **42** (No. RR6): 1–14.

Alfageme I, Vazquez R, Reyes N, Munoz J, Fernandez A, Hernandez M, Merino M, Perez J, Lima J (2005) Clinical efficacy of anti-pneumococcal vaccination in patients with COPD. *Thorax* **61**(3): 189–195.

Department of Health (2005a) Influenza. In Salisbury D, Begg N (eds) *Immunisations against Infectious Disease. The Green Book*. London: The Stationery Office.

Department of Health (2005b) Pneumococcal. In Salisbury D, Begg N (eds) *Immunisations against Infectious Disease. The Green Book*. London: The Stationery Office.

De Roux A, Schmidt N, Rose M, Zielen S, Pletz M, Lode H (2004) Immunogeneity of the pneumococcal polysaccharide vaccine in COPD patients: The effect of systemic steroids. *Respiratory Medicine* **98**(12): 1187–1194.

Driver C (2002) Vaccinations. *Practice Nursing* **13**(3): 120–123.

Fine M J, Smith M A, Carson C A, Meffe F, Sankay S, Weissfeld L A, Detsky A S, Kapoor W N (1994) Efficacy of pneumococcal vaccination in adults: A meta-analysis of randomised controlled trials. *Archives of International Medicine* **154**: 2666–2677.

Fleming D M, et al. (1995) Study of the effectiveness of influenza vaccination in the elderly in the epidemic of 1989/1990 using a general practice database. *Epidemiology and Infection* **115**: 581–589.

Foster D A, Talsam A N, Furumoto-Dawson A, et al. (1992) Influenza vaccine effectiveness in preventing hospitalization for pneumonia in the elderly. *American Journal of Epidemiology* **136**: 296–307.

Garcia-Aymerich J, Monso E, Marrdes R M, Escarrabill J, Felez M A, Sunyer J, Anto J M and the EFRAM investigators (2001) Risk factors for hospitalization for a chronic obstructive pulmonary disease exacerbation: The EFRAM study. *American Journal of Respiratory Critical Care Medicine* **164**: 1002–1007.

George A C, Melegaro A (2000) Invasive pneumococcal infection, England and Wales. *CDR Weekly*: 3–9.

Health Protection Agency (2005a) Seasonal influenza: frequently asked questions. Available at: http://www.hpa.org.uk/infections/topics_as/influenza/seasonal/flufq.htm (accessed 25 Jan. 2006).

Health Protection Agency (2005b) Pneumococcal disease. Available at: http://www.hpa.org.uk/infections/topics_as/pneumococcal/menu.htm (accessed 25 Jan. 2006).

Hedlund J, Christenson B, Lundbergh P, Ortqvist A (2003) Effects of a large scale intervention with influenza and 23-valent pneumococcal vaccines in elderly people: a one year follow up. *Vaccine* **21**(25–26): 3906–3911.

Lipsky B A, Boyko E J, Inui T S, Koepsell T D (1986) Risk factors for acquiring pneumococcal infections. *Archives of Internal Medicine* **146**: 2179–2185.

Lydyard P, Whelan A (2000) *Immunology*. Oxford: BIOS Scientific Publishers Ltd.

Melegaro A, Edmunds W J (2004) The 23-valent pneumococcal polysaccharide vaccine. Part 1 Efficacy of PPV in the elderly: a comparison of meta-analyses. *European Journal of Epidemiology* **19**: 353–363.

Miller K E (2005) Effectiveness of influenza vaccine in patients with COPD. *American Family Physician. Kansas City* **71**(7): 1412–1413.

National Institute for Clinical Excellence (2003) Guidance on the use of zanamivir, oseltamivir and amantandine for the treatment of influenza. Available at: www.nice.org.uk/page.aspx?0=58066 (accessed 10 Mar. 2006).

National Institute for Clinical Excellence (2004) Chronic obstructive pulmonary disease: National Clinical Guideline for the management of chronic obstructive pulmonary disease in adults in primary and secondary care. *Thorax* **59** (Suppl. 1) 1–232.

Nguyen-Van Tam J S, Nicholson K G (1993) Influenza immunization; vaccine offer, request, and uptake in high risk patients during the 1991–1992 season. *Epidemiology Infection* **111**: 347–355.

Nichol K L, Baken L, Nelson A (1999) Relation between influenza vaccination and out-patient visits, hospitalization and mortality in elderly persons with chronic lung disease. *Annals of Internal Medicine* **130**: 397–403.

Nichol K L, Margolis K L, Wuorenma J, Von Sternberg T (1994) The efficacy and cost effectiveness of vaccination against influenza among elderly persons living in the community. *New England Journal of Medicine* **33**: 778–784.

Poole P J, Chacko E, Wood-Baker R W, Cates C J (2005) *Influenza Vaccine for Patients with COPD*. The Cochrane Library (Oxford) no. 4 (ID no CD002733).

Rothbarth P H, Kempen B M, Sprenger M J (1995) Sense and nonsense of influenza vaccination in asthma and chronic obstructive pulmonary disease. *American Journal of Respiratory Critical Care Medicine* **151**: 1682–1686.

Shaprio E D, Berg A T, Austrian R, Schroeder D, Parcells V, Margolis A, Adair R K, Clemens J D (1991) The protective efficacy of polyvalent pneumococcal polysac-charide vaccine. *New England Journal of Medicine* **325**: 1453–1460.

Tata L J, West J, Harrison T, Farrington P, et al. (2003) Does influenza vaccination increase consultations, corticosteroid prescriptions, or exacerbations in subjects with asthma or chronic obstructive pulmonary disease? *Thorax* **58**(10): 835–839.

Torres A, Dorca J, Zalacain R, Bello S, El-Ebiary M, Molinos L, et al. (1996) Community acquired pneumonia in chronic obstructive pulmonary disease: A Spanish multicenter survey. *American Journal of Respiratory Critical Care Medicine* **154**: 2666–2677.

US Department of Health and Human Services (2000) *Health People 2010*. Washington, DC: US Department of Health and Human Services.

Wongsurakiat P, Maranetera K N, Wasi C, Kositanont U, Dejsomritrutai W, Charoen-ratanakul S (2004) Acute respiratory illness in patients with COPD and the effective-ness of influenza vaccination: a randomized controlled study. *Chest* **125**(6): 2011–2020.

6.7 SEXUALITY

Agronin M (2001) Addressing sexuality and sexual dysfunction. *Geriatric Times* **2**: 1.

Carter M (1990) Illness, chronic disease and sexuality. In Fogel C, Lauver D (eds) *Sexual Health Promotion*. Philadelphia, PA: Saunders.

Finger B, Quillen J (2006) Sexuality and chronic illness. AAPA Conference paper, San Francisco, 27 May–1 June.

Gamlin R (1999) Sexuality: a challenge for nursing practice. *Nursing Times* **95**(7): 47–50.

Gift A, McCrone S (1993) Depression in patients with COPD. *Heart Lung* **22**: 289–297.

Gore J, Brophy C, Greenstone M (2000) How well do we care for patients with end-stage chronic obstructive pulmonary disease (COPD)? A comparison of palliative care and quality of life in COPD and lung cancer. *Thorax* **55**: 1000–1006.

Hagherty S (2004) Sex, COPD and nursing's Dr Ruth. *Practice Nursing* **14**(9): 428.

Hordern A, Currow D (2003) A patient-centred approach to sexuality in the face of life-limiting illness. Available at: www.mja.com.au/public/issues (accessed 17 August 2006).

Kochar M, Mazur L, Patel A (1999) What is causing your patient's sexual dysfunction? Available at: www.postgradmed.com/issues/1999/08 (accessed 21 Sept. 2006).

McInnes R (2003) Chronic illness and sexuality. Available at: www.mja.com.au/public/issues (accessed 20 July 2006).

Mooradian A, Greiff V (1990) Sexuality in older women. *Archives of Internal Medicine* **150**: 1033–1038.

Poorman S (1988) *Human Sexuality and the Nursing Process.* Connecticut: Appleton and Lange.

Sadoughi W, Lesher M, Fine H (1971) Sexual adjustment in a chronically ill and physically disabled population; a pilot study. *Archives of Physical Medical Rehabilitation* **52**: 322–417.

Schover L (2000) Sexual problems in chronic illness. In: Leiblum S, Rosen R (eds) *Principles and Practice of Sex Therapy* (3rd edn). New York: Guilford.

Semple P, Beastall G, Brown T, Stirling K, et al. (1984) Sex hormone suppression and sexual impotence in hypoxic pulmonary fibrosis. *Thorax* **58**: 105–106.

Sexton D, Munro B (1985) Impact of a husband's chronic illness (COPD) on the spouse's life. *Respiratory Nurse Health* **8**: 83–90.

Starr B, Weiner M (1981) *On Sex and Sexuality in the Mature Years.* New York: Stein and Day.

Walbroehl G (1992) Sexual concerns of the patient with pulmonary disease. *Postgraduate Medicine* **91**: 455–460.

Webb C (1994) Nurses' knowledge and attitudes about sexuality: Report of a study. *Nurse Education Today* **7**: 209–214.

White K (2003) Sexuality and body image. In O'Connor M, Aranda S (eds) *Palliative Care Nursing: A Guide to Practice* (2nd edn). Oxford: Radcliffe Medical Press Ltd.

Wilson M, Williams H (1988) Oncology nurses' attitudes and behaviours related to sexuality of patients with cancer. *Oncology Nursing Forum* **13**: 49–52.

7 Psychological Needs and Interventions

LINDA FISHER
King's College Hospital, London

The aim of this chapter is threefold. First, to outline the psychological impact of COPD on the individual and those who are important to them. Second, to introduce the principles of both **cognitive behavioural therapy (CBT)** and **motivational interviewing** (MI); and finally, to outline the ways in which these approaches can be used to address common problems encountered by this patient group.

ADJUSTMENT AND CHANGE: LIVING WITH COPD

Emotions such as anger and sadness are often experienced when the diagnosis of a life-limiting condition is made, and form part of the normal response to adversity. Feelings of guilt or remorse about past actions may be particularly acute for some COPD patients, because of the known associations between tobacco use and the development of lung disease. All of these uncomfortable emotions can persist in varying degrees of intensity throughout the illness.

Living with a chronic illness holds challenges that are very different from those involved in coping with an episode of acute ill health. Overall, the emphasis moves away from cure and towards palliation. Uncertainty regarding the exact profile of the disease trajectory is also a prominent feature. Decrements in physical state over time are characteristic and acute exacerbations of COPD may increase the sense of uncontrollability of the illness. Medical or technological intervention has less to offer, and successful management of COPD is heavily reliant on the patient becoming a 'partner' in care. The needs of chronically ill patients also become increasingly complex as co-morbidities develop, age increases and peer support diminishes, and patients with COPD are no different in this respect. Contact with a diverse number of health professionals and a disease-specific service becomes the norm. Severely ill and elderly patients with COPD are known to experience symptoms in excess of the number experienced by cancer palliative care patients (Elofsson & Ohlen 2004), although respiratory care palliative care is less well developed at the

Managing Chronic Obstructive Pulmonary Disease. Edited by L. Blackler, C. Jones and C. Mooney
© 2007 John Wiley & Sons Ltd

present time. For patients who are younger, the decline in health may be accompanied by changes in economic status as employment prospects reduce, and this may also impact upon relatives and carers.

Personal identity can become eroded by an altered appearance: weight loss and physical deconditioning occur in COPD as a result of the primary and secondary effects of disease, although exact aetiologies are complex (Wouters and Schols 2005). Beginning oxygen therapy for breathlessness is also a very visible symbol of increasing frailty. Roles and responsibilities within the family and established social networks may have to be relinquished over time, and it can become increasingly difficult for patients to continue to occupy a position where they feel valued, and as if they are able to make a meaningful contribution to life. Past achievements may be difficult for the patient to remember. Others, new to the patient at this life-stage, may forget to enquire about, or be unaware of, the vitality, qualities and achievements of the patient before the development of COPD. Understandably, the illness experience can begin to eclipse the sense of the former self and cause some degree of existential distress on the part of the patient (Chochinov 2002).

> "My sister and I used to take trips to Oxford Street and go to the theatre, but I can't do that now, my sister misses that and I miss that as well."

THE EFFECTS ON CARERS OF LIVING WITH SOMEONE WHO HAS COPD

Many patients are able to accommodate the demands and effects of chronic illness in their lives, but adjustment is also required on the part of others. Patients are known to be aware that the effects of their illness extend to impact directly on family relationships, and in particular spouses or life partners. Losses that have been cited by couples include social life, shared experiences and the future that they had previously expected together (Seamark et al. 2004). A qualitative study exploring the effects on wives of caring for a husband with COPD found that while some enriching aspects of caring were identified (increased spirituality, satisfaction in caring, and the knowledge that they were able to remain with their life partner until death), most of the themes that emerged for these women involved a sense of loss or a deterioration in their own quality of life (Bergs 2002).

PSYCHOLOGICAL NEED IN PATIENTS WITH COPD: A FRAMEWORK

Psychological need in patients with COPD is most usefully represented as a continuum (see Figure 7.1). This conceptualisation suggests that all staff involved in caring for patients have a part to play in routine *psychological care*,

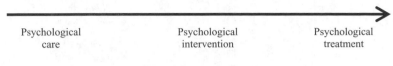

Increasing severity, complexity and persistence of presenting problem

| Psychological care | Psychological intervention | Psychological treatment |

Increasingly expert level of intervention required

Figure 7.1. Continuum of psychological need and intervention in COPD

e.g. offering appropriate reassurance and providing information. Movement along the continuum indicates more complex psychological need with an increasingly expert level of *psychological intervention* necessary for problem resolution, e.g., issues relating to difficulty with coping and adjustment. The far end of the continuum expresses the need for *psychological treatment* to manage psychiatric disorder, e.g. patients who have a clinical depression. The interventions described in this chapter are suitable to be used across the spectrum of psychological need and disease severity.

THE COGNITIVE BEHAVIOURAL THERAPY (CBT) MODEL

Central to the CBT model is the notion that our thoughts or cognitions about any given situation or event have a potent effect on both our feelings (emotional and to a lesser extent physical) and consequent actions. But importantly, the model also outlines the way in which our actions can influence how we feel and what we think, and that our feelings influence our actions and thoughts. Thus the model offers a theoretical framework that integrates both the physical and psychological dimensions of experience in chronic illness (see Figure 7.2).

COGNITIVE BEHAVIOURAL THERAPY: EVIDENCE BASE AND CURRENT USE

Cognitive behavioural therapy is a time-limited, problem-focused and patient-centred talking treatment. It is an evidence-based intervention for the treatment of anxiety, depression and chronic pain (DoH 2001). It is also being used increasingly with a variety of patient populations to help them to cope with the demands and effects of chronic illness. CBT techniques can be used to promote psychological well-being in the face of health-related adversity (Folkman & Greer 2000), and it has been found to be a useful adjunct to

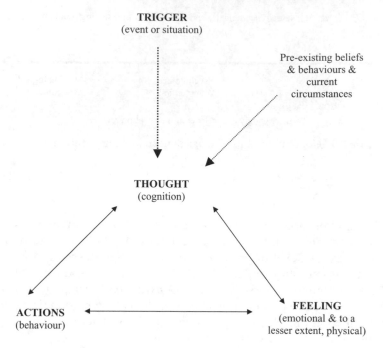

Figure 7.2. The cognitive behavioural model

conventional treatment in cancer care (Moorey et al. 2002). Furthermore, with some adaptation, the techniques are suitable for integration into usual clinical care.

HOW CAN COGNITIVE BEHAVIOURAL THERAPY WORK IN COPD?

Many chronic health problems can be made worse by long-term use of coping strategies that are only appropriate for short-term use, i.e. in the context of acute illness. This is because the strategies themselves become counter-productive if used for protracted periods of time. If we take the example of an acute chest infection in an otherwise healthy adult, a course of action involving time off work to remain at home, reducing activity to limit breathlessness and fatigue and avoiding social contact while waiting to recover would all be appropriate. However, fatigue and breathlessness in COPD are symptoms experienced over the long term and therefore these coping strategies are much less likely to be helpful. Staying at home would begin to make the individual feel cut off and isolated and other problems would ensue. Reduced activity levels would be likely to lead to physical deconditioning, thereby worsening fatigue and breathlessness and increasing the risk of secondary complications. Similarly, reduced social contact over long periods of time can lower mood and contribute to the development of a depressive illness.

Unfortunately, in chronic ill health, many patients become confused about the most useful way to respond to persistent and non-specific symptoms that are only partially ameliorated by the most effective medical interventions available. Entirely understandably, many patients tend to revert to coping strategies that are most appropriately used with acute illness, simply because they are more familiar with these strategies. The strategies themselves usually have their own logic in relation to the symptoms that are experienced (Cameron & Leventhal 2003) but may worsen the symptoms that they are trying to alleviate.

CBT is useful because it helps to identify patterns of thinking and behaviour that contribute to the *maintenance* of problems in chronic illness. Furthermore, CBT interventions can be used to promote thoughts, feelings and actions (behaviours) that are helpful and aid effective coping in the context of chronic illness.

Because the CBT model represents the dynamic interaction of thoughts, feelings and actions, it is possible to begin work with patients on any or all of these dimensions. CBT can be used to help patients in the following ways:

- working on behaviour directly: this is important because it means that it is possible to use CBT to good effect with patients who would not otherwise consider themselves 'psychologically minded'. Changes in behaviour are known to be accompanied by changes in thoughts and feelings;
- working directly with thoughts as a method of reducing distressing feelings and changing unhelpful behaviours;
- working on thoughts and actions together;
- teaching patients to transfer the techniques that they have used in one problem area to apply to other problem areas;
- being used alongside antidepressant medication, or alone.

The two main therapeutic techniques used in CBT are:

1 *Guided discovery* – helping patients to address unhelpful thoughts, feelings and actions through a structured way of talking.
2 *Action experiments* – helping patients to test out new ways of doing things and evaluating the effect that this has on feelings and thoughts, and thus future behaviour.

Understanding the cognitions involved in reluctance to engage in activity or exercise may enable practitioners to work with patients more effectively. Sharing the CBT model with patients and explaining the role of thoughts, feelings and actions in chronic illness can help to educate patients. It also increases the likelihood that they will engage in the active management of their chronic illness.

THE COGNITIVE BEHAVIOURAL THERAPY MODEL: UNPLEASANT SYMPTOMS AND THE EXPERIENCE OF BREATHLESSNESS IN COPD

Within the CBT model, feelings can be divided into emotional and physical and it is thought that there is an interaction between emotions and symptom perception. This idea is an extension of research findings in other areas that have highlighted how an anxious emotional state is associated with an increased perception of 'worrying' bodily sensations, e.g. Ehlers et al. (2000). Alongside this, breathlessness (an innocuous symptom in health) understandably assumes new meaning and increased salience in the context of a chronic and deteriorating respiratory illness. These factors in combination are likely to contribute to an increased preoccupation with, and awareness of, breathlessness for some individuals with COPD. Anecdotal evidence suggests that this can lead to problems with reduced activity, anxiety, loss of confidence, reduced activity to avoid breathlessness, and the excessive use of inhaled bronchodilators that is sometimes seen.

ANXIETY AND BREATHLESSNESS IN COPD

The relationship between emotional states, physiology and breathlessness across the spectrum of respiratory disorders is both unclear and complex (Gardner & Lewis 2005). However, an analysis of the thoughts, feelings and actions of patients who are particularly fearful of becoming breathless and who have responded less well to encouragement to take exercise may be useful.

This analysis of the problem adapts a model of anxiety that has been the impetus behind the development of an effective CBT treatment for panic attacks (Clark et al. 1994; Clark 1996) (Figure 7.3). This framework can be used with patients to identify and record idiosyncratic and problematic thoughts, feelings and actions to establish the focus for a shared understanding of the problem. The model can be used to increase patient awareness of the impact of relevant cognitions, as well as other key physiological and psychological processes that affect the experience of breathlessness itself. It maps onto existing models of understanding the cycle of breathlessness and deconditioning and offers the possibility of an intervention that is closely tailored to patient need, thus fulfilling current guidelines and the requirements of consultation documents outlining good practice in COPD (NCCCC 2004; NHLBI/WHO 2005). Using a CBT model in this way provides an alternative conceptualisation of the problem that appears to resonate with patients and seems to be a first and logical step towards changing behaviour.

The second step towards obtaining behavioural change involves setting a series of simple action experiments to achieve and then reinforce changes in thinking. The aim of an action experiment is to undermine unhelpful beliefs

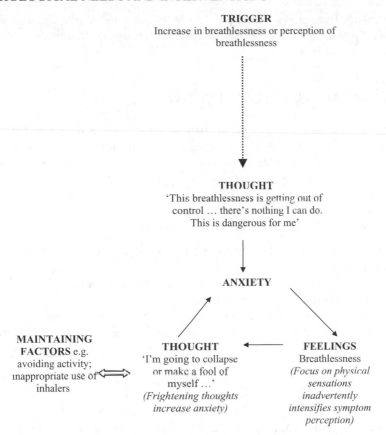

TRIGGER
Increase in breathlessness or perception of
breathlessness

THOUGHT
'This breathlessness is getting out of
control ... there's nothing I can do.
This is dangerous for me'

ANXIETY

**MAINTAINING
FACTORS** e.g.
avoiding activity;
inappropriate use of
inhalers

THOUGHT
'I'm going to collapse
or make a fool of
myself ...'
*(Frightening thoughts
increase anxiety)*

FEELINGS
Breathlessness
*(Focus on physical
sensations
inadvertently
intensifies symptom
perception)*

Figure 7.3. Model of anxiety, breathlessness and maintaining factors in COPD

about breathlessness, e.g. that it is 'dangerous, uncontrollable and should be avoided', and build confidence in more functional beliefs that are consistent with effective coping, e.g. 'exercise is good for me and breathlessness is an important part of keeping well'. The action experiments would involve planned and gradual increases in activity and/or exercise over any given time period. Within a CBT framework, repeated action experiments would also be accompanied by a gradual reduction or planned change in the relevant maintaining factors (e.g. excessive use of bronchodilators): participating in manageable amounts of activity with increasing difficulty, at first in the presence of someone and then alone. These action experiments then *provide persuasive evidence for the patient* in support of a new more adaptive belief. The patient can then learn to tolerate increased breathlessness in a controlled way, and without excessive anxiety in order to continue with activity and exercise and thus limit deconditioning as far as possible. The exact nature of the action experiments that might be negotiated with patients is not covered in this chapter, but would be devised with the intention of acquiring functional gains.

MOTIVATIONAL INTERVIEWING

Motivational interviewing (MI) is also an intervention designed to lead to constructive changes in health-related behaviour by helping patients to explore and resolve ambivalence and thus optimise quality of life (Miller & Rollnick 2002). Crucial to MI is the collaborative spirit or 'tenor' of the intervention that aims to help patients overcome ambivalence and begin the process of change.

The spirit of MI is embodied in the following ideas:

- Motivation to change is nurtured within the patient and not imposed on the patient by the clinician.
- The role of the clinician is to support the patient in expressing and working with the ambivalence experienced.
- Persuasion is not an effective way of dealing with ambivalence.
- Resistance within the therapeutic encounter is a product of the professional 'pushing' the patient too hard in a direction that they are not ready to travel in.
- The relationship between the clinician and the patient in MI is not characterised by the clinician behaving in an 'expert' way.
- The relationship between the clinician and patient is collaborative and the clinician is respectful of the patient's wishes to change or otherwise.

MOTIVATIONAL INTERVIEWING TECHNIQUES TO ENCOURAGE CHANGES IN BEHAVIOUR

It has been found that using interventions of the sort described below will allow professionals to be true to the spirit of MI:

- Using reflective listening to actively elicit and understand the patient's perspective on the situation. For example, 'You were just telling me how hard it seems to be to make that important step. Could you tell me a little more about that, so I can understand where you are coming from?'
- Being non-judgmental and accepting how difficult things are for the patient. For example, 'It sounds as though you feel you have a lot on your plate at the moment, and people are asking you to do even more'.
- Focus on and repeat back to the patient statements that seem to be expressing some recognition of their problem and/or the desire to change. It is thought that articulating the need for change strengthens commitment. For

example, 'You seem to be saying that carrying on as you are gives you a lot of problems, and if you could see a way out of this you would be tempted to try to change things for yourself.'

- Don't rush the patient. For example, 'What you are saying has made me wonder if you are beginning to feel a little more confident about trying to change things. Would I be right in thinking that or am I jumping ahead too much for you?'
- Allow the patient to lead the interaction and be guided by their responses. For example, 'Well, you know that you're in the driving seat with this ... where do you feel we should take this next?'

Using an active and light-handed technique such as MI to facilitate behaviour change has the following advantages:

- It provides an active method of addressing behaviour change with patients that is an alternative to 'nagging' or coercion, and thus minimises clinician frustration.
- Emotions like guilt and blame are avoided and therefore it is easier for patients to return for more help at a later date following a failed attempt at behaviour change.

STRONG EMOTIONS IN CHRONIC ILLNESS

Talking to patients about strong emotions helps to normalise their experience and acknowledge the role of feelings in coping with chronic illness. Specifically, it may be helpful to talk to patients about the following:

- Strong emotions (e.g. fear, anger) are normal responses to difficult circumstances.
- Strong emotions may fluctuate throughout the illness and can feel confusing at times.
- Strong emotions can influence the experience of illness.
- Talking about strong emotions does not mean that medical illness is being ignored.
- Sometimes strong emotions can become overwhelming and extra help is needed to cope.
- Extra help can come in the form of medication, counselling or therapy or self-help material or any combinations of these.
- Patients can choose which sort of extra help they would *like*, once someone has spoken to them about the advantages and disadvantages of each.

Patients may find that sudden deteriorations in health can be difficult to cope with and require periods of rapid adjustment that are taxing both physically and psychologically.

BEING WITH DISTRESSED PATIENTS

Responding appropriately to patients who are very distressed can be both a personal and professional challenge. However, it is important to provide a place and time in which patients can allow themselves to be upset. Many patients wish to conceal how distressed they are from family and friends for fear of burdening them, and so may have limited or no other outlets for emotional expression.

Allowing patients to become upset necessarily involves:

- Suppressing our own desire to try to make things better and learning to tolerate both the patients' discomfort and our own.
- Facilitating emotional expression. For example, 'I can see that you are trying to hold back the tears'; 'This is an ideal place to cry . . .'
- Containing and validating the patients' experience. For example, 'I'm not surprised you are feeling so upset, you have so much to deal with.'

DEPRESSION AND ANXIETY IN COPD

While it has been difficult to measure the prevalence of depression in COPD patients, specifically (van Ede et al. 1999), it is known that depression is twice as common in medical patients in general hospitals as it is in the general population. Depressed medical patients, when compared to non-depressed patients, are more likely to commit suicide, spend more time in hospital and to be more disabled (Royal College of Physicians and Royal College of Psychiatrists 2003). Depression is a reversible complication of chronic illness that further compromises quality of life and therefore it is important that it is detected and then treated appropriately in those whom it affects.

"You get very depressed about what you could do in the past and what you can't do now."

DETECTING DEPRESSION

Depression seems to be more likely in the sickest COPD patients (NCCCC 2004), and is often accompanied by anxiety. Depressive features to assess are:

- Low mood and guilt.
- Diurnal mood variation – typically patients feel worse in the morning, but find that their mood improves over the course of the day
- Insomnia – typically early morning waking, i.e. at a time that is not usual for the patient.
- Impaired enjoyment of life.
- Loss of libido, increase in somatic symptoms and appetite change may be signs of depression, but can also be caused by COPD.

SUICIDE

Patients who express the desire to harm themselves are at high risk of doing so and should be referred for a mental state examination and risk assessment. Suicidal ideas are *always* a sign of an abnormal mental state.

Asking about suicide is perfectly legitimate territory to enter providing the questions are asked appropriately and sensitively and positive responses are followed up promptly. *Asking about suicidal thoughts does not increase the likelihood of suicidal behaviour.*

Ways to ask about suicidal ideas might include the following:

- You just mentioned about 'being better off out of it'. Can you tell me a little bit more about what you mean by that . . .?
- I'm sorry that you are feeling so distressed. I'd like to ask you if it has ever crossed your mind to harm yourself, you describe things as being so bad for you at the moment. I hope you don't feel offended, but I think it is important for me to talk to you about this . . .

ANXIETY

Anxiety often presents with depression and with effective treatment for the depression the anxiety usually resolves. Giving information is a useful strategy to allay anxiety, as are effective communication and appropriate reassurance. If anxiety persists, further assessment may be needed.

MEASURING ANXIETY AND DEPRESSION IN COPD PATIENTS

A useful questionnaire to use is the Hospital Anxiety and Depression Scale (Zigmond & Snaith 1983). It is easy for patients to complete and staff to score. It provides a clear indication of the degree of depression and/or anxiety and can be used as a guideline for referral for assessment of mental state. It is sensitive to change and thus can be used to monitor the effects of treatment.

REFERRAL FOR ASSESSMENT OF MENTAL STATE

Patients are sometimes reluctant to be referred to psychiatrists or psychological services. Optimising the chances that the patient will accept the idea of referral and remain in a position to accept specialist help is important.

Wherever possible, try to prepare the patient by:

- offering to help them make a short list of things to address in the assessment;
- framing the referral in terms of a possible avenue of help that may be taken one step at a time, at a pace that suits them.

USING COGNITIVE BEHAVIOURAL THERAPY TO MANAGE LOW MOOD AND DEPRESSION IN COPD

CBT is an evidence-based psychological intervention for depression and anxiety (DoH 2001), and the available evidence suggests that antidepressants are an effective pharmacological treatment for more severe depression in medical illness (Gill & Hatcher 2001). However, many patients with COPD complain of a low mood that is insufficiently severe to warrant antidepressant medication, and some very depressed patients are reluctant to take medication. Teaching patients to use CBT techniques to deal with unhelpful thoughts as a form of self-management for low mood and treatment for depression can be a useful way of increasing their sense of control over the COPD. It is helpful to explain to patients that just as it is possible for one small incident to trigger a cascade of distressing and overwhelming thoughts that make them feel low and demoralised, it is also possible for small shifts in thinking and modest changes in behaviour to transform mood.

DEFINING UNHELPFUL THINKING IN THE CONTEXT OF CHRONIC ILLNESS

Unhelpful thinking in chronic ill health can be defined as having unpleasant, distressing and overwhelming thoughts. Such thoughts in chronic illness are both common, understandable, and, to some extent, probably inevitable but ultimately unhelpful because they contribute to a low mood and erode the capacity for effective coping. However, importantly, for some people, at least, they seem to be modifiable.

The aim of any cognitive intervention in chronic illness is not to entirely eliminate unhelpful thoughts (as this would be unrealistic) but to attempt to reduce:

- the *frequency* of unhelpful thoughts;
- the *negative impact* of unhelpful thoughts.

There are four steps involved in this process:

1 Helping patients to *identify when they are having unhelpful thoughts.*
2 Helping patients to *identify the content* of unhelpful thoughts.
3 Helping patients to *see the effects* of unhelpful thinking.
4 Helping patients to *generate more helpful thoughts* and thus improve mood and promote actions that are consistent with effective coping in chronic illness.

Helping patients to identify when they are having unhelpful thoughts

Most patients are able to identify the point at which they begin to have unhelpful thoughts by the experience of the associated downward shift in mood.

Helping patients to identify the content of unhelpful thoughts

Crucial in identifying unhelpful thoughts is the notion of establishing the personal meaning of any given event. Any number of patients will interpret the same situation in a slightly different way, depending upon previous experience, established patterns of thinking and behaving and current circumstances.

Interventions to help patients to access and identify the content of unhelpful thoughts include:

- Tell me about the sorts of things that run through your mind when you begin to think about X ...'
- 'If those things were to happen, what would that mean for you?

Changing unhelpful thinking

Distressed thinking is often subject to distinctive distortions. Once patients are able to identify the thoughts that are upsetting them, they can be encouraged to reflect on the distortions that are present. This is the first step towards exploring alternative interpretations of the situation and generating more helpful thoughts.

Some common unhelpful thinking styles with examples are:

- *Black and white thinking*: 'If I can't do all the things I used to do, there's no point in doing anything.'
- *Crystal ball gazing*: 'I'll never be able to enjoy anything again.'
- *Taking feelings as facts*: 'I feel so guilty, I've really let my wife down, it's my fault we can't go on holiday.'
- *Jumping to conclusions*: 'When the doctor came back in the room, he looked so serious ... there's bad news, but they don't know how to tell me.'
- *Discounting the positives in a situation and focusing on the bad*: 'I know my breathing is a bit better and I can do a bit more, what's the point in that? I'm just not the man I used to be.'

Interventions to help patients see the effects of unhelpful thinking: making links between thoughts, feelings and behaviours include:

- 'How does it leave you feeling when you are having these sorts of thoughts ... ?'
- 'Do those "knock-on feelings" help you feel better or worse?'
- 'Do those "knock-on effects" (feelings and actions) help you to cope and get on with the things in life that are important to you, or do they have the opposite effect?'

Interventions to help patients to explore more helpful and alternative thoughts might begin with interventions like: 'Living with a challenging illness like COPD means that there are lots of triggers for unhelpful thoughts ...'. Move on to interventions like these below to 'loosen up' some of the distressing or overwhelming thoughts the patient is having:

- 'Any thought has some truth in it, but I wonder if there is any degree of truth for another perspective of how things are or what might be done?'
- 'What might you say to a good friend if they were in this situation?'
- 'Is there anything that you think you could do about the situation that would help things a little?'

SHARING THE MODEL WITH PATIENTS

As in the case of breathlessness, when using the CBT model, writing out the framework, with examples of problematic feelings, thoughts and actions that have been provided by the patient is a very useful exercise. Figures 7.4 and 7.5 illustrate how, with the use of the talking techniques described above, patients can be helped to make small changes in thinking that then translate into positive changes in mood and behaviour.

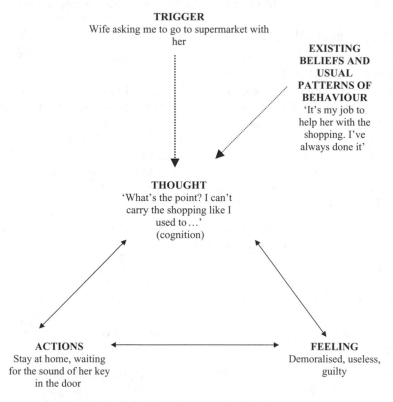

Figure 7.4. Negative mood and behaviour

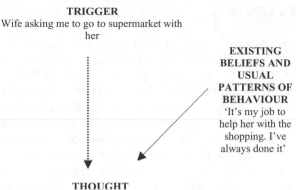

TRIGGER
Wife asking me to go to supermarket with her

EXISTING BELIEFS AND USUAL PATTERNS OF BEHAVIOUR
'It's my job to help her with the shopping. I've always done it'

THOUGHT
'I suppose there is more than one way of helping my wife out ... I'll be company for her, even if I can't carry the shopping any more. Lots of people our age need help with the shopping. We might even meet someone we know...'

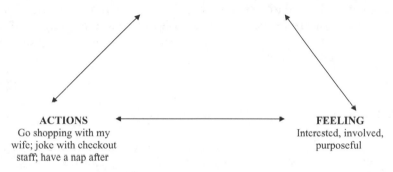

ACTIONS
Go shopping with my wife; joke with checkout staff; have a nap after

FEELING
Interested, involved, purposeful

Figure 7.5. Positive mood and behaviour

USING ACTION EXPERIMENTS TO BUILD ON AND CONSOLIDATE IMPROVEMENT

Facilitating shifts in thinking and thus mood by talking in this structured and purposeful way provides a platform from which to consolidate improvements in mood. One or more action experiments can be planned to test out whether or not doing things differently (i.e. behaviour change) also improves mood. Once the patient has made the connection between mood and behaviour, regular, achievable targets can be negotiated and used to promote regular activities that are consistent with effective coping and thus improved quality of life.

CONCLUSION

Psychological states appear to be increasingly important in the adjustment to and self-management of all chronic illnesses. Because of the pivotal role of collaboration in CBT and MI, and the nature of the problems that patients with COPD encounter, both these interventions seem appropriate to use in this clinical population. Alone or in combination, they provide a flexible approach suitable for use across the spectrum of disease severity in a range of common problems. The interventions are relatively simple, can be brief and are suitable for use in busy clinical settings. They are also easy for non-specialist practitioners to adapt and integrate with routine practice or usual care. Both CBT and MI are derived from evidence-based interventions used in other areas and so need formal evaluation with this patient group. However, intuitive use of these approaches in pulmonary rehabilitation is already common practice. Formalising and enhancing the existing skills of practitioners working with patients with COPD can make a useful contribution to the quality of care delivered to these patients. Finally, and importantly, CBT seems to offer a way forward for patients who wish to be more actively involved in managing the demands and effects of chronic illness, until choice or disease progression dictates otherwise.

REFERENCES

Bergs D (2002) 'The hidden client' – women caring for husbands with COPD: their experience of quality of life. *Journal of Clinical Nursing* **11**(5): 613–621.

Cameron L D, Leventhal H (2003) Self regulation, health and illness: an overview. In: Cameron L D, Leventhal H (eds) *The Self-regulation of Health and Illness Behaviour.* New York: Routledge.

Chochinov H M (2002) Dignity-conserving care: A new model for palliative care. *Journal of the American Medical Association* **287**(17): 2253–2260.

Clark D M (1996) Panic disorder: From theory to therapy. In: Salkovskis P M (ed.) *Frontiers of Cognitive Therapy.* New York: Guilford Press.

Clark D M, et al. (1994) A comparison of cognitive therapy, applied relaxation and imipramine in the treatment of panic disorder. *British Journal of Psychiatry* **164**: 759–769.

Department of Health (2001) *Treatment Choice in Psychological Therapies and Counselling: Evidence-based Clinical Practice Guideline.* London: Department of Health.

Ehlers A, et al. (2000) Psychological and perceptual factors associated with arrhythmias and benign palpitations. *Psychosomatic Medicine* **62**: 693–702.

Elofsson L C, Ohlen J (2004) Meanings of being old and living with a chronic obstructive pulmonary disease. *Palliative Medicine* **18**: 611–618.

Folkman S, Greer S (2000) Promoting psychological well-being in the face of serious illness: when theory, research and practice inform each other. *Psycho-Oncology* **9**: 11–19.

Gardner W N, Lewis A (2005) Hyperventilation and disproportionate breathlessness. In: Ahmedzai S H and Muers F M (eds) *Supportive Care in Respiratory Disease*. Oxford: Oxford University Press.

Gill D, Hatcher S (2001) *Antidepressants for Depression in Medical Illness* (Cochrane Review). In the Cochrane Library 4.

Miller W R, Rollnick S (2002) *Motivational Interviewing: Preparing People for Change* (2nd edn). New York: The Guilford Press.

Moorey S, et al. (2002) *Cognitive Behaviour Therapy for People with Cancer*. Oxford: Oxford University Press.

NCCCC (2004) *Chronic Obstructive Pulmonary Disease: Management of Chronic Obstructive Pulmonary Disease in Adults in Primary and Secondary Care*. London: National Institute for Clinical Excellence.

NHLBI/WHO (2005) Executive Summary: Global strategy for the diagnosis, management and prevention of chronic obstructive pulmonary disease. In: NHLBI/WHO Workshop. 1998. Updated 2005.

Royal College of Physicians and Royal College of Psychiatrists (2003) *The Psychological Care of Medical Patients: A Practical Guide*. London: Royal College of Physicians and Royal College of Psychiatrists.

Seamark D A, Blake S D, Seamark C J (2004) Living with severe chronic obstructive pulmonary disease (COPD): perceptions of patients and their carers. *Palliative Medicine* 18: 619–625.

van Ede L, Yzermans C J, Brouwer H J (1999) Prevalence of depression in patients with chronic obstructive pulmonary disease: a systematic review. *Thorax* 54: 688–692.

Wouters E F, Schols A M (2005) Nutrition and cachexia. In: Ahmedzai S H, Muers F M (eds) *Supportive Care in Respiratory Disease*. Oxford: Oxford University Press.

Zigmond A S, Snaith R P (1983) The Hospital Depression and Anxiety Scale. *Acta Psychiatrica Scandinavia* 67: 361–370.

8 Management of COPD in the Community

PATRICK WHITE

GP and King's College School of Medicine, London

COPD has acquired increasing prominence in health-care policy and in the clinical priorities of primary care teams. This has resulted from a number of influences, among which the efforts of the Global Initiative for Chronic Obstructive Lung Disease (GOLD) and more recently in the National Health Service (NHS), the National Institute for Health and Clinical Excellence (NICE) Guidelines have been significant (Pauwels et al. 2001; Halpin 2004). However, it is not long since the attitude of primary care clinicians to COPD was one of grim resignation to a disease for which there were few useful remedies. Smokers with COPD were widely seen to be reaping the rewards of a lifetime of smoking for which they were responsible.

Attitudes have changed and COPD has leap-frogged asthma to capture the attention of primary care teams, aided by the inclusion of COPD in the incentive targets set for general practitioners (GPs) in their new NHS contract. Nonetheless the perception of COPD in the community setting may still be at odds with its importance for society. The mortality due to COPD, the number of hospital admissions it causes, and its prevalence, demonstrate that COPD is not only a major disease in its consequences for the individuals who have it; it is also a major challenge for society as a whole. But in the community setting and particularly in the primary care team, COPD has not been seen to be such a pressing problem. In the community setting the numbers of people for whom COPD is their major concern, the number of consultations undertaken for the disease, and the persistent belief in some quarters that there are few effective interventions for COPD, have all contributed to the disease being perceived as a less important entity than other diseases with a similar prevalence such as diabetes mellitus. The low prominence of COPD has been compounded by the fact that as people become housebound through the disability of COPD, they are at risk of becoming increasingly invisible to health-care services.

Managing Chronic Obstructive Pulmonary Disease. Edited by L. Blackler, C. Jones and C. Mooney
© 2007 John Wiley & Sons Ltd

BURDEN OF COPD IN THE COMMUNITY

The true prevalence of COPD is uncertain. A representative population survey based on lung function testing in subjects over 35 years of age has not been done in most western countries. A variety of surveys around the world suggest a population prevalence of COPD between 3 and 10 per cent. Smoking causes more than 80 per cent of COPD so the factors that determine the prevalence of COPD are the prevalence of smoking and the susceptibility of smokers to the damaging effects of cigarette smoke. Deprived populations have higher rates of COPD because they have significantly higher rates of smoking. In describing the burden of COPD here I have used as my point of reference United Kingdom GPs because they comprise the basic registration unit in the NHS in the UK, with whom 99 per cent of the population are registered. The average list size of a GP in the UK is about 1,800 patients. The following figures can be extrapolated to other health-care systems using this denominator.

PREVALENCE

In a landmark study in the UK, Soriano and colleagues demonstrated that the prevalence of diagnosed COPD under the care of general practitioners (GPs) was 1.4 per cent in 1999 (Soriano et al. 2000). Based on this prevalence, an average GP in England and Wales with a list of 1,800 patients should have about 27 patients with COPD. *Morbidity Statistics from General Practice* (McCormick 1995) reported that the number of people in general practice who consulted with COPD in 1991–92 was 101 per 10,000 patient years at risk. This is equivalent to about 18 patients with COPD consulting a GP each year and compares to 77 patients consulting with asthma. In the same study, the number of consultations per year for COPD was about 245 per 10,000 persons at risk, or 44 consultations per year per GP for COPD (less than one a week), and compares to 164 per year for asthma, or more than three a week. Community consultations for COPD are likely to be with a GP or practice nurse. There is very little contact with COPD patients by district nurses. Community clinicians can estimate the COPD prevalence and consultation rates in their practices from these figures using the number of patients registered.

Knowledge of prevalence is important to primary care clinicians because their COPD registers are the basic building blocks of COPD care from which workload can be analysed and vulnerable patients identified. Local prevalence rates vary substantially depending on socio-economic status and the urban–rural balance. Segmenting registers by severity will enable primary care services to determine the accuracy of their registers and the effort needed to improve the identification and follow-up of COPD patients. Primary care teams need to know if they are identifying and reviewing the patients who require intervention. Complete prevalence rates may be less useful for clinical practice than the prevalence of moderate and severe asthma because they will include large numbers of patients in whom the role of clinical management is uncertain. Should primary care teams be detecting COPD before it presents with symptoms?

The early diagnosis of COPD has been promoted in some guidelines, but its role is at best uncertain. Using the NICE Guidelines criteria for the diagnosis of COPD, the true prevalence of all COPD is likely to be higher than that of physician-diagnosed or symptomatic COPD. Early diagnosis of COPD is an important issue in the context of primary care because it has the potential to increase the overall workload associated with COPD without improving outcome for patients. The hope was that the earlier COPD was diagnosed, the quicker smoking cessation could be achieved. In fact, only one study has examined the effect of a diagnosis of COPD on rates of smoking cessation. Gorecka and colleagues in 2003 showed no overall improvement in smoking cessation in smokers in whom COPD was diagnosed compared to those who did not have COPD (Gorecka et al. 2003). An effect was seen in sufferers with moderate or severe disease in a sub-group analysis. However, in mild disease the diagnosis of COPD did not improve smoking cessation rates. It seems that the diagnosis of COPD does not improve smoking cessation rates unless the disease is symptomatic. Since smoking cessation is the only useful intervention in mild COPD, it would be more cost effective simply to identify smokers with or without a diagnosis of COPD and offer a smoking cessation intervention with all the benefits it can bring. Since there is no evidence of an additional advantage from seeking to diagnose COPD early in the disease, the possible negative effects of doing so are of increased importance. By expanding the disease register of COPD patients in primary care with patients who have mild asymptomatic disease, the management task for primary care teams is increased with no benefit to patients or to the service. In fact, the effect of having to recall patients with asymptomatic disease in order to assess their status, repeat spirometry and review medication can only dilute the resources available to the management of patients with symptomatic (moderate or severe) COPD. The role of spirometry in detecting asymptomatic mild COPD has now been challenged in the United States because there are no proven advantages to the patient or the services (Boushey et al. 2005).

MORTALITY, MORBIDITY, ADMISSIONS, AND SERVICE USE

More than 30,000 people died from COPD in the UK in 2004. This is equivalent to about one death for every GP. With one death per year from COPD a GP should expect at any time to have two or three patients with COPD who are within two years of dying from the disease. Almost as many people die from COPD as die from lung cancer and there is good evidence that people who die from COPD are likely to have had palliative care needs that are at least as demanding as those of people who die from lung cancer (Gore et al. 2000). Patients with advanced COPD have symptoms that are more severe than patients with lung cancer, and services for COPD with advanced disease are limited with virtually no end-of-life care. Patients' palliative care needs may include uncontrolled symptoms, lack of information about the illness and its prognosis, and lack of choice of the place of care at the end of life.

Estimating the burden of COPD in terms of the morbidity it causes is diffi- cult. There is a lack of good morbidity data. How should the care of people with COPD be evaluated? It should be possible to assess the quality of COPD care in terms of the rate of diagnosis, the access patients have to treatments at different levels of severity (mainly moderate and severe), and disease outcome. However, because there is no reliable measure of COPD outcome, primary care teams are limited to measuring elements of the process of care in attendance rates, treatment, referrals, etc. Admissions are a good indicator of outcome and severity in individuals but the likelihood that a true outcome measure such as the test of glycated haemoglobin in diabetes will be developed for COPD is small. Quality-of-life measures such as the St George's Hospital Respiratory Questionnaire have been used widely in research and evaluation but are relatively unwieldy for clinical practice. There has been some recent interest in using the MRC breathlessness questions to segment COPD patients by severity (Hajiro et al. 1999; Bestall et al. 1999).

Hospital admissions due to COPD are considerably more common than deaths and COPD is currently the largest single cause of emergency admis- sions in the UK accounting for about 300,000 admissions per year (Damiani & Dixon 2004), and 12 per cent of emergency admissions are due to COPD. A GP can expect to have between 7 and 10 admissions for COPD in one year. Admissions for COPD cost the National Health Service more than £600 million per year in 2002. In 2004, Damiani and Dixon found that rates of admission for COPD were highly correlated with social deprivation, being much higher in areas of high social deprivation. Rates of admission for COPD varied hugely from area to area, ranging from 104 admissions per 100,000 population in the wealthiest areas to 932 admissions per 100,000 populations in the poorest areas. However, even between poor and wealthy areas, rates varied considerably. In the fifth poorest health authority areas in the UK between 2000 and 2002, rates of 932 per 100,000 population were found for COPD admissions in north Manchester, compared to rates of 150 per 100,000 in Enfield in north London. Length of stay also varied for COPD admissions, ranging from rates between 10 and 100 days per admission in rural areas of Scotland and Wales, to rates of between 3 and 7 days per admission in East Anglia, Devon and Cornwall.

The relatively low rates of contact associated with COPD belie the seriousness of the condition for patients. In a recent retrospective study of deaths from COPD in 2001, only a third had regular reviews by a chest specialist in the year before they died and more than a third saw their GP less than three monthly or never (Elkington et al. 2005). Less than 5 per cent of the people who died from COPD had any contact with a respiratory nurse specialist (RNS). From these figures it can be assumed that the disease is being under-treated since the rate of receipt of services is less than ideal even in those who have advanced disease.

There is good evidence of under-treatment and under-diagnosis of COPD in many healthcare systems. However, assessing under-treatment is difficult without accurate estimates of prevalence but there are a number of compelling indicators. Among these the most important are access to smoking cessation services, the single most important issue in COPD, regular disease reviews mentioned above, and the use of long-term oxygen therapy (LTOT) in patients with hypoxic respiratory failure. Access to smoking cessation services is low in all ages and disease groups and there is no evidence that this is any different in COPD. People with moderate or severe COPD respond better to smoking cessation counselling than smokers without evidence of lung disease so they should represent an excellent opportunity for primary care team intervention. LTOT is the only therapeutic intervention apart from smoking cessation counselling that increases life expectancy in COPD. In the retrospective study of COPD deaths mentioned above, although oxygen was being used by 40 per cent of those who died in the year before death, more than half of them were using it for less than 15 hours a day. This is an important benchmark for the community care of COPD.

Judging the role of under-diagnosis of COPD is also complicated, not least by the lack of evidence for the usefulness of diagnosing mild disease. There is no evidence that any treatment has a place in mild COPD, mild disease being characterised by an FEV_1 of 60 per cent or more of that predicted for age, height and gender. Recent changes in the NHS contract for GPs have provided incentive payments to GPs for the registration and treatment of people with COPD. In the first year of the new contract, the average prevalence of COPD recorded in GPs' registers was 1.4 per cent, exactly that found by Soriano in the 1990s. Whether this figure will rise as GPs take on primary care-based spirometry, another management strategy that is connected to incentive payments in the UK, remains to be seen.

Although COPD is associated with high morbidity and mortality and high levels of emergency admission to hospital, it is not among the most common long-term conditions in primary care. For that reason persuasive arguments are needed to ensure that it receives the attention it deserves.

GUIDELINES, EVIDENCE, AND AUTHORITY IN THE COMMUNITY MANAGEMENT OF COPD

COPD guidelines are built on a spine of evidence and authority designed to lead clinicians towards optimal therapy. In COPD it is easy to be distracted into the consideration of the drugs that can be prescribed before adequate attention is given to the three key interventions that should be the highest priority in COPD treatment: smoking cessation, pulmonary rehabilitation and long-term oxygen therapy. But there is a range of interventions available in addition to these three essentials. They need to be considered in some sort of order so that the clinician and patient are not paralysed by choice. A stepwise progression of treatment has been offered in the NICE Guidelines, the most recent guidelines in the UK, starting with beta-agonist adrenergic inhalers and ending with oral steroids and mucolytics. In practice, it is difficult to prescribe in an ascending spiral of severity because symptoms are virtually never removed by treatment in moderate and severe disease, only ameliorated. The improvement in lung function offered by the drug treatment of COPD is usually between 10 and 15 per cent so the advantage of treatment in a patient who has less than 60 per cent of expected lung function is not going to be much more than 6 per cent of expected improvement.

In a community setting, clinicians have a dual responsibility for COPD care. They are responsible for the acute management of the individual patient as they present, and also for the long-term management of the whole population of COPD patients. Guidelines for COPD are written mainly with the individual patient in mind. The challenge for the primary care clinician is to ensure that the patient is seen not only during an acute exacerbation, but is also seen when the disease is in its routine, quiet phase. That is when the most important challenge of COPD – smoking cessation – should be met.

The reading of COPD guidelines needs to be done against a background of a clear understanding of the requirements for the organisation of COPD care, the role and priority of different elements of the COPD patient's treatment, and the assurance that the right interventions are being offered at the right time.

The NICE Guidelines suggest that patients with severe disease should be reviewed at least twice a year in primary care, and those with mild or moderate disease at least annually. At the top of the clinical assessment should be smoking status and the need for smoking cessation advice. The understandable tendency of clinicians faced with a patient with COPD symptoms is to seek medication to relieve those symptoms. The role of inhaled medications in COPD is limited, however, and their use needs to be seen in a hierarchy of interventions in which smoking cessation, pulmonary rehabilitation, and long-term oxygen therapy (LTOT) for hypoxic patients are all of greater importance because their impact is likely to be more useful to the patient. Nonetheless, inhaled remedies are effective in COPD, especially in severe disease. The drugs do relieve symptoms, they can improve quality of life, they can reduce the frequency of exacerbations, and they may even reduce the risk of admission to hospital.

TREATMENT STRATEGIES FOR THE INDIVIDUAL PATIENT

Faced with the individual patient, the guidelines help the clinician to stage the disease and to choose a suitable treatment strategy. Patients with mild disease are seen almost exclusively in a community setting. For these patients, treatment consists of smoking cessation and symptom control using broncho dilators. Smoking cessation is by far the more important of these two interventions. A sophisticated and sympathetic approach is needed when the patient is a smoker and presents with symptoms. COPD will be a progressive problem in those who can't stop smoking. Mild disease will disappear as a health issue in those who do succeed in stopping. In mild disease, the goal should be to establish an alliance with the patient through which the main objective of smoking cessation can be addressed. This may require active treatment of symptoms in the first place to respond to the patient's presentation. In responding to the patient's symptoms we have the possibility of engaging the patient in a discussion of smoking. In mild disease inhaled short-acting bronchodilators (beta-agonist or anticholinergic) are the first line of drug treatment. Choice of device is of the same importance as in any other stage of the disease and failure of treatment may be due to poor inhaler technique. Although pulmonary rehabilitation is effective at all grades of severity of COPD, it is a limited resource. In areas where access to pulmonary rehabilitation is limited, people with mild disease should not be a priority for this treatment until those with moderate and severe disease have been considered for referral.

In moderate or severe disease the treatment plan should address the following interventions in order of importance:

- smoking cessation
- pulmonary rehabilitation
- assessment of hypoxia and the role of LTOT
- inhaled bronchodilator medication
- inhaler technique
- inhaled steroids in frequent exacerbations
- self-management plan for exacerbations with home supply of steroids and antibiotics
- mucolytics in selected patients.

The principles of COPD treatment in mild disease apply equally to moderate and severe disease with smoking cessation the priority closely followed by pulmonary rehabilitation. Drug treatment of COPD is limited in its effectiveness so it is particularly important to consider the disease as a whole, particularly its complications and their management. The complications of COPD are dominated by acute exacerbations especially in severe disease in which exacerbations can be life-threatening. Of great importance but less frequently considered are the patient's nutritional state, the development of right heart failure due to pulmonary hypertension (commonly referred to as cor pulmonale), and particularly in severe disease the presence of low mood and pain. Low mood and pain are unexpected but common symptoms in advanced disease (Elkington et al. 2005). Research evidence does not provide a guide for how best to respond to these issues in COPD, but acknowledging their importance is a good first step. Poor nutritional status is a predictor of premature death in COPD so its role may reflect some hidden aspect of disease severity.

The drug treatment of COPD has been discussed in Chapter 3. In moderate and severe disease all patients should be on a long-acting bronchodilator (beta-agonist or anti-cholinergic). It is not clear if these are synergic, so dual therapy should be considered (van Noord et al. 2005). The most difficult decision is the initiation of inhaled corticosteroids. Inhaled corticosteroids should be considered in patients whose FEV_1 is less than 50 per cent predicted and who have had two or more exacerbations requiring antibiotics or oral steroids in the previous year (NICE 2004).

Patients with moderate or severe COPD may only be seen during acute exacerbations of the disease unless arrangements are made for formal review by their primary care teams. During an acute exacerbation the priority is to assess the severity and to make a decision about acute management. If the patient is still smoking, the clinician must ensure that the patient is seen again after the exacerbation to review their overall management. The review appointment is the opportunity to assess the potential for a smoking cessation intervention. It is commonly the case that the demands of the acute exacerbation make the discussion of smoking difficult, if not inappropriate. Furthermore, smoking may be an embarrassing subject for the patient to raise, especially if he or she feels that it is smoking that has led to the need to demand help. A conspiracy of silence can prevent the most important COPD intervention of all from being considered. Recovery from the exacerbation may lead to loss of motivation to return for review.

A number of dilemmas remain for primary care teams, which are not resolved by the guidelines. How can limited resources be best used in a community setting, and which elements of the guidelines should be prioritised? This challenge can be divided into two elements. In the first place, the patient who presents with symptoms has to be treated effectively and this should invariably include a review appointment after the cause of the initial presentation has resolved, either spontaneously or with medication. The second element is the strategy for reviewing patients on the COPD disease register. The coordination of COPD care is discussed later in this chapter.

THE ROLE OF LUNG FUNCTION TESTING IN PRIMARY CARE

The provision of lung function testing is complicated in a community setting. The diagnosis of COPD and an accurate assessment of disease progression require spirometry. Spirometry can be done by primary care teams, or patients may be referred to a specialist centre, based either in the locality or in a local respiratory centre. In most countries direct access to a spirometry service is not available to primary care clinicians. In these circumstances, either spirometry has to be done within primary care or referral has to be made to a respiratory physician in secondary care. Cost may be an important obstacle to specialist referral.

Spirometry can be done to a high standard in primary care as has been demonstrated in Holland (Schermer et al. 2003). However, it may not be done adequately, and the problem of poorly executed tests may be compounded by inadequate interpretation. Modern electronic spirometers are now cheap enough that cost should not be the main hurdle to overcome. Effective spirometry requires adequate training, both for the operator and for the interpreter. The role of the interpreter is crucial because it is the feedback of interpretation on both the spirometry indices (FEV_1, FVC and FEV_1/FVC) and the spirometry curves (flow–volume loop and time–volume curve) that informs the operator whether the test has been done to an adequate standard. A number of possible approaches can be taken in the primary care provision of spirometry for COPD:

- Spirometry done by the primary care team with high-quality training of an operator and test reporter with some form of long-term quality control.
- Spirometry done by the primary care team but tests reported remotely by a primary care clinician with a special interest, or by a respiratory specialist.
- Spirometry done in a locality primary or intermediate care setting with reporting by a primary care clinician with a special interest, or by a respiratory specialist.
- Spirometry done entirely in secondary care.

In the United Kingdom, the National Health Service has provided incentive payments for the conduct of spirometry in COPD patients by primary care teams. These incentive payments have increased significantly the number of patients with COPD who have spirometry carried out. The risk of this approach is that the spirometry tests will be done inadequately by primary care teams, with no control over the quality of the tests.

Primary care teams have used peak expiratory flow (PEF) recording in the assessment of asthma for many years. Although PEF is not adequate for the diagnosis and assessment of disease progression in COPD, it is widely used for the assessment of short-term changes in COPD when spirometry is not available. It may be more acceptable in some circumstances to use PEF in the assessment of COPD where the PEF is performed well than to encourage the conduct of spirometry when that is done badly. This is a difficult dilemma for primary care teams, especially in the context of guideline advice that PEF is unsuitable for COPD.

CO-ORDINATION OF COPD MANAGEMENT IN THE COMMUNITY

Health-care systems that have a primary care service as the first point of contact will find the most accurate prevalence of diagnosed COPD in their primary care registers. The NHS, in which 99 per cent of the UK population is registered with a GP, offers an exceptional opportunity to undertake a whole system approach to COPD care. The key to such an approach is in the COPD disease registers of primary care teams. The pivotal position of primary care in any chronic disease management programme in the NHS comes from these registers. The potential of a disease register in a system where almost the whole population is registered with a GP derives from the possibility of identifying and following people with a diagnosed condition. If the register of diagnosed COPD is augmented by spirometry-based segmentation into severity groups, the efficiency of the register is enhanced. Additional information about smoking status provides an unparalleled opportunity to intervene where the need is greatest. It should be no surprise that disease registers have been targeted in the New Contract for NHS GPs. This contract offers incentive payments to GPs who compose disease registers, an example of which is the COPD register. The disease register is the opening to a whole system approach to COPD care.

We have already discussed the potential for missing both the key intervention of smoking cessation, and the other important elements of a routine COPD review in a system of COPD care that is dominated by the response to acute exacerbations. Establishing an effective system of review allows for complex interventions at every level of severity of COPD, targeting in particular those who are vulnerable. Effective co-ordination of COPD management in the community changes the balance of care from one dominated by the 'fire fighting' of treating acute exacerbations, to the proactive management culture characterised by patient education, early intervention in acute exacerbations, self-management, and mastery over the disease. To achieve such effective co-ordination of COPD management, the system of care requires:

- a dynamic register;
- lung function testing;
- pulmonary rehabilitation;
- a multidisciplinary team;

- access to specialist services;
- preparation for the palliative phase of the disease.

The NICE Guidelines have outlined the components of the routine reviews of mild or moderate disease, and of severe disease (NICE 2004). These reviews are underpinned by four principles:

1 Patient education/empowerment
2 Rigorous assessments of need (i.e. smoking cessation, etc.)
3 Optimisation of treatment
4 Identification of management priorities.

The identification of management priorities is a challenge, because the needs of people with severe COPD can be complex. Two groups vie for attention: the established severely affected patients who have already required hospital admission; and moderately affected people who have had acute exacerbations managed entirely in primary care. In both these groups other diseases may co-exist and raise the overall severity level because of the impairment caused by the second disease. Common examples of co-morbidity in COPD include chronic heart failure, osteoarthritis and depression.

COMMUNITY IMPLICATIONS OF INTERVENTIONS IN ACUTE SEVERE EXACERBATIONS

The high cost of COPD admissions has stimulated the interest of health-care planners in strategies that might reduce COPD admissions and length of hospital stay. Savings that can be achieved by reducing the cost of COPD admissions could be used to develop services that maintain lower rates of admission or further reduce admissions. This area of work has appeal for hospital administrators and health-care commissioners across all medical specialties. Interventions that prevent the need for admission are usually disease-altering treatments that limit exacerbations of the disease or interrupt disease progression. Interventions that divert patients home in the early phase of hospital presentation are called supported discharge or early discharge. Interventions that enable an exacerbation of a condition to be managed at home where previously it would have been treated in hospital are collectively called 'hospital at home'.

The latter stages of COPD are often characterised by acute exacerbations that lead to admission. Exacerbations are associated with accelerated deterioration of the disease. Interventions that limit exacerbations may have the benefit of improving life expectancy in addition to the advantages to both the patient and the service of avoiding the admission itself. Four points of intervention in acute severe exacerbations present themselves: self-management; early clinical intervention; supported discharge; and hospital at home.

Self-management of the disease refers to patient-led intervention at the beginning of acute exacerbations in which high dose bronchodilators are accompanied by early use of antibiotics and oral steroids. The aim is to abort the attack at the earliest possible stage. Frequent use of oral steroids that might be required for two weeks out of four in the winter months demands consideration of **bisphosphonates** and calcium to reduce the risk of osteoporosis. Early clinical intervention during an exacerbation may use the same strategy of high dose bronchodilator (e.g. salbutamol 100 mcg metered-dose inhaler, 6 puffs 3–4 hourly in a spacer), high dose oral steroids (prednisolone 40 mg daily in one dose for at least one week) and antibiotics (e.g. amoxicillin 500 mg three times daily for seven days). One of the difficult elements of COPD exacerbations for patients is that of tolerating breathlessness alone in the dark of night. A comprehensive service may offer telephone support to such patients whose COPD symptoms would ordinarily trigger a house call or ambulance, especially out of hours. Current organisation of out-of-hours and emergency services in the NHS means that it is difficult not to respond to the symptoms of an exacerbation of increasing breathlessness in COPD without automatically arranging a transfer to A&E, despite the fact that a telephone consultation with a clinician known to the patient may actually prevent the transfer simply through patient-specific reassurance.

Supported early discharge in COPD may take many forms. In essence, it is the discharge of patients home with nurse specialist and/or community support with the understanding that readmission can be arranged immediately should the patient need it. To be most effective, this service must be available at night. Follow-up at home on the following day may be provided as part of the package. The advantage of early discharge of a COPD exacerbation lies in the return of the patient to his or her own environment with the reduction in the physiological stress that an admission would have implied. Hospital admissions bring the risks of hospital-acquired infections, they can promote dependence in the patient and they set the pattern for future episodes. Bucking that trend may reduce the compounding effect of repeated exacerbations, promote self-reliance in acute episodes and lead to increasing confidence that acute exacerbations do not inevitably lead to hospital admission. The disadvantage of early discharge is largely the risk of readmission, worsening of the disease by poor control of exacerbations and undermining the confidence of the patient in self-management.

Hospital at home is treatment provided at home for patients whose conditions would normally require admission to hospital. The concept of hospital at home has been used for a wide range of conditions and current research is equivocal about its role (Shepperd & Iliffe 2005). Much optimism has been expressed about the possibility of treating people with acute exacerbations of severe COPD at home, rather than in hospital. The mainstay of hospital treatment of acute exacerbations of severe COPD consists of high dose bronchodilators delivered by nebulisation with continuous oxygen. Patients are usually nursed in bed and given oral antibiotics and high dose oral steroids. Some patients will require non-invasive ventilation (NIV), which is sometimes called NIPPV or 'NIPPY' (non-invasive positive pressure ventilation), and less frequently patients in respiratory failure will require mechanical ventilation with intubation. Hospital at home is unlikely to be suitable for most patients who are admitted to hospital (Ram et al. 2004). Factors that make hospital at home inappropriate include the need for ventilation, lack of continuous support at home, severe co-morbidity (e.g. chronic heart failure), unsuitable home environment, anxiety, and unwillingness of the patient to accept discharge to the hospital at home scheme. Hospital at home schemes vary in their designs. All offer higher levels of home care than is routinely available. Most offer the option of immediate transfer back to hospital at the request of the patient or of the attending staff. Initial continuous monitoring and nursing care for periods of 8 to 24 hours are usually followed by daily or more frequent home visits by specialist nursing staff.

The advantage of hospital at home care of COPD includes less disruption and more satisfactory care for the patient, with reduced hospital costs and an equally effective clinical outcome. The conclusion of Ram et al.'s (2004) systematic review of hospital at home for COPD was that hospital at home may be suitable for one in four patients presenting to hospital emergency departments with acute exacerbations of COPD who can be successfully and safely treated with support from respiratory nurses (Ram et al. 2004). There were no differences between hospital at home patients and hospital in-patients in terms of outcome, and hospital at home was preferred by patients and carers. Two years later a more general review was carried out by Shepperd and Iliffe which looked at hospital at home across a range of conditions (Shepperd & Iliffe 2005). They included 22 trials compared to the 7 trials assessed by Ram et al. (2004), of which 6 were trials examined by Ram et al. One of the drawbacks of the more recent review was the lack of uniform outcome measures between the studies included. Shepperd and Iliffe found no difference between hospital at home and hospital inpatient treatment in outcome or costs, and noted that the burden on carers can be greater in the hospital at home schemes.

No conclusion can be drawn at present from evidence of hospital at home studies of COPD, but the increasing experience in published studies and unpublished local hospital experiments has generated much new understanding about the care of acute exacerbations of COPD and the interventions that might reduce the need for admission, or reduce length of stay in patients who have been admitted.

Most exacerbations of COPD present first to primary care teams and in the early stages of the disease these are relatively simple to manage, have a short course, and respond well to antibiotics and high dose inhaled bronchodilators. As the disease progresses, the implications of the exacerbation become more serious both for the progression of the disease and for the immediate risk it may pose to the patient. At the same time the interplay of primary and secondary care becomes more important. Patients need to be well versed in self-management, knowing how and when to use antibiotics and oral steroids. The response to calls for help out of hours requires a more specific and tailored response than simply sending the patient to A&E. Patients who are seen at A&E may be discharged if the facilities for care at home are suitable and adequate support is available. Ultimately the capacity to treat patients at home who might otherwise be treated in hospital is a marker of a system in which the integration and confidence between primary and secondary care of COPD have been optimised.

END-OF-LIFE CARE

The palliative care of COPD is discussed in Chapter 11. From a community perspective the register of COPD patients may enable primary care teams to identify patients whose COPD management needs have become largely palliative. The palliative care of non-malignant disease is a new consideration for most clinical services. Its role in COPD is emphasised by the considerable unmet needs of COPD sufferers in the last year of life. It is virtually impossible to make an accurate prognosis for COPD at the end of life so clinicians have to be vigilant for patients whose symptoms are not controlled, or who want to talk about their future with respect to COPD, or for whom an admission to an acute hospital and the possibility of high-tech treatment generates dread. In the last year of life of people who died from COPD, only a third saw a specialist for check-ups and more than a third saw their GP less than three monthly or never (Elkington et al. 2005). People with advanced COPD are clearly at risk of being neglected between acute exacerbations of their disease.

REFERENCES

Bestall J C, Paul E A, Garrod R, Garnham R, Jones P W, Wedzicha J A (1999) Usefulness of the Medical Research Council (MRC) dyspnoea scale as a measure of disability in patients with chronic obstructive pulmonary disease. *Thorax* **54**(7): 581–586.

Boushey H, Enright P, Samet J (2005) Spirometry for chronic obstructive pulmonary disease case finding in primary care? *American Journal of Respiratory Critical Care Medicine* **172**(12): 1481–1482.

Damiani M, Dixon J (2004) *COPD Medical Admissions in the UK*. Newmarket: Hayward Medical Publications.

Elkington H, White P T, Addington-Hall J, Higgs R, Edmonds P (2005) The healthcare needs of chronic obstructive pulmonary disease patients in the last year of life. *Palliative Medicine* **19**(6): 485–491.

Gore J M, Brophy C J, Greenstone M A (2000) How well do we care for patients with end stage chronic obstructive pulmonary disease (COPD)? A comparison of palliative care and quality of life in COPD and lung cancer. *Thorax* **55**(12): 1000–1006.

Gorecka D, Bednarek M, Nowinski A, Puscinska E, Goljan-Geremek A, Zielinski J (2003) Diagnosis of airflow limitation combined with smoking cessation advice increases stop-smoking rate. *Chest* **123**(6): 1916–1923.

Hajiro T, Nishimura K, Tsukino M, Ikeda A, Oga T, Izumi T (1999) A comparison of the level of dyspnea vs disease severity in indicating the health-related quality of life of patients with COPD. *Chest* **116**(6): 1632–1637.

Halpin D (2004) NICE guidance for COPD. *Thorax* **59**(3): 181.

McCormick A F (1995) *Morbidity Statistics from General Practice. Fourth National Study: 1991–2*. London: Office of Population Censuses and Surveys.

National Institute for Clinical Excellence (2004) *Chronic Obstructive Pulmonary Disease. Management of Chronic Obstructive Pulmonary Disease in Adults in Primary and Secondary Care. Clinical Guideline 12*. London: National Institute for Clinical Excellence.

Pauwels R A, Buist A S, Calverley P M, Jenkins C R, Hurd S S (2001) Global strategy for the diagnosis, management, and prevention of chronic obstructive pulmonary disease. NHLBI/WHO Global Initiative for Chronic Obstructive Lung Disease (GOLD) Workshop summary. *American Journal of Respiratory Critical Care Medicine* **163**(5): 1256–1276.

Ram F S, Wedzicha J A, Wright J, Greenstone M (2004) Hospital at home for patients with acute exacerbations of chronic obstructive pulmonary disease: systematic review of evidence. *British Medical Journal* **329**(7461): 315.

Schermer T R, Jacobs J E, Chavannes N H, Hartman J, Folgering H T, Bottema B J, et al. (2003) Validity of spirometric testing in a general practice population of patients with chronic obstructive pulmonary disease (COPD). *Thorax* **58**(10): 861–866.

Shepperd S, Iliffe S (2005) Hospital at home versus in-patient hospital care. Cochrane Database Systematic Review (3): CD000356.

Soriano J B, Maier W C, Egger P, Visick G, Thakrar B, Sykes J, et al. (2000) Recent trends in physician diagnosed COPD in women and men in the UK. *Thorax* **55**(9): 789–794.

van Noord J A, Aumann J L, Janssens E, Smeets J J, Verhaert J, Disse B, et al. (2005) Comparison of tiotropium once daily, formoterol twice daily and both combined once daily in patients with COPD. *European Respiratory Journal* **26**(2): 214–222.

9 Management of Acute Exacerbations in Hospital

JACQUI FENTON
King's College Hospital, London

INTRODUCTION

The National Institute for Health and Clinical Excellence (NICE) is an independent organisation responsible for providing national guidance on the promotion of good health and the prevention and the treatment of ill health in the UK. In 2004 they issued a set of guidelines on the care and management that should be available from the NHS to patients with COPD (NICE 2004). These guidelines define a COPD exacerbation as 'a sustained worsening of the patient's symptoms from their usual stable state which is beyond normal day-to-day variations, and is acute in onset'.

Although there is no clear consensus on a definition of COPD, there is a clear set of symptoms, which will increase or worsen bringing the patient to the attention of health-care providers. These include:

- increasing dyspnoea;
- decreased exercise tolerance;
- increased sputum purulence;
- increased sputum volume;
- cough;
- wheeze/chest tightness.

AETIOLOGY

Exacerbations of COPD have been related to a number of aetiological factors including pollution and infection (Table 9.1). The most common precipitant to an exacerbation of COPD is an upper respiratory tract infection. The winter months bring with them an increased susceptibility to infection and hospital admission for COPD patients and it is at this time that educational initiatives could prevent the severity of exacerbations experienced by this patient group.

Managing Chronic Obstructive Pulmonary Disease. Edited by L. Blackler, C. Jones and C. Mooney
© 2007 John Wiley & Sons Ltd

Table 9.1. Causes of COPD exacerbations

Cause	Effect
Viruses	Rhinovirus (common cold)
	Influenza
	Parainfluenza
	Adenovirus
	RSV
	Chlamydia pneumoniae
Bacteria	Haemophilus influenzae
	Streptococcus pneumoniae
	Branamella catarrhalis
	Staphylococcus aureus
	Pseudomonas aeruginosa
Common pollutants	Nitrogen dioxide
	Particulates
	Sulphur dioxide
	Ozone

Source: Brewis (1991)

PATHOPHYSIOLOGY OF A COPD EXACERBATION

Relatively little information is available on pathological changes in the airways during an exacerbation of COPD. In patients with moderate and severe COPD, the performance of the respiratory muscles is reduced. The airflow obstruction experienced leads to hyperinflation, and a reduction in the function of the inspiratory muscles, this in turn creating reduced inspiratory pressure.

Hypoxia in COPD usually occurs due to a combination of ventilation/ perfusion mismatching and **hyperventilation**. This causes increases in pulmonary artery pressures, which can lead to water and salt retention and the development of oedema.

DIFFERENTIAL DIAGNOSIS

Due to the physical presentation of a patient during an exacerbation of COPD, i.e. dyspnoea, chest pain, cough, their symptoms may mask another underlying pathophysiology so a differential diagnosis should be considered in each patient:

- pneumonia
- pneumothorax
- left ventricular failure/pulmonary oedema
- pulmonary embolus
- lung cancer
- upper airways obstruction.

INVESTIGATIONS ON ADMISSION TO A&E

Investigations undertaken on admission to A&E can provide the clinician with a better indicator of the causative factor of the exacerbation and reinforce the treatment regimes decided.

CHEST RADIOGRAPH

A normal chest X-ray will show:

- rib cage
- diaphragm
- bony structures
- shape and size of heart
- lung fields and pleura
- soft tissue of the breast.

A chest X-ray in a mild to moderate COPD patient can be non-remarkable; as the COPD worsens, there is evidence of hyperinflation and flattened diaphragm. At the time of an exacerbation, radiography may be useful in identifying areas of infection, or if a pneumothorax is present.

ARTERIAL BLOOD GAS TENSIONS (ABGs)

Blood gas analysis is performed to evaluate the adequacy of ventilation, oxygenation, the oxygen-carrying capacity of the blood and acid-base levels. It will identify the following issues:

- the presence and severity of hypoxaemia and hyper/hypocapnia and the amount of **metabolic compensation**;
- changes in **acid–base homeostasis**, which might need further investigation and intervention.

Arterial blood gases should be repeated regularly to ascertain the patient's response to treatment. If there has been an increase in the amount of supplemental oxygen the patient is receiving, it is advisable to wait at least 30 minutes before taking another ABG (Table 9.2).

TYPE II RESPIRATORY FAILURE

In some individuals, an exacerbation of COPD may lead them to experience type II respiratory failure; this is caused by reduced ventilatory drive and the inability to 'blow off' their carbon dioxide. The features of type II respiratory failure (Table 9.3) are:

Table 9.2. Diagnostic inference

	Normal	Increased values	Decreased values
PaO_2	12–14 kPa	–	hypoxia
$PaCO_2$	4.6–6.0 kPa	respiratory acidosis (if pH decreased)	respiratory alkalosis (if pH increased)
pH	7.35–7.45	alkalosis hyperventilation	acidosis CO_2 retention
HCO_3	22–26 mmol/L	metabolic alkalosis	metabolic acidosis
Base excess	−2 to +2	metabolic alkalosis	metabolic acidosis

Source: Brewis (1991)

Table 9.3. Definition of type I and type II respiratory failure

ABG results	Normal	Type I	Type II
pH	7.35–7.45	7.35–7.45	7.35–7.45 or <7.35
PaO_2	12–14 kPa	<8 kPa	<8 kPa
$PaCO_2$	4.6–6 kPa	4.6–6 kPa	>6 kPa
SaO_2	95% +	<92%	<92%

Source: Esmond (2001)

- ventilatory failure
- PaO_2 low/**$PaCO_2$** high (>7 kPa)
- the patient is hypoxic and hypercapnic.

ECG

An ECG should be recorded to exclude any co-morbidities or acute cardiac events.

BLOOD TESTS

According to NICE (2004), all patients experiencing an exacerbation of their COPD should have a full blood count, electrolytes and urea concentrations should be measured (Table 9.4). The elevation of blood urea will be suggestive of dehydration or renal failure that can be associated with cardiac failure. A blood test can help detect:

- infection
- inflammatory markers
- polycythaemia.

If the patient is pyrexial, a set of blood cultures should be sent.

Table 9.4. Results of tests performed after COPD exacerbation

Cell type/test performed	Normal values	Increased values	Decreased values
White blood cell	4–11×10^9/L	Bacterial infections Malignancy	Viral infections Overwhelming bacterial infection
Neutrophil	2.5–7.5×10^9/L	Bacterial infections Malignancy	Viral infections Overwhelming bacterial infection
Eosinophil	0.04–0.44×10^9/L	Pneumonia Allergic reactions	Steroid therapy
Monocyte	0.2–0.8×10^9/L		Chronic infection
Lymphocyte	1.5–4.0×10^9/L	Infection TB	TB
C-reactive protein	<4 mg/L	Acute infection – inflammation	
Urea	2.5–6.7 mmol/L	>7 mmol/L indicates a poor prognosis in pneumonia	
Potassium	3.5–5.00 mmol/L		B-agonists
ACE	10–70 U/L	Sarcoidosis	
Calcium	2.12–2.65 mmol/L	Malignancy	
Glucose	3.5–5.5 mmol/L	Long-term steroid use	

Source: Jefferies and Turley (1999)

SPUTUM SAMPLE

Sputum can be a problem for many patients with COPD. A British study of COPD exacerbations in primary care has demonstrated that green (purulent) sputum is a good indicator of a high bacterial load and that patients with lack of purulence will improve without antibiotic therapy (Stockley et al. 2000). It is recommended that the health-care practitioner does the following:

- Look at the colour, consistency and quantity of the sputum.
- Where sputum purulence is present and antibiotic treatment is intended, obtain a sputum culture.

If overnight analysis is not available, proceed with a broad spectrum antibiotic until you have the results, if appropriate (SIGN 2005).

THEOPHYLLINE LEVEL

On presentation, a patient being pharmacologically managed on theophylline should have a blood level done to check if they are within the therapeutic range (10–20 mg/L). Medication, diet and underlying diseases can alter the theophylline narrow therapeutic window.

DECISION TO ADMIT

The NICE Guidelines list the factors to be taken into account when deciding whether a patient should be admitted or discharged. The algorithm in Table 9.5 allows a clinician to make an informed decision in regard to the management of the patient. This algorithm should be used alongside a good clinical assessment of the patient and not as a 'stand-alone tool'.

Over the last few years, models of community management have arisen for patients with COPD. COPD accounted for more than 100,000 hospital admissions in England in 2000/2001, the most common cause of admission to hospital with a respiratory illness (Britton 2003). The financial burden this places on the NHS is huge and with a predicted increase in prevalence over the next ten years or so, other means of management must be explored as a matter of urgency.

An increase in Acute Respiratory Assessment Services (ARAS) or supported discharge schemes have been seen as a must in many acute care settings as a means of providing appropriate assessment and treatment for patients with COPD in their homes. Two studies have explored the effectiveness of such a service, both Cotton and colleagues in 2000 and Skwarska and colleagues in 2000. Both undertook randomised controlled trials comparing the difference between conventional hospital management and supported

Table 9.5. Algorithm to decide management of the patient

Factor	Treat at home	Treat in hospital
Able to cope at home	Yes	No
Breathlessness	Mild	Severe
General condition	Good	Poor/deteriorating
Level of activity	Good	Poor/confined to bed
Cyanosis	No	Yes
Worsening of peripheral oedema	No	Yes
Level of consciousness	Normal	Impaired
Already receiving LTOT	No	Yes
Social circumstances	Good	Living alone/not coping
Acute confusion	No	Yes
Rapid rate of onset	No	Yes
Significant co-morbidity (particularly cardiac disease and insulin-dependent diabetes)	No	Yes
$SaO_2 < 90\%$	No	Yes
Changes on chest radiograph	No	Present
Arterial pH level	>7.35	<7.35
Arterial PaO_2	>7 kPa	<7 kPa

Source: NICE (2004)

discharge at home. Their results mirrored each other in that there was a reduction in mean hospital length of stay, there were no differences in readmission rates or any increases in visits to primary care physicians by the group managed at home. There was also a significant cost saving found between the two groups.

INDICATIONS FOR ITU ADMISSION

In some cases, in an exacerbation of COPD there may be the development of severe hypoxaemia. In order to deliver a sufficient amount of oxygen, intubation and mechanical ventilation may be necessary.

The utilisation of mechanical ventilation in patients with obstructive lung disease is not without its risks. Of patients admitted to ITU, between 4 and 58 per cent will require mechanical ventilation and of these there will be a mortality rate of between 6–30 per cent (Seneff et al. 1995). Complications of mechanical ventilation (GOLD 2005) include **barotrauma**, infection and effects on cardiac output. These complications can lead to:

- severe dyspnoea that responds inadequately to initial emergency therapy;
- confusion, lethargy, coma;
- persistent or worsening hypoxaemic ($PaO_2 < 5.3\,kPa$) and/or severe/worsening hypercapnia ($PaCO_{2^-} > 8\,kPa$) and/or a severe worsening **respiratory acidosis** (Ph < 7.25) despite supplemental oxygen and NIPPV (GOLD 2005).

MANAGEMENT OF AN ACUTE EXACERBATION IN HOSPITAL

OXYGEN THERAPY

The role of oxygen therapy is to treat hypoxia. Oxygen should be given to patients with COPD to maintain their saturations above 90 per cent. The NICE Guidelines (2004) point out that it is not desirable for the oxygen saturations of this patient group to go over 93 per cent. In most people, respiratory drive is largely initiated by PCO_2 but in COPD hypoxia can be a strong driving force and so if there is an excess of supplemental oxygen, the respiratory drive reduces with a build-up of carbon dioxide and acidosis. Patients who develop hypercapnia or acidosis should be considered for non-invasive ventilation. Titration of oxygen in the presence of type II respiratory failure must be made in response to arterial blood gas results (Bateman and Leach 1998).

OXYGEN DELIVERY

Due to the risks associated with the over-use of supplemental oxygen in an exacerbation of COPD, it is important to give controlled oxygen at all times. This is done: (1) by ensuring the oxygen is always prescribed; (2) by monitoring its effects; and (3) by delivering it in an appropriate device.

The device that is chosen to administer oxygen to the patient can greatly influence the amount that they receive. In COPD, accuracy is the key. The following oxygen delivery devices are safe for use in patients experiencing an exacerbation of COPD.

Nasal cannulae

Nasal cannulae are shown in Figure 9.1, and have advantages and disadvantages:

- Suitable for patients in type I and type II respiratory failure.
- Deliver low O_2 concentration between 24 and 35 per cent.
- Comfortable and easily tolerated, patient able to eat, drink and communicate.
- No re-breathing.
- Low cost product.
- Not suitable for patients with nasal obstructions
- Remember: 2 l/min, via nasal cannulae, may deliver up to 40 per cent O_2 in some people, therefore monitoring is important.

VENTURI MASK SYSTEM

The Venturi mask system is shown in Figure 9.2:

- Ideal for patients with type II respiratory failure.
- Venturi jets can be changed to deliver fixed oxygen concentrations (24–28–31–35–40–60 per cent).

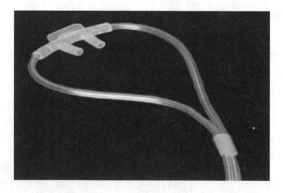

Figure 9.1. Nasal cannulae

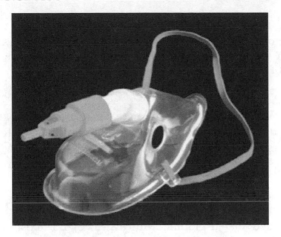

Figure 9.2. The Venturi mask system

- Delivers prescribed O_2 concentrations irrespective of respiratory pattern.
- Guidance for flow written on all devices.
- No re-breathing.
- But can be noisy, claustrophobic and interferes with eating and drinking.

HUMIDIFIED OXYGEN SYSTEM

- Most systems provide controlled oxygen therapy at levels of 28, 35, 40 and 60 per cent.
- Not suitable for 24 per cent oxygen.
- Guidance provided on flow rates.

BRONCHODILATORS

Inhaled beta$_2$ agonists should be administered as soon as possible in an acute exacerbation of COPD to provide relief to the patient. The delivery of the drug is dependent on the severity of the exacerbation but the clinician must ensure the patient is able to use or manage the delivery system. This is especially important in clinical areas utilising spacer devices and pressurised metered dose inhalers. Nebulised therapy is the therapy of choice in secondary care when treating a COPD exacerbation. Nebulised therapy is discussed in Section 3.3. Inhaled anticholinergics (e.g. ipratropium) have been shown to have the same or greater bronchodilation properties as salbutamol for patients with COPD (GOLD 2005). They are generally used in conjunction with beta$_2$ agonists in the emergency setting.

SYSTEMIC CORTICOSTEROIDS

In the absence of significant contraindications, oral corticosteroids should be used, in conjunction with other therapies, in all patients admitted to hospital with an exacerbation of COPD.

(NICE 2004)

The dose of prednisolone to be administered in an exacerbation should be 30 mg for 7–14 days only. Therapy should be discontinued at fourteen days as there is no benefit from continuing the therapy (NICE 2004).

WITHDRAWAL OF CORTICOSTEROIDS

It is recommended that a gradual withdrawal of corticosteroids should be considered in those whose disease is unlikely to relapse and who fulfil the following conditions:

- have recently received repeated courses (particularly if taken for longer than three weeks);
- have received more than three weeks' treatment;
- have taken a short course within 1 year of stopping long-term therapy;
- have other possible causes of adrenal suppression;
- have received more than 40 mg daily prednisolone (or equivalent);
- have been given repeat doses in the evening (BNF 2006).

Systemic corticosteroids may be stopped abruptly in those whose disease is unlikely to relapse *and* who have received treatment for 3 weeks or less *and* who are not included in the patient groups described above (BNF 2006).

Glucocorticoid side effects include osteoporosis which is a danger, particularly in the elderly and diabetes. Mental disturbances may occur; a serious paranoid state or depression with risk of suicide may be induced, particularly in patients with a history of mental disorder. Euphoria is frequently observed. Muscle wasting (proximal myopathy) may also occur. High doses of corticosteroids may cause **Cushing's syndrome**, with moon face, striae, and acne; it is usually reversible on withdrawal of treatment.

As a guide, long-term treatment, that is more than three months in duration with doses of more than 7.5 mg of prednisolone per day (or equivalent doses of hydrocortisone 2 mg per day or dexamethasone 50 mg per day), increases the risk of osteoporosis. In addition, if other risk factors for osteoporosis, such as being postmenopausal, are present, then the effects of corticosteroid medication on the bones can be severe (RCP 2002). Osteoporosis prophylaxis therapy should be considered in patients requiring frequent prednisolone courses (NICE 2004).

INHALED CORTICOSTEROIDS

All patients admitted to hospital with an exacerbation of COPD should have oral corticosteroids. This is the same for patients in the community who are experiencing debilitating shortness of breath that is preventing them from undertaking their usual daily activities. Patients should be placed back on their regular inhaled corticosteroid as soon as possible in order to ensure they have adequate levels of their 'preventer' medication in their system when they stop the oral corticosteroids. Failure to do so could lead to increased airway inflammation and relapse.

THEOPHYLLINES AND METHYLXANTHINES

The use of methylxanthines and theophyllines in acute COPD exacerbations is rather contentious. Although they have been shown to be of some help in diaphragmatic function, there is little evidence to support their use, and they also have a narrow therapeutic and toxic range and, as such, serious side effects are a risk (BNF 2006).

IV aminophylline in the treatment of COPD continues to be used when the patient is not responding to other bronchodilators. The dose of IV aminophylline is a calculation involving the patient's weight. Correct calculation is imperative due to the risk of side effects and a therapeutic range of 10–20 mg per ml is required for the drug to be beneficial. Box 9.1 presents information on aminophylline.

Box 9.1. Aminophylline information

Drug name:	Theophylline/Aminophylline
Laboratory:	Clinical Biochemistry
Sample Requirements:	2 mL clotted blood
Sampling Time:	Oral therapy: Pre-dose or 4–6 hours after dose if giving slow release preparation
	IV therapy: Before treatment if patient has history of theophylline ingestion, preferably at 6 hours and 18 hours
Therapeutic Range:	10–20 mg/L
Half Life:	6–12 hours
Time to Steady State:	2 days

Note: Half life is decreased in smokers, chronic alcoholism. Aminophylline is metabolised to theophylline. Serum drug levels may be used to forewarn of impending serious toxicity.

The following medicines may increase blood levels of aminophylline: aciclovir, allopurinol, calcium channel blockers, nifedipine, methotrexate, isoniazid, flu vaccine, quinoline-type antibiotics, macrolide-type antibiotics, oral contraceptives, propranolol.

The following medications may decrease the blood levels of aminophylline: barbiturates, St John's Wort, anti-epileptic medicines, rifampicin.

DOSING

Patients not previously treated with theophylline/aminophylline will require a loading dose which is by slow intravenous infusion over 20 minutes (with close monitoring), 250–500 mg (5 mg/kg). For patients previously on oral theophylline/aminophylline or after the loading dose: 500 mcg/kg/hour, adjusted according to plasma concentrations. To avoid excessive dosage in obese patients, dose should be calculated on the basis of ideal weight for height (BNF 2006).

ANTIBIOTICS

According to NICE Guidelines (2004), antibiotics should be used when the patient presenting with an exacerbation of COPD has a history of increased purulent sputum. With this, those patients presenting with an exacerbation who have not got an increased level of purulent sputum should only be started on antibiotics if there is consolidation on the chest X-ray or there are clinical signs of pneumonia. For guidance on the antibiotic of choice, prescribers should take guidance from their local microbiologists.

RESPIRATORY STIMULANTS

Doxapram hydrochloride is the only respiratory stimulant to be recommended by the NICE (2004) COPD Guidelines. It is only recommended when non-invasive ventilation is contra-indicated or not being tolerated by the patient. Doxapram is a stimulant of the central nervous system (analeptic agent). It can be administered to patients in acute hypercapnic type II respiratory failure where intubation or ventilation is deemed unsuitable. Doxapram is given intravenously and causes an increase in respiratory and tidal volume. This in turn increases the minute volume with an associated fall in $PaCO_2$ and a rise in PaO_2. It is not a stand-alone therapy and should be used in conjunction with nebulised bronchodilators, controlled oxygen therapy, physiotherapy and anti-biotics as required. Side effects of doxapram include agitation and confusion; also, the patient can become less drowsy and more aware of their condition, causing anxiety which may exacerbate the dyspnoea.

CARE OF THE PATIENT ON A WARD WITH AN EXACERBATION OF COPD

The following issues are important during an exacerbation of COPD:

- *Positioning* – The positioning of a patient experiencing difficulty in breathing is vital to reduce the work of breathing and increase patient comfort. High sitting with pillow support allows better diaphragmatic movement and better depth of breathing. If in doubt, liaise with your physiotherapy service for advice.
- *Chest clearance/Physiotherapy* – Due to the very nature of COPD, patients can have retained purulent sputum, which is often very distressing to them. Always ensure the patient has a receptacle to expectorate into: often patients find this embarrassing so the provision of tissues is essential. Hydration is important to the viscosity of the sputum; patients will find it difficult to expectorate if dehydrated. For further advice on sputum clearance, speak to your physiotherapy service.
- *Nutrition* – Increased respiratory rate, infection, etc. in COPD can all contribute to an increased amount of energy being expended. Meals for patients with COPD should be small, frequent and high in energy-giving properties. Counsel your patient on their diet when at home in order to maintain their well-being.
- *Hydration* – Inconsequential loss from mouth breathing, sweating, etc. can lead to COPD patients becoming dehydrated. Ensure your patient is drinking adequately and blood results are reviewed daily to ensure the renal function is adequate. Hydration is also important in allowing the patient to expectorate effectively.
- *Energy conservation* – Nearly all patients with COPD want to stay as independent as possible but they often find the smallest tasks are very tiring such as maintaining their own hygiene. When managing a patient during an exacerbation, place all necessary implements, clothing, etc. within reach, and actively adapt any strenuous activity or action that will increase the patient's shortness of breath.
- *Mobilisation* – Mobilisation should be encouraged as soon as the patient's condition allows. The complications of immobility include DVT, PE and pneumonia. The patient may lack confidence and need encouragement. They should be encouraged to mobilise at their own pace regardless of how long it may take. Reassurance is key to the confidence of the patient.
- *Anxiety* – Shortness of breath is a very frightening symptom of COPD. Anxiety is a common 'side effect' of difficulty in breathing and many patients exacerbate their perception of breathing difficulties by becoming tense and scared. Anxiety is not a symptom to be dismissed, as the patient is unable to control it without support and sometimes pharmacological management. The first line of management is to reassure your patient when undertaking

an activity or feeling tense. The physiotherapy service is often able to assist in breathing control and breathing techniques to reduce anxiety. If all else fails, the patient may be prescribed anti-anxiolytics such as diazepam. These medications need to be used with great care as they may reduce respiratory drive and make the patient more unwell.

- *Discharge planning* – Discharge planning should commence as soon as the patient is admitted to ensure a thorough and safe service. There are many reasons why patients with COPD are admitted to hospital, primarily infection, but often there are social circumstances and family difficulties that give rise to increased levels of shortness of breath and admission to hospital. A concise history will allow you to establish the cause of admission and ascertain if there is anything that can be done to decrease the risk of future admissions. Social isolation is a large precursor to hospital admission: linking your patient to social groups such as Breathe-Easy or day centres may be of benefit to the future health of your patients.

CONCLUSION

The acute management of COPD involves a varied and skilled mix of health professionals who work side by side to ensure the best possible patient management. The journey from A&E to home is often a traumatic and frightening experience for the patient and as such every opportunity should be taken to allay any fears or concerns the patient has. The extended journey around the total management is mind-boggling when put into the context of time, cost and burden on the NHS. One true feature of a COPD exacerbation is that the patient often has forewarning of it by worsening symptoms over the space of a few days or so. One key element to patient management is to encourage earlier presentation, and earlier utilisation of prednisolone and antibiotics in order to stave off an exacerbation requiring hospitalisation. There is very much an ethos with the older population of COPD sufferers that they try to cope alone and 'not bother' their doctor; this is a mentality we need to address if we are to manage COPD appropriately in the future.

End-stage COPD and prognosis are a difficult topic for any physician or health-care provider to address (Table 9.6). Historically patient knowledge about their condition has dictated that many patients were not aware that they had a terminal disease process. Today we have many more resources targeted at educating our COPD patients and empowering them to make decisions re their own care. Hospice beds have now become more freely available to patients with chronic respiratory problems, and specialist palliative staff are more geared up to address symptom control and patient comfort.

End-of-life decision-making is never an easy concept for any human being to address. Decisions should always be made jointly with the patient, relatives and health-care staff. These decisions can take two forms:

Table 9.6. Factors influencing survival in patients with COPD

Risk factor	Effect on survival
Rate of FEV_1 decline	Decreases mortality with slower decline: $FEV_1 < 1\,L$ generally considered severe disease.
History of atrophy	Decreases mortality with slower decline
Higher diffusion capacity	Decreases mortality with slower decline
	Decreases mortality with increased level
PaO_2 level	$PaO_2 < 55\,mmHg$
	Increases mortality
Age	Increases mortality in older patients
Cigarette smoking	Increases mortality with continued use and greater consumption
Hypercapnia ($PaCO_2 > 45\,mmHg$)	Increases mortality
Right-sided heart failure	Increases mortality
Malnutrition	Increases mortality
Resting tachycardia	Increases mortality

FEV_1 – forced expiratory volume in one second; PaO_2 – partial pressure of arterial oxygen; $PaCO_2$ – partial pressure of carbon dioxide

1 Each patient, following discussion, should have a resuscitation form completed and its contents communicated to all health-care providers involved in the care of that patient. Legally speaking, the resuscitation status of the patient is a medical decision and the doctor's decision overrides that of the patient and relative. This can create a difficult situation for all parties involved, and every step should be taken to obtain a consensus on the decision.

2 In an age where patients are far more aware of their rights in regard to the health care they are entitled to, and information is more freely on hand than ever before with the advent of the internet, advanced directives are more and more frequently seen. There is no legislation in England and Wales governing advanced directives but they are frequently recognised by case law. Advanced directives are a general statement of wishes and views. They allow patients to state their preferences and indicate what forms of medical treatment they would or would not like to receive in the future if they became unable to communicate them directly. It is worth bearing in mind that we are now empowering our COPD patients, we are arming them with knowledge and skills in regard to the management of their disease and as such we should actively promote the use of advanced directives so we are able to support their wishes throughout the whole of the patient journey.

REFERENCES

Bateman N, Leach L (1998) ABC of oxygen: Acute oxygen therapy. *BMJ* **317**(7161): 798–801.
BNF (2006) British National Formulary No. 51 – March 2006 edition.
Brewis R A L (1991) *Lecture Notes on Respiratory Disease* (4th edn). London: Blackwell.
Britton M (2003) The burden of COPD in the UK: results from the confronting COPD survey. *Respiratory Medicine* 571–579.
Cotton M M, et al. (2000) Early discharge for patients with exacerbations of COPD: a randomised trial. *Thorax* **55**: 902–906.
Esmond G (2001) *Respiratory Nursing*. Edinburgh: Baillière Tindall.
GOLD (2005) www.goldcopd.org (accessed 13 April 2007).
Jefferies A, Turley A (1999) *Mosby's Crash Course Respiratory System*. London: Mosby.
NICE (2004) *Chronic Obstructive Pulmonary Disease: Management of Chronic Obstructive Pulmonary Disease in Adults in Primary and Secondary Care*. London: DOH.
Royal College of Physicians (2002) Bone and Tooth Society, National Osteoporosis Society, Royal College of Physicians. *Glucocorticoid-induced Osteoporosis: Guidelines for Prevention and Treatment*. London: Royal College of Physicans.
Seneff M G, et al. (1995) Hospital and one year survival of patients admitted to ICU with exacerbations of COPD. *JAMA* **274**: 1852–1857.
SIGN (2005) *Scottish Intercollegiate Guidelines on the Management of COPD*. Available at: www.sign.ac.uk (accessed 13 April 2007).
Skwarska E, et al. (2000) A randomised controlled trial of supported discharge in patients with exacerbations of COPD. *Thorax* **55**: 907–912.
Stockley R A, et al. (2000) Relationship of sputum colour to nature and out-patient management of acute exacerbations of COPD. *Chest* **117**: 1638–1645.

10 Non-Invasive Ventilation

TRACEY MATHIESON
King's College Hospital, London

Standard medical therapy (as described in Chapter 9) may not always be successful in reversing an acute hypercapnic exacerbation of COPD. In such situations, ventilatory support may be required and the use of non-invasive ventilation (NIV) should be considered. This chapter will discuss the role of NIV in the management of acute hypercapnic COPD, including national and international recommendations, and evidence for the use of NIV in COPD. The practicalities of NIV delivery will also be addressed.

WHAT IS NIV?

Non-invasive ventilation (NIV) is a method of providing respiratory support that does not require the placement of an endotracheal tube (NICE 2004). NIV is an all-encompassing term which includes both **positive pressure** ventilation, where air is pushed into the patient's lungs through the patient's upper airway using a mask or similar device (BTS Guidelines 2002), and negative pressure ventilation (e.g. iron lungs) which is applied externally to the chest wall. The term NIV may also be used to refer to **continuous positive airway pressure (CPAP)**, although technically CPAP does not ventilate (i.e. increase tidal volume), but provides respiratory support by increasing the functional residual capacity (FRC).

Non-invasive positive pressure ventilation (NIPPV) has developed as a treatment for acute hypercapnic COPD over the past 20 years or so, and rapidly in the past 12–15 years. Numerous ventilators are now available and range from ITU ventilators with an NIPPV mode to portable units suitable for home use. The sheer range of ventilators available (e.g. NIPPY, Breas, Harmony, Synchrony, Bi-PAP) can make terminology confusing. In essence, two types of ventilators are used: volume-cycled ventilators and **pressure-cycled ventilators**.

The BTS recommends bi-level pressure-cycled ventilators for COPD patients as the majority of randomised controlled trials of NIV (especially the most recent) have used this type of ventilator (BTS 2002). These ventilators

Managing Chronic Obstructive Pulmonary Disease. Edited by L. Blackler, C. Jones and C. Mooney
© 2007 John Wiley & Sons Ltd

deliver a variable volume of air to the patient to achieve a pre-set pressure and are able to compensate for mask leaks. Breaths are delivered when 'triggered' by the patient. Many machines are now very sensitive to the patient's ventilatory pattern and demands and this provides a greater degree of comfort for the patient. A back-up rate can be set so that a mandatory number of breaths per minute can be delivered should the patient fail to trigger the machine; however, NIV should not be used to provide life support.

HOW DOES NIV WORK?

During an exacerbation of COPD the inflammatory process in the airways further impairs the respiratory mechanics as well as further challenging the gas exchange process (see Chapter 1 on pathophysiology). Patients with severe disease may no longer be able to maintain effective ventilation as they are working at the top end of hyperinflation, and respiratory acidosis develops as a result of alveolar hypoventilation. Acidosis itself may further reduce the function of the respiratory muscle pump and a vicious cycle of worsening acidosis causing further impairment of respiratory muscle function develops (Elliott 2005).

Delivery of NIV allows the patient to take deeper breaths with less effort (Brochard 2003). Bi-level pressure-cycled ventilators deliver two levels of positive pressure to the patient via a mask or similar interface; a higher level during inspiration compared to a lower level during expiration (Figure 10.1).

IPAP (inspiratory positive airway pressure) is delivered as the patient begins to breathe in and is comparable to pressure support on a conventional ITU ventilator. This increases tidal volume and facilitates the removal of carbon dioxide from the lungs, thus reversing the acidosis.

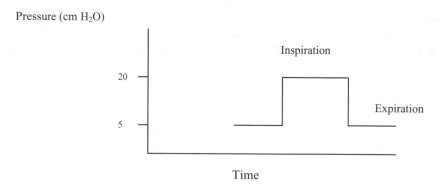

Figure 10.1. Pressure profiles of bi-level pressure support ventilation

EPAP (expiratory positive airway pressure) or PEEP (positive end expiratory pressure) at a low level (4–6 cm H_2O) is thought to assist lung deflation by preventing airway collapse as the patient breathes out. This increases the expiratory time, allowing for the emptying of lung units. This lowers the patient's end expiratory volume (i.e. the effects of intrinsic PEEP and dynamic hyperinflation are counterbalanced). With less air in the lungs at the end of expiration, the diaphragm returns to a more effective position at which to generate power for the next breath.

Together, the two levels of ventilation work optimally to reduce the patient's work of breathing, allowing the breathing pattern to normalise and alveolar hypoventilation to be reversed.

WHY USE NIV?

NIV as a treatment option for acute hypercapnic COPD has been extensively researched. The recent NICE Guidelines (2004) report the findings of randomised controlled trials and meta-analysis reviews that show that NIV, when compared to usual medical care, can reduce:

- mortality;
- the need for endotracheal intubation;
- in turn, this reduces associated complication rates (especially ventilator associated pneumonia);
- length of stay.

Such is the strength of evidence for NIV in acute COPD that several consensus documents and guidelines have advocated its use:

> Non-invasive ventilation has been shown to be an effective treatment for acute hypercapnic respiratory failure, particularly in COPD. Facilities for NIV should be available 24 hrs per day in all hospitals likely to admit such patients.
>
> (BTS Guidelines 2002)

Non-invasive ventilation (NIV) should be used as the treatment of choice for persistent hypercapnic ventilatory failure during exacerbations of COPD not responding to medical therapy (NICE 2004). There is extensive evidence that NIPPV increases pH, reduces $PaCO_2$, reduces the severity of breathlessness in the first 4 hours of treatment, and decreases the length of hospital stay (Global Initiative for Chronic Obstructive Lung Disease, updated 2005). Additional benefits of NIPPV, compared to intubation and mechanical ventilation, are that patients may be able to eat, drink and communicate, and participate with physiotherapy, especially if they are able to tolerate short periods off the ventilator.

Indications for NIV are acute hypercapnic respiratory failure (pH < 7.35 and $PaCO_2$ > 6.0 kPa) not responding to medical therapy.

GOALS OF NIV

The BTS Guidelines (2002) identify three situations in which NIV may be beneficial:

1 As a holding measure to assist ventilation at an earlier stage than that at which tracheal intubation would be considered.
2 As a trial with a view to intubation if NIV fails.
3 As a ceiling of treatment in patients who are not candidates for intubation.

EARLY USE OF NIV

Results from RCTs and their subsequent meta-analysis suggest that instituting NIV at an earlier stage of respiratory failure may improve outcome (Light-owler et al. 2003). Plant et al. (2000a) conducted a prospective multicentre randomised controlled study to compare NIV with standard therapy in patients with mild to moderate acidosis (mean pH 7.32). They found that NIV reduced the need for intubation, reduced in-hospital mortality and led to more rapid improvement of physiological variables such as pH and respiratory rate.

TRIAL OF NIV

Using NIV as a trial provides an opportunity to avoid endotracheal intubation and its risk of associated complications. Clinicians have raised concerns that delaying intubation by using NIV inappropriately may have serious conse-quences for the patient. A recent study by Squadrone et al. (2004) found that NIV had a high failure rate in patients with advanced hypercapnic acute respi-ratory failure (40/64 patients required intubation). Importantly, however, sub-group analysis suggested that the delay in intubation was not deleterious in the patients who failed NIV, and patients who avoided intubation had fewer complications. Careful monitoring of patients undergoing a trial of NIV is clearly advisable, with a low threshold for intubation if the trial fails.

Ideally, clinicians would be able to identify those patients in whom NIV is unlikely to be of benefit. This would allow appropriate management to be initi-ated at the earliest opportunity, whether that is intubation and mechanical ventilation, continuation of medical management, or palliative care.

A recent prospective study of 1,033 consecutive patients affected by COPD and respiratory acidosis identified risk factors associated with failure of NIV (Confalonieri et al. 2005). Patients presenting with the following variables had a risk of failure of >70 per cent:

- Glasgow Coma Score < 11;
- acute physiology and chronic health evaluation (APACHE) II ≥ 29;
- respiratory rate ≥ 30;
- pH < 7.25.

A pH of <7.25 after two hours of NIV greatly increased the risk of failure (>90 per cent). The authors developed a risk failure chart as a tool to assist clinical decision-making in identifying patients who are unlikely to benefit from NIV. Analysis of this chart showed good sensitivity and specificity and the authors suggest that it could be used as an aid to clinical decision-making.

An additional benefit of using NIV as a trial is that it may also 'buy time' for collecting valuable information regarding the patient's pre-morbid status, co-morbidities and importantly, patients' and relatives' wishes regarding invasive treatment. This will facilitate clinical decision-making should non-invasive ventilation fail to reverse the deterioration in the patient's respiratory status or the patient does not tolerate NIV.

CEILING OF TREATMENT

There will be a group of patients in whom endotracheal intubation and mechanical ventilation are not appropriate and for whom NIV would be considered the ceiling of treatment. A study by Benhamou et al. (1992) suggested that NIV could be a possible alternative in the treatment of acute respiratory failure in elderly patients who were not considered suitable candidates for invasive ventilation. More recently, a study by Levy et al. (2004) found that just over 50 per cent of patients with COPD and do not intubate orders, treated with NIV, survived to hospital discharge. NIV may also have a role in palliation to reduce breathlessness (Meduri et al. 1994) if the patient finds its use beneficial.

CONTRA-INDICATIONS TO NIV

The BTS Guidelines (2002) suggest that the only absolute contra-indications to NIV are fixed airway obstruction, facial trauma and vomiting. Several other contra-indications have been suggested but may be attributable to exclusion criteria for controlled trials (BTS 2002). Clinical judgement should be applied in all cases as to whether or not NIV is contra-indicated and whether or not NIV is to be the 'ceiling' of treatment. Table 10.1 shows areas where caution is required.

WHERE SHOULD NIV BE USED?

NIV for acute hypercapnic respiratory failure has been successfully used in a variety of settings, i.e. A&E, ICUs, HDUs and general wards (Bott et al. 1993; Brochard et al. 1995; Wood et al. 1998; Plant et al. 2000a). There have been no studies comparing the efficiency of NIV between ICU, HDU, general wards and respiratory wards (BTS Guidelines 2002; Elliott 2002).

Table 10.1. Considerations of clinical judgement

Relative contra-indication	Considerations
Imminent cardio-respiratory arrest/life-threatening hypoxaemia	Intubation should not be delayed if considered appropriate as NIV takes time to set up
	The presence of advance directives or 'do not resuscitate orders' may allow for a trial of NIV
Inability to protect airway	Increased risk of chest infections secondary to aspiration of saliva
Undrained pneumothorax	Use of positive pressure may increase size of pneumothorax. Should be drained wherever possible
Copious respiratory secretions	Consider chest physiotherapy first as use of NIV may dry out secretions and prevent expectoration
	Physiotherapists may use NIV as an adjunct to airway clearance techniques
Haemodynamic instability	Cardiac output may fall as positive pressure applied but rare
Severe co-morbidity	May not be appropriate to use NIV
Impaired consciousness	Unless secondary to CO_2 narcosis
Confusion/agitation	Patient may not tolerate wearing a tight-fitting mask
Bowel obstruction	Distended abdomen may splint the diaphragm and should be investigated/treated prior to starting NIV – air may be forced into the stomach causing further distension
Focal consolidation on CXR	

The BTS guidelines (2002) state:

The clinical area in which a patient is treated with NIV will be influenced by several factors including their clinical state, whether they will be intubated if NIV fails, and the availability of beds. Taking into account the overall clinical picture, patients with more severe acidosis (pH < 7.30) should be managed in a higher dependency area such as an ICU or HDU, as should those in whom improvement in clinical state and arterial blood gas tensions is not seen after 1–2 hours of NIV on a respiratory ward.

The location chosen to deliver NIV will vary from hospital to hospital. Using NIV outside of the ICU is an attractive option in terms of demands on ICU beds and cost (Elliott 2005).

The NICE Guidelines (2004) recommend that: 'NIV should be delivered in a dedicated setting with staff who have trained in its application, who are experienced in its use and are aware of its limitations.' With those recommendations in mind, the following should be considered:

- *A&E* – A significant proportion of patients (in a one-year prevalence study, 20 per cent) presenting with acute respiratory failure will correct their acidosis with standard medical therapy alone, and, importantly, controlled oxygen therapy (Plant et al. 2000b). Patients may also present requiring immediate intubation and ventilation and this should not be delayed. However, this may not be considered an appropriate intervention for some patients and so NIV could be started in A&E (Elliott et al. 2002).
- *Wards* – A large prospective multicentre randomised trial by Plant et al. (2000a) looked at the use of NIV in 14 centres in the UK. This simple protocol-driven trial found that NIV could be used effectively in the ward setting, reducing the need for intubation, and reducing mortality. However, sub-group analysis suggested that the outcome in patients with ph < 7.30 after initial treatment was inferior to that in studies performed in the ICU. Additionally, intensive staff training was provided prior to and during the study.

The clinical experience of staff involved in providing an NIV service cannot be underestimated as undoubtedly NIV delivery improves. Commitment is required from all personnel involved in providing training and maintaining competency and this may be easier to achieve in one or two dedicated settings.

ESTABLISHING PATIENTS ON NIV

Local policy will determine the exact procedure for establishing patients on NIV, i.e. location, personnel, monitoring; however, the following factors should always be taken into account:

- *Consent* – as with any treatment, consent for initiating NIV should be sought. This may not always be possible, however, especially if the patient is confused or drowsy, and thus a medical decision must be taken to start ventilation. The use of advanced directives is becoming more common in the UK and may cover patients' informed decisions regarding the use of NIV as well as endotracheal intubation and ventilation. Many patients with advanced COPD may have used NIV in the past and made decisions based on that experience, or discussed NIV during educational sessions in pulmonary rehabilitation.
- *Procedure* – wherever possible, the rationale behind using NIV, along with possible complications should be discussed with the patient before starting ventilation. Additionally, a clear decision regarding further treatment should be documented if NIV were not to correct the clinical situation (NICE 2004). This should include a decision regarding resuscitation and endotracheal intubation and ventilation. Ideally, NIV should be started in a calm environment, allowing the patient to have control over the situation. Clear

explanations and instructions are essential if the patient is to have confidence in the procedure and this is especially important when it comes to actually fitting the mask. Often, allowing the patient to feel the pressure from the ventilator on the back of the hand or arm will prepare them for the sensation on the face.

- *Mask fitting* – choosing the correct interface for a patient can often prove the most crucial factor in determining the success of NIV. A poorly selected interface may make a patient less likely to tolerate NIV (Elliott 2005). A wide range of interfaces are available and include full-face masks, nasal masks, nasal pillows and, currently being investigated, helmets (Antonelli et al. 2004). Unfortunately, cost is likely to be a major factor in determining those available locally. As patients with acute exacerbations of COPD often mouth-breathe, full face masks may be the best interface with which to start. These cover the nose and mouth but can be difficult to fit comfortably to minimise leak around the eyes or cheek area. A common error is to fit the mask too tightly, causing discomfort, a feeling of claustrophobia and possibly tissue necrosis, especially over the bridge of the nose. Pressure-cycled ventilators are able to compensate for leaks somewhat, although large leaks will reduce the efficiency of the ventilator. Additionally, patients are less able to communicate and secretion clearance may be more difficult if using a full-face mask. If prolonged NIV use is required, it may be possible to change the interface to a nasal mask once the acute phase has resolved, although a chin strap may be necessary to prevent the mouth from opening and pressure being lost, especially during sleep.
- *Oxygen entrainment* – Oxygen can be entrained into the ventilator for those patients who are hypoxic. Care with entraining oxygen is essential as many patients with acute exacerbations of COPD are sensitive to the amount of oxygen they receive. A prospective prevalence study by Plant et al. (2000b) established that for hypercapnic patients a higher PaO_2 was associated with more significant acidosis. Guidelines for supplementing oxygen will differ locally; however, titrating the oxygen to achieve saturations in the range of 85–92 per cent (equivalent to PaO_2 7.3–10 kPa) should provide adequate oxygenation while minimising the risk of acidosis (Plant et al. 2000b). This range may be higher for patients with additional cardiac involvement (e.g. acute myocardial infarction).

MONITORING PATIENTS ON NIV

The BTS Guidelines (2002) provide comprehensive details of the level of monitoring required for patients receiving NIV. It is recommended that all patients receive a regular clinical assessment, as shown in Table 10.2.

Regular and well-documented observations allow the team to assess the effectiveness of NIV and make informed decisions regarding continuation of ventilation, adjustments to ventilator settings and weaning strategies from

Table 10.2. Clinical assessment and procedures for patients receiving NIV

Clinical assessment	Rationale
Chest wall movement	Should improve with NIV, indicating improved alveolar ventilation Asymmetrical movement could indicate a pneumothorax
Coordination of respiratory effort with the ventilator	Patient less likely to tolerate NIV if ventilator settings are not synchronised appropriately Ventilation may be ineffective
Accessory muscle recruitment	Should reduce as work of breathing reduces and hyperinflation lessens Continued accessory muscle use may indicate ventilator pressures inadequate to provide sufficient respiratory support
Heart rate	Should reduce as acidosis reverses
Respiratory rate	Should reduce if sufficient respiratory support provided
Patient comfort	Discomfort may result in patient intolerance to NIV Breathlessness should improve in first 1–2 hours
Mental state	Anxiety/claustrophobia could be heightened by use of NIV Confusion secondary to hypoxia or hypercapnia should resolve as gases normalise with NIV

Pulse oximetry and arterial blood gas tension monitoring

Oxygen saturation monitoring	Continuous in first 24 hours aiming for saturations >85% with supplemental oxygen if necessary (see oxygen entrainment above)
ABG monitoring • Initial assessment	ABG assessment is a prerequisite for starting NIV – see indications
• 1–2 hours post-initiation of NIV	Initial aim is to stabilise $PaCO_2$ and prevent further deterioration in pH Ventilator settings can be adjusted to increase ventilation if gases show insufficient improvement
• 1–2 hours post-ventilator setting changes	Necessary to evaluate effectiveness of ventilation
• Subsequent measurements	Will depend on the patient's progress: – If improving rapidly, then frequent ABG analysis may be unnecessary – If slow or no improvement, then more frequent measurements required and an arterial line should be considered for access and patient comfort

NIV. While there are no hard and fast rules regarding optimal use of NIV, it is generally accepted that the first 24 hours are critical if NIV is to be successful and so NIV use should be maximised during this time. Once the patient has stabilised clinically and ABGs have normalised, then weaning may commence. Time spent off NIV should be increased during the day first. Last to be weaned is night-time use as ventilation reduces during sleep.

Some patients may remain in established respiratory failure. While there is currently little evidence to support the long-term ventilation of patients with COPD with home NIV, a proportion of patients with other co-morbidities which may contribute to respiratory failure such as **obesity hypoventilation**, obstructive sleep apnoea or thoracic cage deformity, should be considered for home ventilation. This generally requires referral to a specialist ventilation unit for assessment.

REFERENCES

Antonelli M, Pennisi M A, Pelosi P, et al. (2004) Noninvasive positive pressure ventilation using a helmet in patients with acute exacerbation of chronic obstructive pulmonary disease: a feasibility study. *Anesthesiology* **100**: 16–24.

Benhamou D, Girault C, Faure C, et al. (1992) Nasal mask ventilation in acute respiratory failure: experience in elderly patients. *Chest* **102**: 912–917.

Bott J, Carroll M P, Conway J H, et al. (1993) Randomised controlled trial of nasal ventilation in acute ventilatory failure due to chronic obstructive airways disease. *Lancet* **341**: 1555–1557.

British Thoracic Society Standards of Care Committee (2002) NIPPV Non-Invasive Ventilation in acute respiratory failure. *Thorax* **57**: 192–211.

Brochard L, Mancebo J, Wysocki M, et al. (1995) Noninvasive ventilation for acute exacerbations of chronic obstructive pulmonary disease. *New England Journal of Medicine* **333**: 817–822.

Confalonieri M, Garuti G, Cattaruzza M S, Osborn J F, et al. (2005) A chart of failure risk for noninvasive ventilation in patients with COPD exacerbation. *The European Respiratory Journal* **25**(2): 348–355.

Elliott M W (2002) Non-invasive ventilation in acute exacerbations of chronic obstructive pulmonary disease: A new gold standard? *Intensive Care Medicine* **28**: 1691–1694.

Elliott M W (2005) Non-invasive ventilation for acute respiratory disease. *British Medical Bulletin* **72**(1): 83–97.

Elliott M W, Confalonieri M, Nava S (2002) Where to perform non-invasive ventilation? *European Respiratory Journal* **19**(6): 1159–1166.

Global Initiative for Chronic Obstructive Lung Disease (2005) Update: Workshop Report, Global Strategy for Diagnosis, Management, and Prevention of COPD. Available at: www.goldcopd.org/GuidelineItem.asp?intId=991 (accessed 15 Feb. 2007).

Levy M, Tanios M A, Nelson D, Short K (2004) Outcomes of patients with do-not-intubate orders treated with noninvasive ventilation. *Critical Care Medicine* **32**(10): 2002–2007.

Lightowler J V, Wedzicha J A, Elliott M W, et al. (2003) Non-invasive positive pressure ventilation to treat respiratory failure resulting from exacerbations of chronic obstructive pulmonary disease: Cochrane systematic review and meta-analysis. *British Medical Journal* **326**: 185–187.

Meduri G U, Fox R C, Abou-Shala N, et al. (1994) Noninvasive mechanical ventilation via face mask in patients with acute respiratory failure who refused endotracheal intubation. *Critical Care Medicine* **22**: 1584–1590.

NICE Guidelines (2004) *Chronic Obstructive Pulmonary Disease: Management of Chronic Obstructive Pulmonary Disease in Adults in Primary and Secondary Care. Clinical Guideline.* London: HMSO.

Plant P K, Owen J L, Elliott M W (2000a) Early use of non-invasive ventilation for acute exacerbations of chronic obstructive pulmonary disease on general respiratory wards: A multicentre randomised controlled trial. *Lancet* **355**: 1931–1935.

Plant P K, Owen J L, Elliott M W (2000b) One year period prevalence study of respiratory acidosis in acute exacerbations of COPD: Implications for the provision of non-invasive ventilation and oxygen administration. *Thorax* **55**: 550–554.

Squadrone E, Frigerio P, Fogliati C, Gregoretti C, et al. (2004) Noninvasive vs invasive ventilation in COPD patients with severe acute respiratory failure deemed to require ventilatory assistance. *Intensive Care Medicine* **30**(7): 1303–1310.

Wood K A, Lewis L, Von Harz B, Kollef M H (1998) The use of noninvasive positive pressure ventilation in the Emergency Department. *Chest* **113**: 1339–1346.

11 End-of-Life Care

FLISS MURTAGH
King's College Hospital, London

MARY PRESTON
King's College Hospital, London

CLAUDIA BAUSEWEIN
King's College Hospital, London, University Hospital, Munich

WHAT IS PALLIATIVE CARE?

Palliative care is an approach that improves the quality of life of patients and their families facing life-threatening illness, through the prevention, assessment and treatment of pain and other physical, psychosocial and spiritual problems (World Health Organisation 2002) (Box 11.1). It aims to optimise care and quality of life, by switching the main focus from controlling or curing the disease to improving the illness experience and addressing the needs of patient and family.

THE EXTENSION OF PALLIATIVE CARE TO NON-MALIGNANT DISEASE

Palliative care has traditionally focused on end-of-life care for patients suffering from advanced cancer. Since the 1990s, however, there have been increasing calls for palliative care to be provided on the basis of need, not diagnosis (Higginson & Addington-Hall 1999). This encouraged hospices and specialist palliative care providers to increasingly recognise their role of caring for and promoting wider awareness of the needs of patients with non-malignant diseases towards the end of life. This change has been acknowledged by the new World Health Organisation definition of palliative care (World Health Organisation 2002), which now relates to all with 'life-threatening illness', not just those with cancer as in the earlier definition, and the National Council for Palliative Care in the UK has announced that their focus of care has broadened to include patients with any terminal diagnosis. The government has also recognised the needs of non-cancer patients by incorporating palliative care

Managing Chronic Obstructive Pulmonary Disease. Edited by L. Blackler, C. Jones and C. Mooney
© 2007 John Wiley & Sons Ltd

Box 11.1. What palliative care involves

Palliative care:

- Provides relief from pain and other distressing symptoms.
- Affirms life and regards dying as a normal process.
- Intends neither to hasten nor postpone death.
- Integrates the psychological and spiritual aspects of patient care.
- Offers a support system to help patients live as actively as possible until death.
- Offers a support system to help the family cope during the patient's illness and in their own bereavement.
- Uses a team approach to address the needs of patients and their families, including bereavement counselling if indicated.
- Will enhance quality of life, and may also positively influence the course of illness.

into some of its recent National Service Frameworks, including those for coronary heart disease and renal disease (Department of Health 2000, 2005). Despite this increased recognition, a recent UK survey has shown that cancer patients still make up the vast majority of those cared for by specialist palliative services. Just 5.9 per cent of patients admitted to hospices, and 10.7 per cent of patients seen by hospital specialist palliative care teams have non-malignant diagnoses; overall, about 24 per cent of these non-cancer patients will have respiratory diseases (The National Council for Palliative Care 2005).

Some authorities distinguish between general and specialist palliative care, where the 'general' palliative care approach is adopted by a wide variety of professionals in different disciplines and specialities, and 'specialist' palliative care is provided by professionals trained in and working predominantly or exclusively in palliative care (National Council for Hospice and Specialist Palliative Care Services 2001). This may be a somewhat artificial distinction, but it is important to recognise both the need for general and respiratory nurses to acquire palliative skills in the care of end-stage COPD patients, and for specialist palliative services to be involved in care of end-stage COPD patients with more complex needs. Specialist services also have a role in education; facilitating skill development in those adopting the general palliative and supportive approach.

Whether care is provided by respiratory teams with palliative knowledge and skills, by specialist palliative services, or (most likely) by some combination of these services, it is paramount that the palliative needs of patients with end-stage COPD are recognised and effectively addressed.

THE NEEDS OF COPD PATIENTS APPROACHING THE END OF LIFE

According to Blackler et al. (2004), as well as equitable access to care, these patients have extensive needs, including:

- *Informational/educational needs*, about the incurable nature of their illness, prognosis, likely trajectory, management options (including information about non-invasive ventilation when appropriate), and help with advance planning. All information giving and education needs to take individual patient preferences for information and involvement into account.
- *Physical needs*, including symptom management (see below), but also detailed consideration of functional impairment, appropriate aids, services and support.
- *Psychosocial and emotional needs*, including screening for anxiety and depression, active management of identified psychological problems, help in dealing with uncertainty, and attention to the social impact of illness, such as social isolation.
- *Spiritual needs*, as patients face impending mortality.
- *Need for privacy and dignity*.

In addition to patient needs, family and carers also will have considerable informational, educational and support needs (Elkington et al. 2005).

There are some specific considerations in COPD. Evidence shows that in COPD, symptom control is currently poor, and services from both primary and secondary care are limited and often fail to meet needs (Skilbeck et al. 1998; Elkington et al. 2005). COPD patients have been described as 'socially invisible' until acute care is required, which leads to fragmented and inadequate services, especially outside the acute setting (Guthrie et al. 2001).

Other considerations include the uncertain illness trajectory – both in terms of overall prognosis and in predicting acute-on-chronic episodes. Patients may follow a fluctuating course as they experience, and recover from, acute exacerbations. This can make it particularly difficult for professionals to recognise and facilitate the switch to palliative management, and for patients and families to comprehend the true severity of illness. It also has extensive implications for planning care in the end-of-life period (Murtagh et al. 2004). Patients with COPD are also often elderly, and their needs encompass being old and ill, as well as having a progressive disease (Elofsson & Ohlen 2004).

These considerations call for an integrated and holistic approach to end-of-life care in COPD, with all professionals adopting palliative care principles and working towards an integrated approach (Skilbeck et al. 1998; Elofsson & Ohlen 2004).

COMMUNICATION WITH PATIENT AND FAMILY

Skilled and detailed communication with the patient and their family is important to achieve, but challenging in practice. COPD patients recognise the importance of understanding their disease, including prognosis and the terminal nature of advanced COPD (Curtis et al. 2002), but they experience limited information giving and explanation. They want to understand their illness better and to talk about death, dying, and future plans, but rarely have this opportunity (Curtis et al. 2002). There are both patient and professional factors contributing to this poor communication. Patients are often reluctant to initiate talk about getting sicker and dying, and are unsure about what kind of care they may want in the future, and who will deliver that care, while professionals are concerned about limited time, removing hope from patients, or prompting patients to talk when they are not ready (Knauft et al. 2005).

Communication needs to be clear, timely and matched to patient preferences. Nurses need to be aware of the high prevalence of anxiety in COPD patients, which will affect communication, and to bear in mind the reluctance of patients to initiate discussions about sensitive areas of future care and disease progression. Professionals need to take the initiative and make it clear to patients that it is acceptable (and sensible) to talk about these issues, if they wish. They need to signal their willingness to discuss such issues using open questions, such as 'Have you thought about the future?' or 'Do you worry about what might happen?' while remaining sensitive to each patient's responses and reactions to such 'openers'.

SYMPTOM PREVALENCE

Patients with COPD suffer from a variety of symptoms. The mean number of symptoms reported in the final year of life is seven, with 1.6 symptoms being classified as very distressing. In the last week of life, patients still complain of an average of six symptoms (Edmonds et al. 2001). Breathlessness is the most dominant symptom with up to 90 per cent of patients experiencing it (Edmonds et al. 2001). In the SUPPORT study, around 70 per cent of patients with COPD experienced moderate to severe breathlessness in the last six months of life with an increase towards death (in the last three days) to more than 80 per cent (Lynn et al. 2000). However, breathlessness is not the only respiratory symptom in COPD patients; cough and wheeze are often directly related to breathlessness. The second most common symptom is pain, occurring in 77 per cent of patients (Edmonds et al. 2001). Patients also suffer from anxiety, weakness, fatigue, sleep disturbances, confusion and depression (Skilbeck et al. 1998). Furthermore, patients experience gastrointestinal symptoms such as anorexia, nausea, vomiting, constipation and mouth problems.

The illness and the symptoms have a big impact on patients' daily life. Many patients are not able to leave the house and require help with washing, dressing and getting to the toilet. As well as physical symptoms, a low level of functioning leads to negative effects on the family and social life, with associated social isolation and emotional distress (Skilbeck et al. 1998).

SYMPTOM ASSESSMENT AND MANAGEMENT

Thorough symptom assessment is crucial in selecting the right management approach, and requires several steps:

1 Evaluation
2 Explanation
3 Individual management plan.
4 Re-evaluation.
5 Careful attention to detail throughout.

The first step is the *evaluation* of the patient and the situation. The patient has to be asked regularly about the presence of symptoms, their frequency, duration and severity. The various dimensions of a symptom should be considered: there is usually a psychosocial and spiritual dimension that will influence the patient's perception. It is also important to find out what helps to relieve the symptom and what aggravates it. Possible causes have to be considered: is the symptom caused by the disease, the treatment or independent from the illness? Are there reversible causes? Physical examination of the patient related to the symptom is an important part of the evaluation and will often establish the underlying cause of any particular symptom.

The next step, which is often overlooked, is the *explanation* to the patient and the relatives. They should know what is going on, why the symptom is causing trouble and what can be done to relieve it. A clear and realistic aim should be defined for all parties. Complete freedom from a symptom is often difficult to achieve, but some degree of relief is nearly always possible.

Depending on the likely cause of the symptom and the situation of the patient, an *individual management plan* needs to be decided on. This should include the decision on drugs, their dose and application, the frequency of use, and rescue doses. Close *re-evaluation* is necessary to check whether the treatment is successful or consider any changes, e.g. dose escalation, addition of new drugs or change of the medication. *Attention to detail* is paramount in symptom management. Is the patient taking the medication regularly? Are the doses right? Are the psychosocial issues being addressed?

For the measurement of breathlessness, the symptom most complained of by patients with COPD, various tools are available. Uni-dimensional measures such as the visual analogue scale (VAS) or the Modified Borg Scale (Wilson and Jones 1989) help to assess changes in breathlessness between outpatient visits, or with change in medication. These uni-dimensional scales are also helpful where breathlessness is being measured at one point in time, e.g. exercise testing or general assessment of breathlessness in the previous 24 hours. If quality of life is the focus of measurement, a multidimensional tool is essential. The most used disease-specific scales are the Chronic Respiratory Disease Questionnaire (Guyatt et al. 1987) and the St George's Respiratory Questionnaire (Jones et al. 1991).

SPECIFIC SYMPTOMS

BREATHLESSNESS

The terms 'breathlessness' and 'dyspnoea' can be used interchangeably (Roberts et al. 1993) but the first is more often used by patients whereas the latter is more medical. Breathlessness is a very distressing symptom for patients, and challenging for carers, as it is difficult to treat. It is a multidimensional symptom with psychosocial and spiritual components, and defined as 'a subjective experience of breathing discomfort that consists of qualitatively distinct sensations that vary in intensity' (American Thoracic Society 1999). The actual experience of breathlessness results from a complex interaction between breathing abnormalities and perception of these abnormalities that the patient interprets and reacts to (Ripamonti & Bruera 1997). The degree of breathlessness experienced does not correlate with lung function tests or other laboratory parameters. Various causes can lead to breathlessness or aggravate breathlessness caused by COPD (see Table 11.1). Treatment of reversible causes is the first step to successful symptom management.

To relieve breathlessness sufficiently, a combination of non-pharmacological and pharmacological treatment is usually necessary (see Table 11.2).

The pharmacological treatment of patients with COPD plays an important role throughout all stages of the disease. Inhaled and oral bronchodilators, corticosteroids and other anti-obstructive drugs aim to reduce airways obstruc-

Table 11.1. Causes of breathlessness and specific treatments

Cause	Treatment
Airways obstruction	Bronchodilators
Acute infection	Antibiotics
Chronic infection	Antibiotics
Left ventricular heart failure	Angiotensin converting enzyme (ACE) inhibitors, diuretics
Pleural effusion	Pleural tapping
Pneumothorax	Drainage
Anaemia	Transfusion

Table 11.2. Symptomatic treatment of breathlessness in advanced stages

Intervention	Treatment
Non-pharmacological interventions	Relaxation
	Positioning
	Fan or hand-held fan
	Education, coping strategies
	Nursing intervention
	Physiotherapy
Pharmacological interventions	Opioids
	Benzodiazepines
	Oxygen

tion, correct hypoxia and reduce breathlessness (see Chapter 6). If these regimens are not successful in relieving breathlessness further symptomatic treatment should be considered. Opioids play a major role in the reduction of breathlessness especially in patients who are breathless at rest and in the last days of life (Corner et al. 1996). The mechanisms by which opioids relieve breathlessness are not fully understood: both central and peripheral mechanisms are suggested (Jennings et al. 2001). The dose necessary to relieve breathlessness is normally lower than for analgesia but, similar to pain reduction, the dose should be titrated gradually against the effect. Inhaled morphine has been used but the evidence is conflicting; therefore it cannot be recommended. The use of benzodiazepines and phenothiazines will be discussed later in this chapter.

As the sole use of drugs will not be sufficient to relieve breathlessness in many cases, non-pharmacological interventions play an important role in the management of breathlessness. A variety of measures are available. They can be as simple as a hand-held fan, where a draft of cool air relieves the sensation of breathlessness. Physiotherapy offers the patient help in living with breathlessness, through breathing techniques and diaphragmatic breathing. To support the patient in managing breathlessness, an integrated nursing intervention has been developed and successfully validated over the past few years including behavioural, cognitive and psychotherapeutic strategies and management of panic and anxiety (Bredin et al. 1999). Patients are supported in exploring the meaning and significance of the illness and other symptoms, as well as the impact of the illness on work and relationships. They are introduced to breathing control exercises, relaxation and visualisation techniques. Goal setting, prioritisation and activity pacing play an important role.

Long-term oxygen therapy extends the life expectancy of patients with advanced hypoxic COPD and improves symptoms such as breathlessness. Patients should use the oxygen at least 12–15 hours per day (Medical Research Council Working Party 1981). Both oxygen concentrators and oxygen cylinders, with or without a conserver device, are available for the delivery of oxygen. The latter are less practical for long-term use and are more expensive. Liquid oxygen is an alternative but not as widely available at present. High flows of oxygen have to be used with considerable caution in COPD patients, because low O_2 may be the only respiratory drive patients have; removing it gives rise to the danger of CO_2 retention with subsequent narcosis.

ANXIETY

Breathlessness is aggravated by anxiety and panic attacks which are part of a vicious circle: breathlessness causing more anxiety, which causes more breathlessness, and so on. Patients should be taught how to cope with panic attacks: relaxation of shoulders and chest wall muscles, slow expiration as long as possible, staying calm.

The above-mentioned nursing interventions help the patients to manage these attacks. However, some patients need anxiolytic drug therapy. Benzodiazepines such as diazepam and lorazepam have both anxiolytic and muscle relaxant effects. Their use is controversial, especially in patients with COPD, because of the side effects of sedation and drowsiness, and associated reduction of respiratory drive. Promethazine is therefore sometimes used as an alternative.

COUGH

Cough is a common and distressing symptom in COPD affecting the patient by interrupted sleep, disturbed communication, and social isolation. Cough aims to support muco-ciliary clearing in chronic bronchitis. The most common causes are smoking, acute or chronic infection, left ventricular failure, interstitial fibrosis, oesophageal reflux or drugs (e.g. ACE inhibitors). Gastrointestinal reflux should be excluded as it can cause cough or aggravate it. Smoking cessation will reduce cough in 50 per cent of cases (Irwin et al. 1990). Treatment of the underlying cause is essential. Chronic productive cough should be improved by adequate hydration, physiotherapy and pharmacological treatment to increase secretion clearance. For the latter, inhaled saline or oral cysteine derivatives (N-acetylcysteine) are available. If there are no reversible causes and the impact on the patient's quality of life is high, suppressive therapy should be started. Various opioids can be given to suppress the cough reflex centrally. Codeine and dextromethorphan are common ingredients in cough preparations (Twycross et al. 2002). If these drugs are ineffective, a strong opioid such as morphine should be prescribed. Alternatively, nebulised local anaesthetics can be used. However, they are of limited value as they cause an unpleasant taste, oropharyngeal numbness and risk of bronchoconstriction (Twycross et al. 2002), and their effect only lasts 10–30 minutes.

PAIN

There are several causes of pain in patients with COPD. Chest wall pain is due to localized muscular tenderness or rib fractures mainly caused by cough. This can lead to hypoventilation. Oral analgesics including strong opioids or local nerve blocks may be necessary for adequate pain control. Pain connected to breathing may be caused by pleural inflammation (pleurisy). Anti-inflammatory drugs (e.g. diclofenac) will bring quick relief. Sharp and burning pain mainly behind the sternum and worse when coughing is often caused by tracheo-bronchitis that will also respond to anti-inflammatory drugs.

ANOREXIA, NAUSEA AND VOMITING

Anorexia is a common symptom in advanced disease. Potentially reversible causes are breathlessness, pain, constipation, nausea and vomiting, drugs, delayed gastric emptying, anxiety and depression. First, assess whether the patient is suffering from the symptom or whether it is in fact the relatives who want him or her to eat. If the relatives are pressurising the patient to eat, careful explanation may be most helpful. Patients should be offered small meals in a pleasant atmosphere; unpleasant smells should be avoided. If drugs are necessary, steroids can bring a transient effect. Some patients respond positively to cannabinoids.

Nausea and vomiting occur often but not necessarily together. A patient can be nauseated without vomiting or vomit without feeling nauseated. Causes such as constipation, gastritis, hepatomegaly, side effects of drugs and uraemia should be excluded or, if present, treated. Anti-emetics should be given regularly to prevent recurrence, rather than on an 'as required' basis. Metoclopramide acts mostly in the gastrointestinal tract, to increase gastric emptying, whereas haloperidol, levomepromazine and cyclicine predominantly work via central pathways. Choice between these depends therefore on assessment of the underlying cause of the nausea or vomiting.

CONSTIPATION

Patients with advanced disease often complain of constipation due to decreased mobility, reduced fluid intake and loss of privacy. Many drugs necessary for symptom control, such as opioids, anticholinergics, sedatives, diuretics and others, aggravate or are the main cause of constipation. Management includes, if possible, increased fluid intake (encouraging fruit juice), critical review of prescribed drugs, and creation of privacy for the patient when using the toilet. However, in advanced disease, laxatives are often necessary, especially when the patient is on opioids. A variety of laxatives are available. Most useful is either a combination of stimulants (e.g. bisacodyl, senna) and faecal softener (e.g. docusate) or the prescription of an osmotic laxative (e.g. Movicol®). If the regular use of laxatives is not sufficient, rectal measures with suppositories or enemas may be necessary. Depending on the patient's usual bowel habit, bowel opening at least every three days should be aimed at.

TERMINAL SYMPTOMS (DEATH RATTLE, DELIRIUM)

Symptoms may change towards the terminal phase. Some symptoms become less prominent, others develop especially in this phase. Death rattle is a typical symptom in the last days and hours of cancer patients. However, there is no data available for COPD patients. Death rattle is a rattling noise with inspiration and expiration in dying patients, who have lost the ability to swallow or cough, and who produce secretions that then pool in the oropharynx, the trachea and the bronchi. It is not known how stressful it is for the patient, but it often causes distress for relatives, carers and professionals. Positioning of the patient on the lateral side is suggested to help the secretions drain. The use of suctioning is limited, as it will only bring short relief because of recurrent secretions that are produced continuously. Parenteral fluids will increase the rattling and should therefore be restricted in the terminal phase. Pharmacological treatment includes the use of anticholinergics such as hyoscine butylbromide or glycopyrrolate. All anticholinergics used for relief of death rattle are best started early because they do not clear existing secretions. When first signs of rattling are noticed, drug therapy should be started.

Delirium is a common symptom in the terminal phase with restlessness and hallucinations due to uncontrolled symptoms, anxiety, infections, dehydration or drug side effects. Important for the management are a quiet atmosphere, familiar surroundings, and not too many new faces. Touch, massage, or aromatherapy can help to reassure the patient. Drugs may be necessary if simple measures are ineffective. When the patient is hallucinating, haloperidol is the drug of choice. Restlessness can be relieved by benzodiazepines. However, they should not be given alone in delirium as they may aggravate it, but are best combined with neuroleptics such as haloperidol. With good symptom control most patients will achieve a peaceful death.

PSYCHOSOCIAL AND SPIRITUAL CARE

As patients approach the end of their disease trajectory, it is increasingly important to consider a holistic approach to care, and to move away from a disease-focused, towards a person-focused approach (Murtagh et al. 2004). Many COPD patients have a high degree of social isolation, along with low physical functioning and high levels of emotional distress (Skilbeck et al. 1998). Gore and colleagues also found that 86 per cent of patients with COPD were housebound compared with 36 per cent of cancer patients (Gore et al. 2000), and Almagro et al. (2002) found that unmarried patients had a notably shorter prognosis.

These patients therefore need considerable social care, and may need specialist palliative care support as well. Gore et al. (2000) compared two groups of patients, 50 with severe COPD, 50 with non-small cell lung cancer, to examine the differences in provision of care. Some 36 per cent of COPD patients were dissatisfied with their social care arrangements compared to 12 per cent of those with lung cancer. None of the patients with COPD had been offered access to a specialist palliative care service. Thorough patient assessment, and liaison with specialist palliative care teams for those with complex needs, in addition to more generic health and social services, may enhance care substantially.

It is not only the patient who will have psychosocial needs, but also the family and carers. Living and dying with a chronic disease affects not only the patient, but takes a considerable toll on their carer and wider family members. Carers play an important and multifaceted role, which can be burdensome at times, and cause tensions within relationships. Regular support from health care professionals, which can be provided by any member of the team, is important and reassuring for carers (Seamark et al. 2004).

Spiritual and religious needs are often closely linked, yet it is important to understand their differences. Spirituality is to do with meaning within one's life, but not necessarily through any formal religious beliefs, while religion is an expression of spiritual beliefs through a more formal framework (Speck et al. 2004). The importance of provision of spiritual care for patients is important; especially for those nearing the end of their lives. Patients may be distressed for many different reasons, and are likely to reflect on their life as their illness progresses. They may also feel angry at their situation, which can manifest in spiritual distress.

Providing spiritual care for patients can feel threatening and uncomfortable for staff (McSherry 2005). It can feel frightening to raise issues that may be challenging. It is important to remember that there are not always answers to patients' questions, but that listening and being present are important. Patients who display signs of spiritual distress can show altered behaviour and/or mood, they may be tearful, angry, anxious and/or withdrawn. Patients who have a formal religion may re-examine their belief system (National Institute for Clinical Excellence 2004). Patients can be very distressed, and may have many questions about identify, self worth, and the meaning of life. Having an awareness of people's needs and showing respect for individual religious beliefs is helpful, but asking questions if you are unsure, and taking the time to listen is invaluable.

The NICE guidelines for supportive and palliative care (National Institute for Clinical Excellence 2004) have highlighted spiritual support for cancer patients. One of their key recommendations is that patients and their carers should have access to staff that are sensitive to their spiritual needs. This need for spiritual care obviously extends to patients with diseases other than cancer. Patients with COPD face many difficulties; they may have experienced a long and fluctuant illness trajectory, and faced a number of losses. Their spiritual needs are likely to be at least as great as those with advanced cancer.

ADVANCE PLANNING

When caring for patients with end-stage COPD, it is essential to anticipate and plan for the future to ensure patients' and carers' wishes are met. To ensure this happens, it is important to examine the role of advanced directives, planning for acute hospital admissions and prevention of inappropriate admissions, cardiopulmonary resuscitation (CPR) and patient preferences.

ADVANCE DIRECTIVES

Advance directives or statements, sometimes known as living wills, are a means for individuals to state in advance how they would wish to be treated in the future should they suffer loss of mental capacity (British Medical Association 1995). Sections that clearly refuse interventions may be legally binding, and should therefore be respected (British Medical Association 1995). At the time that a directive is prepared, an adult must be competent and should specify all or some forms of medical treatment that they would find unacceptable, and under which circumstances. Treatment that may be deemed clinically inappropriate cannot be demanded. Advance statements are usually written documents, and ideally should be signed by the patient and witnessed. They should be regularly updated and reviewed. The forthcoming Mental Capacity Bill in the UK (due to become law in 2007) will formalise advance statements and also allow for patients to elect a person to legally represent their preferences once they lose capacity.

An example of good practice is to ask patients what their wishes might be in the event of future deterioration. Relatively few patients choose to write a formal advance directive, but all should be offered the chance to discuss preferences for future care and management. These discussions should be carefully documented, re-visited at intervals (preferences may change), and made available to relevant team members for appropriate future use. Gaber et al. (2004) surveyed the attitudes of 100 patients with COPD towards artificial ventilation and CPR, and found that an overwhelming 98 per cent agreed that these sensitive issues should be discussed with all patients.

ADVANCE PLANNING AND PREVENTION OF INAPPROPRIATE ADMISSIONS

Patients are sometimes admitted with increasing frequency due to deteriorating lung function (Gore et al. 2000). It has been shown that patients requiring increasingly frequent hospitalisation have higher mortality (Almagro et al. 2002). If it is observed that a particular patient is being admitted with increasing frequency, this may be an appropriate time to discuss plans for future care. The hospital setting is not always the most appropriate environment to care for patients with end-stage COPD who are close to their terminal phase, and other options may be suggested, such as care at home, nursing home or hospice admission. Specialist palliative care teams in the community may provide additional advice and support at home, beyond that provided by primary care and respiratory services; referral may be appropriate in more complex cases.

Various studies have explored patients' preferences about future treatment options, including ventilation and CPR (Dales et al. 1999; Gaber et al. 2004). In the study by Gaber et al. (2004) 100 patients were surveyed, 48 wanted all additional treatments to be attempted, and 12 wanted none. These studies conclude that discussions with patients, when they are well and able to make decisions about future treatments, are beneficial to patients, relatives and staff. In the event of patients becoming too unwell to express themselves, knowing what their preference for care is can prevent unnecessary interventions that may cause distress.

Yeager (1997) takes this one step further and proposes that patients who decline intubation and ventilation be referred to palliative care services. This may be helpful, but needs consideration on an individual basis, and according to knowledge of locally available services. Patients at home with increasing symptom severity, who have expressed a wish not to be actively managed, need to be actively supported at home by community professionals, in conjunction with palliative care professionals where appropriate, and in liaison with hospital physicians, thus ensuring seamless patient-focused care. The exact configuration of services will depend on local provision, but it should be clear to the patient, family and professionals exactly who has responsibility and involvement at each stage.

CARDIOPULMONARY RESUSCITATION

CPR continues to be a much-debated treatment in both medical and nursing journals and in the wider media. Often inappropriately portrayed on the television in hospital dramas, there continues to be much confusion around what CPR means for patients who are terminally ill, and whether this sensitive subject needs discussion with patients (Manisty & Waxman 2003). CPR in this group of patients is often inappropriate, as in this group of patients the cessation of cardiac and respiratory function is part of the dying process (British

Medical Association, Resuscitation Council (UK) and Royal College of Nursing 2002). It is also important to recognise that there is no ethical obligation to discuss CPR with terminally ill patients, if this treatment is judged to be futile and therefore would not be provided. Good practice includes timely support and communication, individualised decision-making and sensitive discussion that is not forced. If the clinical team are as certain as they can be that CPR will not be successful, it should not be offered (BMA/RCN/RC 2002).

PLANS OF CARE FOR PATIENT AND FAMILY

Planning future care for patients and their families is part of the foundation of palliative care. *Building on the Best: Choice, Responsiveness and Equity in the NHS* (Department of Health 2003) identified that patients want a high quality service, which meets their needs, is personal and equitable. In order to meet this need, a national programme was set up in 2004 (the End of Life Care Initiative), enabling the principles of end-of-life care for cancer patients to be spread into other disease groups by widening numbers of generalist staff trained in palliative care. This programme promotes three end-of-life tools, co-ordinated at national level by the End of Life Care Programme. These may help improve care on the ground for COPD patients approaching the end of life, and are explained in more detail below.

The Gold Standards Framework (GSF)

This model was developed by Thomas (2005) for use within primary care. Patients are identified as approaching their palliative phase, and then appropriate plans for their needs are agreed and implemented. There are seven key areas, which include: communication, continuity of care, advanced care planning, patient and carer support and team working. Further details are available at the designated website www.goldstandardsframework.nhs.uk.

Preferred Place of Care (PPC)

This tool was developed to promote discussion around patients' preferred place of death, enabling completion of a patient-held record, which documents their preferred wishes. Originally developed for cancer patients as part of a palliative care education programme, it is now a nationally recognised tool (Pemberton et al. 2003) to help facilitate care planning.

Liverpool Care Pathway (LCP)

Originally developed to translate the excellence of hospice care to acute settings, the Liverpool Care Pathway (LCP) has been developed to provide a framework to direct care during the last few days of life and thus enabling delivery of high quality, standardised care for patients (Ellershaw et al. 2001). Key aspects relating to communication between patients, carers and professionals are incorporated, as are clinical guidelines, which can be used as an education tool. Any deviance from the LCP is documented as a variance, analysis of which can provide a tool for audit. Its use has now spread nationally, and it is now promoted in all care settings including hospital, hospice, community and care homes. Although it was originally developed as a tool for cancer patients, it focuses specifically on symptoms at the end of life and can also be used for patients with any terminal diagnosis, including those patients with end-stage COPD.

BEREAVEMENT FOLLOW-UP

Grief is a usual response to loss, and facing bereavement provides many challenges for those who are left behind. There are a number of theoretical models which examine bereavement phenomena (Kissane 2004). Most people do find a way to adjust to an altered way of life without formal support; however, some require specific interventions by services (National Institute for Clinical Excellence 2004). Bereavement support encompasses understanding and recognising the need for psychological support (Melliar-Smith 2002).

Most services offering bereavement support are provided by the voluntary sector, and 90 per cent of this support by volunteers (Bereavement Care Standards UK Project 2001). Generally services across England and Wales are poorly developed and services fragmented, although specialist palliative care services provide more established services (National Institute for Clinical Excellence 2004). It is useful to have an understanding of services operating locally in order to ensure ongoing support for bereaved carers. If patients are linked to palliative care services, their family may automatically be offered bereavement support. If this is not the case, many local and national organisations exist which can be accessed, including Cruse Bereavement Care, which is the leading charity in the United Kingdom specialising in bereavement support.

Bereavement care should be an integral part of care. There are a number of tools that may provide an indication of increased risk of a complex grief reaction (Kissane 2004). Previous losses, medical history, including psychiatric history and mode of death, are some examples of bereavement risk factors that have been identified. Assessing the levels of risks for each factor may have a bearing on a person's outcome in the bereavement phase. Early and targeted interventions may prevent complex and unresolved grief reactions (Melliar-Smith 2002). Bereavement can also give rise to wider concerns, including: practical and financial issues, as well as emotional and psychosocial needs (Bereavement Care Standards UK Project 2001), and these should not be neglected.

REFERENCES

Almagro P, Calbo E, Ochoa d Echaguen A, Barreiro B, Quintana S, Heredia J L, Garau J (2002) Mortality after hospitalization for COPD. *Chest* **121**(5): 1441–1448.

American Thoracic Society (1999) Dyspnea, mechanisms, assessment, and management: a consensus statement. *American Journal of Respiratory and Critical Care Medicine* **159**(1): 321–340.

Bereavement Care Standards UK Project (2001) *Standards for Bereavement Care in the UK*. London: Bereavement Care Standards UK Project.

Blackler L, Mooney C, Jones C (2004) Palliative care in the management of chronic obstructive pulmonary disease. *British Journal of Nursing* **13**(9): 518–521.

Bredin M, Corner J, Krishnasamy M, Plant H, Bailey C, A'Hern R (1999) Multicentre randomised controlled trial of nursing intervention for breathlessness in patients with lung cancer. *British Medical Journal* **318**(7188): 901–904.

British Medical Association (1995) Advance statements about medical treatment – code of practice. Available at: www.bma.org.uk/ap.nsf/Content/codeofpractice (accessed 10 Apr. 2006).

British Medical Association, Resuscitation Council (UK), and Royal College of Nursing (2002) *A Joint Statement from the British Medical Association, the Resuscitation Council (UK) and the Royal College of Nursing*. London: British Medical Association.

Corner J, Plant H, A'Hern R, Bailey C (1996) Non-pharmacological intervention for breathlessness in lung cancer. *Palliative Medicine* **10**(4): 299–305.

Curtis J R, Wenrich M D, Carline J D, Shannon S E, Ambrozy D M, Ramsey P G (2002) Patients' perspectives on physician skill in end-of-life care: differences between patients with COPD, cancer, and AIDS. *Chest* **122**(1): 356–362.

Dales R E, O'Connor A, Hebert P, Sullivan K, McKim D, Llewellyn-Thomas H (1999) Intubation and mechanical ventilation for COPD: Development of an instrument to elicit patient preferences. *Chest* **116**(3): 792–800.

Department of Health (2000) *Coronary Heart Disease: National Service Framework for Coronary Heart Disease – Modern Standards and Service Models*. London: HMSO.

Department of Health (2003) *Building on the Best: Choice: Responsiveness and Equity in the NHS*. London: HMSO.

Department of Health (2005) *National Service Framework for Renal Services – Part 2*. London: HMSO.

Edmonds P, Karlsen S, Khan S, Addington-Hall J (2001) A comparison of the palliative care needs of patients dying from chronic respiratory diseases and lung cancer. *Palliative Medicine* **15**(4): 287–295.

Elkington H, White P, Addington-Hall J, Higgs R, Edmonds P (2005) The healthcare needs of chronic obstructive pulmonary disease patients in the last year of life. *Palliative Medicine* **19**(6): 485–491.

Ellershaw J, Smith C, Overill S, Walker S E, Aldridge J (2001) Care of the dying: setting standards for symptom control in the last 48 hours of life. *Journal of Pain Symptom Management* **21**(1): 12–17.

Elofsson L C, Ohlen J (2004) Meanings of being old and living with chronic obstructive pulmonary disease. *Palliative Medicine* **18**(7): 611–618.

Gaber K A, Barnett M, Planchant Y, McGavin C R (2004) Attitudes of 100 patients with chronic obstructive pulmonary disease to artificial ventilation and cardiopulmonary resuscitation. *Palliative Medicine* **18**(7): 626–629.

Gore J M, Brophy C J, Greenstone M A (2000) How well do we care for patients with end stage chronic obstructive pulmonary disease (COPD)? A comparison of palliative care and quality of life in COPD and lung cancer. *Thorax* **55**(12): 1000–1006.

Guthrie S J, Hill K M, Muers M E (2001) Living with severe COPD: A qualitative exploration of the experience of patients in Leeds. *Respiratory Medicine* **95**(3): 196–204.

Guyatt G H, Berman L B, Townsend M, Pugsley S O, Chambers L W (1987) A measure of quality of life for clinical trials in chronic lung disease. *Thorax* **42**(10): 773–778.

Higginson I J, Addington-Hall J M (1999) Palliative care needs to be provided on basis of need rather than diagnosis. *British Medical Journal* **318**(7176): 123.

Irwin R S, Curley F J, French C L (1990) Chronic cough: The spectrum and frequency of causes, key components of the diagnostic evaluation, and outcome of specific therapy. *American Review of Respiratory Disease* **141**(3): 640–647.

Jennings A L, Davies A N, Higgins J P, Broadley K (2001) *Opioids for the Palliation of Breathlessness in Terminal Illness*. Cochrane Database of Systematic Reviews (4): CD002066.

Jones P W, Quirk F H, Baveystock C M (1991) *The St George's Respiratory Questionnaire. Respiratory Medicine* **85** Suppl B: 25–31.

Kissane D W (2004) Bereavement. In Doyle D, et al. (eds) *Oxford Textbook of Palliative Medicine*. Oxford: Oxford University Press.

Knauft E, Nielsen E L, Engelberg R A, Patrick D L, Curtis J R (2005) Barriers and facilitators to end-of-life care communication for patients with COPD. *Chest* **127**(6): 2188–2196.

Lynn J, Ely F W, Zhong Z, McNiff K L, Dawson N V, Connors A, Desbiens N A, Claessens M, McCarthy E P (2000) Living and dying with chronic obstructive pulmonary disease. *Journal of the American Geriatrics Society* **48** Suppl 5: S91–S100.

Manisty C, Waxman J (2003) Doctors should not discuss resuscitation with terminally ill patients. *British Medical Journal* **327**(7415): 614–615.

McSherry W (2005) Spirituality in palliative care. In: Nyatanga B and Astley-Pepper M (eds) *Hidden Aspects of Palliative Care*. London: Quay Books.

Medical Research Council Working Party (1981) Long-term domiciliary oxygen therapy in chronic hypoxic cor pulmonale complicating chronic bronchitis and emphysema: Report of the Medical Research Council Working Party. *Lancet* **1**(8222): 681–686.

Melliar-Smith C (2002) The risk assessment of bereavement in a palliative care setting. *International Journal of Palliative Nursing* **8**(6): 281–287.

Murtagh F E, Preston M, Higginson I (2004) Patterns of dying: Palliative care for non-malignant disease. *Clinical Medicine* **4**(1): 39–44.

National Council for Hospice and Specialist Palliative Care Services (2001) *What Do We Mean by Palliative Care?* London: National Council for Hospice and Specialist Palliative Care Services.

National Council for Palliative Care (2005) *National Survey of Patient Activity Data for Specialist Palliative Care Services: Full Report for the Year* 2003–4. London: The National Council for Palliative Care.

National Institute for Clinical Excellence (2004) *Improving Supportive and Palliative Care for Adults with Cancer*. London: National Institute for Clinical Excellence.

Pemberton C, Storey L, Howard A (2003) The Preferred Place of Care document: an opportunity for communication. *International Journal of Palliative Nursing* **9**(10): 439–441.

Ripamonti C, Bruera E (1997) Dyspnea: Pathophysiology and assessment. *Journal of Pain and Symptom Management* **13**(4): 220–232.

Roberts D K, Thorne S E, Pearson C (1993) The experience of dyspnea in late-stage cancer: Patients' and nurses' perspectives. *Cancer Nursing* **16**(4): 310–320.

Seamark D A, Blake S D, Seamark C J, Halpin D M (2004) Living with severe chronic obstructive pulmonary disease (COPD): perceptions of patients and their carers: An interpretative phenomenological analysis. *Palliative Medicine* **18**(7): 619–625.

Skilbeck J, Mott L, Page H, Smith D, Hjelmeland-Ahmedzai S, Clark D (1998) Palliative care in chronic obstructive airways disease: a needs assessment. *Palliative Medicine* **12**(4): 245–254.

Speck P, Higginson I, Addington-Hall J (2004) Spiritual needs in health care. *British Medical Journal* **329**(7458): 123–124.

Thomas K (2005) Gold Standards Framework: A programme for community palliative care. www.goldstandardsframework.nhs.uk (accessed 14 Sept. 2005).

Twycross R, Wilcok A, Charlesworth S, Dickman A (2002) *Palliative Care Formulary 2* (2nd edn). Abingdon: Radcliffe Medical Press.

Wilson R C, Jones P W (1989) A comparison of the visual analogue scale and modified Borg scale for the measurement of dyspnoea during exercise. *Clinical Science* **76**(3): 277–282.

World Health Organisation (2002) Definition of Palliative Care. www.who.int/cancer/palliative/definition/en/ (accessed 14 Sept. 2005).

Yeager H Jr. (1997) Is hospice referral ever appropriate in COPD? *Chest* **112**(1): 8–9.

12 The Future for the Care and Management of Individuals with COPD

LAURA BLACKLER
Guy's and St Thomas' Hospital, London

CAROLINE MOONEY
Luton Treatment Centre, Luton

CHRISTINE JONES
Kings College Hospital, London

CHRONIC DISEASE MANAGEMENT

Chronic disease management has become a key focus in both primary and secondary care. The increased incidence of long-term conditions is a major challenge for the NHS, and it is estimated that there are around 17.5 million people in Great Britain living with a long-term condition. By 2030, it is expected that the number of people over the age of 65 years with a long-term condition will double. Therefore, this has become a priority for the Department of Health, the NHS and social services because of the impact this will have on the provision of services for this population.

Under the General Medical Services (GMS) contract that came into force in April 2004, the Quality and Outcomes Framework (QOF) is a component of this. The QOF rewards practices for the provision of quality care and helps to fund further improvements in the delivery of care. GP practices receive financial rewards if a full assessment of a patient with a chronic disease is undertaken to determine their diagnosis; if this is recorded on the appropriate disease register, and they are being actively managed (Booker 2004). This is a major incentive to improve primary care COPD management. It has been suggested by Rudolf (2000) that a substantial number of patients are not diagnosed with COPD, and also once there is a correct diagnosis guidelines on the management are not always followed in both community and hospital settings (Roberts et al. 2001; Feifer et al. 2002; Barr et al. 2005).

Managing Chronic Obstructive Pulmonary Disease. Edited by L. Blackler, C. Jones and C. Mooney
© 2007 John Wiley & Sons Ltd

QOF is made up of four domains: clinical domain, organisational, patient experience domain and additional services. COPD and smoking information are both indicators within the clinical domain (Table 12.1).

Some of the criticisms of QOF are that it could become a 'box ticking' exercise that says little about quality of care, and that the current targets are a measure of process rather than outcome (Booker 2005). There are also incongruencies between the NICE Guidelines for the diagnosis and management of COPD and the QOF targets. The two main areas are reversibility

Table 12.1. Indicators for QOF for 2006

Indicator	Points	Payment stages (%)
Records		
COPD 1. The practice can produce a register of patients with COPD	3	
Initial diagnosis		
COPD 9. The percentage of patients with COPD in whom diagnosis has been confirmed by spirometry including reversibility testing	10	40–80
Ongoing management		
COPD 10. The percentage of patients with COPD with a record of FEV1 in the previous 15 months	7	40–70
COPD 11. The percentage of patients with COPD receiving inhaled treatment in whom there is a record that inhaler technique has been checked in the previous 15 months	7	40–90
COPD 8. The percentage of patients with COPD who have had influenza immunisation in the preceding 1 September to 31 March	6	40–85
Smoking ongoing management		
Smoking 1. The percentage of patients with any or any combination of the following conditions: coronary disease, stroke or TIA, hypertension, diabetes, COPD or asthma whose notes record smoking status in the previous 15 months. Except those who have never smoked where smoking status need only be recorded once since diagnosis	33	40–90
Smoking 2. The percentage of patients with any or any combination of the following conditions: coronary heart disease, stroke or TIA, hypertension, diabetes, COPD or asthma, who smoke whose notes contain a record that smoking cessation advice or referral to a specialist service, where available, has been offered within the previous 15 months	35	40–90

testing and routine monitoring of FEV_1. However, despite the differences, the QOF scheme is seen as an important starting point for managing patients with COPD and has served to raise the profile in primary care.

One of the stated aims of the GMS contract was to provide a framework for continuing improvements in the standards of care that patients receive. In the future other aspects of quality care as stated in NCCCC (2004), for example, details of impairment, monitoring for anxiety or depression, weight monitoring, pulse oximetry, could be used in the QOF data to further improve standards.

Linked to this within the NHS Plan (2000) self-care was put forward as a key objective in a patient-centred health service. There is growing evidence that supporting self-care has a significant impact on both the patient and the care services (DoH 2005). The concept of self-care is based on a spectrum that ranges from 100 per cent self-care to 100 per cent professional care, and in between this is shared care where individuals and/or families work in partnership with health-care professionals. Within the concept of self-care is self-management which is specifically related to chronic disease management and has been defined by the DoH as 'The individual's abilities to manage the symptoms, treatments, physical and psychosocial consequences and lifestyle changes inherent in living with a long term disorder' (Tomkins and Collins 2005).

There is evidence to support the fact that self-management has a significant impact on the number of times a patient contacts their GP or attends hospital. In a Canadian study, patients with COPD had weekly visits for two months from a health-care professional and then monthly telephone follow-up calls. The self-care management and education was linked with a 40 per cent reduction in hospital visits (Bourbeau et al. 2003). These results were similar in a study carried out in Norway which showed an 85 per cent reduction in visits to the GP, a decrease in the use of reliever medication and an increase in patients' satisfaction with the care provided by their GP (Gallefoss 2004).

There are a variety of types of support that increase the capacity, confidence and efficacy of the individual using a wide range of options (Figure 12.1).

The National Service Framework (NSF) (DoH 2006) supports people with long-term conditions. Although the NSF focuses on people with neurological conditions the framework can be tailored to any long-term condition. The self-care triangle means most people living with long-term conditions able to manage their condition with minimal input from service providers, provided they are given appropriate support and information to enable them to take care of their condition and have a good quality of life (Figure 12.2).

People with COPD will fall into this category while they are in the mild to moderate phases of the disease process; however, they will move into the middle and top stages as the disease moves into the moderate to severe stages.

Case management is a system of managing complex patients with a focus on meeting the needs of individuals, not populations. It is a collaborative

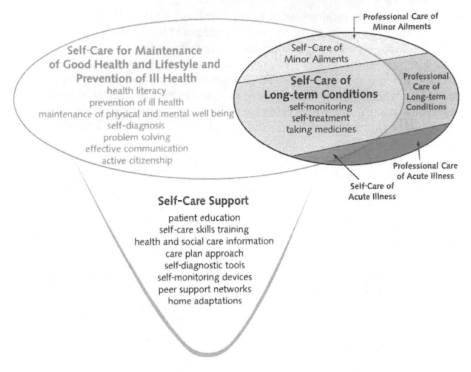

Figure 12.1. Self-care types of support. *Source*: DOH (2005)

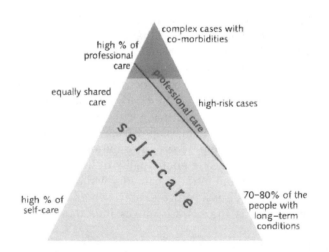

Figure 12.2. The self-care triangle. *Source*: DOH (2005)

process between the patient and case manager to provide a co-ordinated approach to ensuring their needs are met (Huston 2002). It promotes continuity of care and improved communication between patient and health-care providers. Case management systems have been shown to be effective in chronic disease management according to Debusk et al. (1999).

Taylor et al. (2005) conducted a systematic review of randomised controlled trials of chronic disease management interventions for COPD and concluded that the evidence generally failed to detect any benefits using the case management approach. They recommended that early discharge schemes for patients with COPD should be prioritised over other types of nurse-led models of chronic disease management that have been studied to date.

CONCLUSION

COPD has been the 'Cinderella' of respiratory disease and in the past it has not always been one of the main priorities for health-care professionals, and the general public has limited awareness about it. It is often mistakenly viewed as untreatable (Sciurba 2004). Over the years the body of knowledge regarding COPD has increased substantially. It is recognised that COPD is not only a pulmonary disease but also one that affects all systems. Early diagnosis and effective interventions, i.e. smoking cessation, can prevent further accelerated decline in lung function. Other interventions that have been shown to impact significantly on morbidity and mortality include long-term oxygen therapy, non-invasive ventilation for acute exacerbations and lung volume reduction surgery for selected patients with emphysema. In addition, pulmonary rehabilitation, pharmacological therapy, and lung transplantation can improve patients' quality of life, sensation of breathlessness, exercise tolerance and hospital admissions (Celli 2006).

Education of the general public will help to raise awareness of COPD. By alerting people to the factors that may increase their risk of developing COPD and what the symptoms are, individuals should be prompted to seek medical attention at an earlier stage in the disease process.

The future for patients with this disease is more positive as awareness and recognition of COPD is growing. This will have an impact on the standards of care expected by patients and help drive innovations in primary and secondary care. At the time of writing a National Service Framework for COPD is being developed, the first one for a respiratory disease, which can only raise the profile further.

REFERENCES

Barr R, Celli B, Martinez F, Ries A, et al. (2005) Physican and patient perceptions in COPD: the COPD resource network needs assessment survey. *The American Journal of Medicine* **118**(12): 1415.

Booker R (2004) COPD and the new GMS: Part 1. *Practice Nursing* **15**(1): 41–43.

Booker R (2005) COPD, NICE and GMS: getting quality from QOF. *Primary Health Care* **15**(9): 33–36.

Bourbeau J, Maltasis J, et al. (2003) Reduction of hospital utilization in patients with chronic obstructive pulmonary disease: a disease-specific self management intervention. *Archives of Internal Medicine* **163**(5): 585–591.

Celli B R (2006) Chronic obstructive pulmonary disease: From unjustified nihilism to evidence-based optimism. *Proceedings of the American Thoracic Society* **3**(1): 58–65.

Debusk R, West J, Houston-Miller N, Taylor C (1999) Chronic disease management: treating the patient with disease(s) vs. treating disease(s) in the patient. *Archives of Internal Medicine* **159**: 2739–2742.

Department of Health (2000) *NHS Plan.* London: HMSO.

Department of Health (2005) *Self Care: A Real Choice.* London: COI.

Department of Health (2006) *National Service Framework for Supporting People with Long Term Conditions.* London: HMSO.

Feifer R, Aubert R, Verbrugge R, et al. (2002) Disease management opportunities for chronic obstructive pulmonary disease: gaps between guidelines and current practice. *Disease Management* **5**(3): 143–156.

Gallefoss F (2004) The effects of patient education in COPD in a 1-year follow-up randomised controlled trial. *Patient Education Counselling* **52**(3): 259–266.

Huston C (2002) The role of the case manager in a disease management programme. *Lippincotes Case Management* **7**: 221–227.

National Collaborating Centre for Chronic Conditions (NCCCC) (2004) Chronic obstructive pulmonary disease; National clinical guideline for management of chronic obstructive pulmonary disease in adults in primary and secondary care. *Thorax* **59** Suppl. 1: 1–232.

Roberts C, Ryland I, Lowe D, Kelly Y, et al. (2001) Audit of acute admissions of COPD: standards of care and management in the hospital setting. *European Respiratory Journal* **17**: 343–349.

Rudolf M (2000) The reality of drug use in COPD: The European perspective. *Chest* **117**: 29–32.

Sciurba F (2004) Diagnosing and assessing COPD in primary care: the elephant in the room. *Advanced Studies in Medicine* **4**(10A): S750–S755, S779–S781.

Taylor S, Candy B, et al. (2005) Effectiveness of innovations in nurse-led chronic disease management for patients with chronic obstructive pulmonary disease: systematic review of evidence. *British Medical Journal* **331**: 485–491.

Tomkins S, Collins A (2005) *Promoting Optimal Self Care.* London: HSMO.

Glossary

Acid–base homeostasis/Acid–base balance – balance between carbonic acid and bicarbonate in the blood, constant ratio must be maintained to keep the hydrogen ion concentration (pH) of plasma at a constant value.

Acinus – this is the working part of the lung where oxygen/carbon dioxide exchange takes place – respiratory bronchioles, alveolar ducts, and alveolar sacs.

Active cycle of breathing – this comprises a cycle of breathing control, thoracic expansion exercises and forced expiration.

Addiction – a state of dependence on something.

Adrenal suppression – a potential complication of treatment with corticosteroids in which the normal adrenal response is suppressed.

Aerobic respiration – cellular respiration where carbohydrates are completely oxidised by atmospheric oxygen to produce maximum chemical energy.

Air-trapping – abnormal retention of air in the lungs after expiration.

Allograft (Homograft) – a living tissue or organ graft between two members of the same species.

Alpha-1-antitrypsin deficiency – genetic defect which causes a severe reduction in hepatic production of the major antiprotease in lung parenchyma and leaves the lung susceptible to the destructive effects of neutrophil elastase and other endogenous proteases resulting in severe basal panacinar emphysema.

Alveolar hypoventilation – ventilation is inadequate to enable gas exchange.

Anabolism – the synthesis of complex molecules, such as proteins or fats, from simpler ones by living things.

Anaemia – a reduction in the quantity of the oxygen-carrying pigment haemoglobin in the blood.

Anticholinergic – block the cholinergic receptors of the parasympathetic nervous system, preventing narrowing of the airways in response to vagal stimulation.

Antigenic drift – accumulation of mutations in the genetic make-up of influenza virus.

Managing Chronic Obstructive Pulmonary Disease. Edited by L. Blackler, C. Jones and C. Mooney
© 2007 John Wiley & Sons Ltd

Antigenic shift – process by which two different strains of influenza combine to form a new sub-type.

Antimuscarinics – type of anticholinergic.

Antiproteases – protect against the digestion of elastin, and other structural proteins.

Atelectasis – collapse by absorption of air of a segment or lobe of the lung due to an obstruction to its supplying airway, e.g. thick mucus, a foreign body or a tumour.

Atrophy – the wasting away of a normally developed organ or tissue due to degeneration of the cells.

Barotrauma – physical damage to body tissues caused by a difference in pressure between an air space in the body and the surrounding gas or liquid.

Basement membranes – separate the epithelium from the submucosa.

Beta$_2$ agonists – act on the beta$_2$ receptors of the sympathetic nervous system which when stimulated relax bronchial smooth muscle and dilate the bronchi.

Beta$_2$ receptors – sympathetic adrenergic receptors on the surface of the muscle cells, found mainly in the airways.

Bisphosphonates – a class of drug that inhibits the re-absorption of bone.

Breathing control – major aim of treating the breathless patient must be to minimise the work of breathing and encourage the return of a normal pattern of respiration by teaching the patient 'Breathing Control' or gentle breathing.

Bronchi – airways with cartilage in their walls.

Bronchiectasis – a chronic disease characterised by irreversible dilatation of the bronchi.

Bronchioles – small airways 2 mm in diameter with no cartilage, dividing off the bronchi.

Bronchoconstriction – smooth muscle contraction causing narrowing of the airways.

Bronchospasm – spasmodic contraction of the smooth muscle of the bronchi.

Buccal mucosa – moist membranes in the mouth.

Bulla – a thin walled air-filled space within the lung, arising congenitally or in emphysema.

Bullectomy – removal of a localised large compressive bulla, commonly performed with video-assisted thoracoscopic surgery.

Cachexia – a condition of abnormally low weight, weakness and general bodily decline associated with chronic disease.

Candidiasis – an infection with a yeast-like fungus occurring in moist areas of the body, such as the skin folds, mouth, respiratory tract, and vagina.

Cartilage – a dense connective tissue, consisting chiefly of chondronitin sulphate, which is capable of withstanding considerable pressure.

Catabolism – the chemical decomposition of complex substances by the body to simpler ones accompanied by the release of energy.

Cell proliferation – reproduction or multiplication of cells.

Centrilobular emphysema – most common cause of cigarette-induced emphysema in COPD, resulting in the dilatation and destruction of the respiratory bronchioles.

Chronic bronchitis – hypersecretory disorder diagnosed if there is a production of phlegm on most days for three months during any two consecutive years.

Chronic obstructive pulmonary disease (COPD) – airflow obstruction that is usually progressive, not fully reversible and does not change markedly over several months.

Cilia – tiny 'hairs' which beat constantly and in synchrony at about 100 beats a minute.

Circadian rhythm – the periodic rhythm, synchronised approximately to the 24 hour day/night cycle, seen in various metabolic activities of most living organisms.

Cognitive behavioural therapy (CBT) – a form of psychotherapy used to treat depression, anxiety disorders, etc.

Collagen – a protein that is the principal constituent of white fibrous connective tissue.

Continuous positive airway pressure (CPAP) – method of respiratory ventilation which provides a constant pressure that causes a 'pneumatic splint' which blows open the pharynx to allow unobstructed breathing, often used for sleep apnoea.

Cor pulmonale – development of pulmonary hypertension and right ventricular hypertrophy as a consequence of the chronic hypoxaemia associated with chronic lung disease or thoracic cage disease.

Cough – a defensive reflex which aims to eject foreign material from the bronchial tree.

Crico–sternal distance – distance between the cricoid cartilage (forms the lower and back parts of the larynx) and the sternal notch.

Cushing's syndrome – the condition resulting from excess amounts of corticosteroid hormones in the body.

Cytokines – used extensively for inter-cell communication and play a major role in a variety of immunological, inflammatory and infectious diseases.

Diaphragm – a dome-shaped muscle that separates the thoracic and abdominal cavities, and plays an important role in breathing.

Diurnal variation – occurring during the day.

Diverticular disease – diverticula (sacs or pouches formed at weak points in the walls of the alimentary canal) in the colon associated with lower abdominal pain and disturbed bowel habit.

Dynamic hyperinflation – caused by progressive air trapping, a major cause of dyspnoea on exertion.

Dynamometry – the recording of the force of a muscle contraction.

Dyspnoea – the subjective awareness of the increased work of breathing.

Elastase – enzyme found mainly in the pancreatic juice.

Elastic recoil – the ability of a stretched object or organ to return to its resting position.

Elastic recoil pressure – force required to open the airways.

Elastin – protein forming the major constituent of elastic tissue fibres.

Emphysema – a destructive process in which the airspace walls are destroyed. In the severe form the destruction involves both the small airways from which the alveoli arise as well as the alveoli themselves.

Endogenous – arising from within or derived from the body.

Endothelium – the single layer of cells that lines the heart, blood vessels and lymphatic vessels.

EPAP – expiratory positive airway pressure.

Epithelium – the tissue that covers the external surface of the body and lines hollow structures (except blood and lymphatic vessels).

Erythema – relates to the abnormal flushing of the skin caused by dilatation of the blood capillaries.

Exacerbation – a sustained worsening of a patient's symptoms from their usual stable state that is beyond normal day-to-day variation, and is acute in onset.

Exhalation/Expiration – the diaphragm relaxes and the ribs fall back to their original position, the natural elastic recoil of the lungs provides an additional driving force behind exhalation.

External respiration – gas exchange that takes place in the lungs.

FEV_1 (forced expiratory volume in one second) – volume of air that can be exhaled in the first second of a forced exhalation.

FEV_1/FVC per cent – ratio of forced expiratory volume in one second to forced vital capacity.

Fibrosing alveolitis – there are two components of this disease – alveolar inflammation and subsequent fibrosis.

Fibrosis – thickening and scarring of connective tissue, and most often a consequence of inflammation or injury.

FiO_2 – fraction of inspired oxygen (FiO_2 of 0.4 = 40 per cent inspired oxygen).

Forced vital capacity (FVC) – the total volume of air that can be exhaled from maximum inhalation to maximum exhalation.

Functional residual capacity (FRC) – volume of air left in the lungs at the end of tidal breath.

Goblet cells – lie within the epithelium and get their name from their shape, produce mucus which lines the surface of the airway.

Granulation – the growth of small rounded outgrowths, made of small blood vessels and connective tissue, on the healing surface of a wound.

Haemoptysis – coughing up blood.

Hydrocarbons – class of chemical compounds only consisting of hydrogen and carbon.

Hypercapnia – the presence in the blood of an abnormally high concentration of carbon dioxide.

Hyperinflation – airflow limitation develops, the rate of lung emptying is slowed and the interval between expiratory efforts does not allow expiration of the relaxation volume.

Hyperplasia – the increased production and growth of normal cells in a tissue or organ.

Hypertrophy – an increase in the size of an organ brought about by the enlargement of its cells rather than by cell multiplication.

Hyperventilation – increased ventilation in excess of that required for metabolic needs and quite often has a psychogenic component.

Hypokalaemia – the presence of abnormally low levels of potassium in the blood.

Hypotonia – a state of reduced tension on muscle.

Hypoventilation – breathing at an abnormally slow rate, which results in an increased amount of carbon dioxide in the blood.

Hypoxaemia – the presence in the blood of an abnormally low concentration of oxygen.

Hypoxia – a deficiency of oxygen in the tissues.

Inflammatory factor – an agent or element that contributes to the inflammatory process.

Inflammatory mediator – a substance that causes a specific response, in COPD these include leukotriene B_4, interleukin, growth-related oncogene-alpha, monocyte chemotaxic protein 1 alpha.

Inhalation/Inspiration – muscles attached to the ribs (intercostal muscles) contract, pulling the ribs upwards and outwards; at the same time the muscles of the diaphragm contract causing it to flatten and descend. This has the effect of increasing the volume of the chest cavity. This reduces the pressure of air in the lung to below atmospheric pressure so that the air is sucked in.

Intima – the inner layer of the wall of an artery or vein, composed of a lining of endothelial cells and an elastic membrane.

Intra-luminar – inside a cavity or tube.

Intrinsic – exclusive to a part or body.

Intrinsic PEEP (IPEEP) – intrinsic positive end expiratory pressure.

Isokinetic – maintaining constant tension as muscles shorten or lengthen.

Isometric – of or denoting muscular contraction that does not cause muscle shortening.

Isotonic muscles – describes muscles that have equal tonicity.

KCO – a figure derived from the transfer factor correlated for alveolar volume.

Lactic acid – a compound that forms in the cells as the end product of glucose metabolism in the absence of oxygen.

Left ventricular failure – congestive heart failure whereby the heart is unable to pump the blood around the body effectively.

Leukotrienes – mediators involved in the inflammatory process.

Lung compliance – distensibility of the lungs.

Lung recoil pressure – produced when the lungs retract from the chest.

Lymphocytes – colourless cell formed in the lymphoid tissue involved in the development of immunity.

Macrophage – a large scavenger cell present in connective tissue, and many major organs and tissues.

Metabolic compensation – mechanism to return to homeostasis.

Metaplasia – an abnormal change in the nature of a tissue.

Methylxanthine – a group of drugs comprising theophylline, aminophylline and choline theophyllinate.

Mitochondria – structures in varying numbers in the cytoplasm of every cell.

Motivational interviewing – counselling approach seeks to help clients think differently about their behaviour and ultimately to consider what might be gained through change.

Mucous glands – lie below the epithelium; airway mucus traps small particles of dust in the air and prevents them from penetrating further into the lungs.

Myalgia – pain in the muscles.

Nasal ventilation – avoids the use of endotracheal tube and uses a tight-fitting face mask with headgear.

Negative pressure – pressure is less than that of the surrounding fluid, e.g. air.

Neuropathies – a functional disturbance or pathological change in the peripheral nervous system.

Neutrophil – a variety of granulocyte capable of ingesting and killing bacteria.

Noradrenaline – a hormone closely related to adrenaline, causes constriction of blood vessels leading to an increase in blood pressure, increase in rate and depth of breathing and relaxation of the smooth muscle in the intestinal walls.

Noradrenergic – activated by or secreting noradrenaline.

Non-rapid eye movement (NREM) – a stage of sleep divided into four stages, stages 3 and 4 represent the deeper levels of sleep thought to 'refresh' the brain and are known as slow wave sleep.

Obesity hypoventilation syndrome – combination of severe obesity and obstructive sleep apnoea causing hypoxia and hypercapnia.

Obstructive sleep apnoea – a period of absent breathing of 10 seconds or longer occurring five or more times per hour of sleep.

Orthopnoea – shortness of breath when lying flat.

Osteoporosis – a loss of bony tissue resulting in bones that are brittle, and liable to fracture.

Oxidative stress – damage to cells caused by an imbalance between free radicals and antioxidants.

Oxygen saturation – is a measure of the percentage of oxygenated haemoglobin to total haemoglobin in the circulation.

Ozone – a poisonous gas containing three oxygen atoms per molecule, is a very powerful oxidising agent.

$PaCO_2$ – Partial pressure of arterial carbon dioxide.

Panacinar emphysema/Panlobular emphysema – characteristic lesion seen in alpha-1-antitrypsin deficiency, extends throughout the entire acinus, involving the dilatation and destruction of the alveolar ducts and sacs as well as the respiratory bronchioles.

PaO_2 – Partial pressure of arterial oxygen.

Paradoxical breathing/costal margin paradox – an important sign in patients with severe airways obstruction, and high inspiratory impedance in hyperinflated lungs. Expansion of the lower rib cage is assessed by spreading the hands with the fingers directed along the ribs and the thumbs near to the midline. With paradoxyical breathing on inspiration there is movement of the thumbs together and movement apart on expiration which is opposite to what happens with normal quiet breathing.

Parenchyma – the functional part of an organ.

Parietal pleura – lining the thoracic cavity.

Paroxysmal nocturnal dyspnoea – breathlessness that occurs in the night is characteristically described in left heart failure.

Particulate particles – tiny particles of solid (a smoke) or liquid (an aerosol) suspended in a gas.

Peak expiratory flow – peak expiratory flow is the maximum flow achieved in the first 10th of a second of a forced exhalation starting from a full breath in.

PEEP – positive end expiratory pressure.

Peripheral airways resistance – increased resistance to air flow occurs during disease in the respiratory bronchioles.

Pleural cavity – potential space between the parietal and visceral layers.

Pneumonia – accumulation of infecting organisms, white blood cells and exudates in the alveolar spaces sufficient to fill them (consolidation) and impair gas exchange.

Pneumonitis – refers to small areas of infection, often multiple and has generally replaced the term 'bronchopneumonia'.

Pneumothorax – the presence of air in the pleural cavity between the chest wall and the lung.

Polycythaemia – a compensatory process whereby more red blood cells are produced.

Polymorphonuclear leukocytes – see neutrophil.

Positive pressure – pressure within a system that is greater than the environment that surrounds that system.

Pressure-cycled ventilation – patient breathing is supported by a constant inspiratory pressure that is delivered for a set time.

Protease – a digestive enzyme that causes the breakdown of protein.

Pulmonary embolism (thrombo-embolism) – emboli originate from thrombi in the venous system, thrombo-emboli lodge in the arteries of the lung because they are too large to pass through the pulmonary capillaries into the left side of the heart. Extensive blockage with emboli impedes the flow of blood from the right side of the heart through the lungs into the left, and so pulmonary artery blood pressure arises.

Pulmonary hypertension – normal mean pressures in the pulmonary artery are around 20 mmHg (2.5 kPa) compared to 90 mmHg (12 kPa) in the systemic circulation. Pressure can rise in the pulmonary vascular system either because parts of it are blocked or because muscles in the walls of the blood vessels constrict, narrowing their lumen, this is commonly the result of hypoxia, but can occur for no apparent reason – primary pulmonary hypertension.

Pulmonary vasculature – lung circulation system.

Rapid eye movement (REM) – a stage of sleep where there is generalised inhibition of skeletal muscles including the intercostals, accessory and pharyngeal dilators) but not the diaphragm. Thus ventilation during REM sleep is more dependent on diaphragmatic function than during slow wave sleep and upper airway function is more precarious.

Residual volume – small amount of air left in the lungs after expiration.

Respiratory acidosis – reduction in alveolar ventilation causes an increase in arterial PCO_2 – low pH and normal bicarbonate.

Respiratory alkalosis – alveolar hyperventilation causes a fall in PCO_2, raised pH and normal bicarbonate.

Respiratory drive – the stimulus to breathe.

Segmental bronchi – within each lung the bronchi divide into 10–19 further generations of smaller branches. The larger bronchi have cartilaginous rings; the smaller bronchi have cartilage plates.

Serotonin – a compound widely disturbed in the tissues, particularly in the blood platelets, intestinal wall, and central nervous system. It is thought to play a role in inflammation similar to that of histamine and it also acts as a neurotransmitter.

Smooth muscle – occurs between cartilages in the trachea and bronchi, and on its own in the bronchioles. Two sets of muscle fibres wind down the airways in a double spiral.

Spirometry – measurement of the volume of air forced out of the lungs against the time taken to blow out all the air.

Sputum – a visco-elastic liquid because it is rather sticky when still but becomes more liquid when a force is applied to it, consists of 95 per cent water and the rest is mucus and various cells and proteins.

Squamous cell – an epithelial cell that is flat like a plate and forms a single layer of epithelial tissue.

Submucosa (lamina propria) – connective tissue that supports the network of capillaries and nerve fibres which supply the lung.

Tachypnoea – rapid shallow breathing.

Terminal bronchioles – bronchioles that are immediately proximal to the alveoli.

Thoracoscopy – the technique of opening the pleura under local anaesthesia and using specifically designed optical instruments to look into the pleural cavity.

Tidal breathing – the amount of air breathed in or out during normal breathing.

Tissue respiration – gas exchange that takes place in the tissues.

Trachea – this consists of a fibrous tube kept open by horseshoe-shaped cartilage rings, it is lined with ciliated epithelium containing goblet cells and mucous glands.

Transfer factors (TICO)/Diffusing capacity (DICO) – this test assesses gaseous diffusion across the membrane separating the alveoli from the blood capillaries.

Urticaria – an acute or chronic allergic reaction in which red round wheals develop on the skin, ranging in size from small spots to several inches across.

Vascular tone – normal degree of vigour and tension.

Vasoconstriction – a decrease in the diameter of blood vessels, especially arteries.

Venous stasis – impairment or cessation of venous flow.

Ventilation–perfusion ratio (V/Q) – it is essential that in each alveolus there is an appropriate amount of ventilation with air and a matched amount of perfusion with blood. This matching is expressed as a ratio of ventilation to perfusion (V/Q) and ideally the ration should be 1.0.

Venturi valve/fixed percentage masks – oxygen is forced through a narrow orifice entraining air from the surroundings and the percentage oxygen in the mixture will vary with: the flow rate, the size of the orifice through which it passes, and the size of the gap through which the air is entrained.

Visceral pleura – covers the surface of the lung and dips into its fissures. The smooth surfaces face one another and are moistened by a film of fluid, so that as the lungs fill and empty with air, they glide smoothly and quietly over one another.

VO_2 – uptake of oxygen.

Appendix Useful Organisations

Age Concern England
Astral House
1268 London Road
London
SW16 4ER
Tel (Freephone Age Concern Information Line (UK)): 0800 00 99 66
Web: www.ageconcern.org.uk
Age Concern is the leading movement in the UK working with and for older people. Age Concerns are independent charities that work together in agreed ways, sharing the name and a commitment to making later life fulfilling, enjoyable and productive. They do this by providing as little or as much help as older people need to continue living independently in their own homes and to maintain their emotional well-being.

ASH – Action on Smoking and Health
102 Clifton Street
London
EC2A 4HW
Tel: 020 7739 5902
Fax: 020 7613 0531
Web: www.ash.org.uk
ASH is a campaigning public health charity working for a comprehensive societal response to tobacco aimed at achieving a sharp reduction and eventual elimination of the health problems caused by tobacco.

Befriending Network
Claremont
24–27 White Lion Street
London
N1 9PD
Tel: 020 7689 2443

Managing Chronic Obstructive Pulmonary Disease. Edited by L. Blackler, C. Jones and C. Mooney
© 2007 John Wiley & Sons Ltd

Web: www.befriending.net
Best time to telephone: 24 hour answerphone available.
The Befriending Network provides trained volunteers to offer practical and emotional support in the home to those who have terminal or life-threatening disease.

Benefit Enquiry Line – For People with Disabilities
Room 901
Victoria House
Ormskirk Road
Preston
Lancashire
PR1 2QP
Tel (Helpline – Voice): 0800 882200
Tel (Helpline – Text): 0800 243355
Fax: 01772 238953
Web: www.direct.gov.uk
The Benefit Enquiry Line (BEL) is a benefits helpline for people with disabilities, carers and representatives. BEL is part of the Department for Work and Pensions. It offers confidential advice and information on benefits and how to claim them. In addition to giving advice it is also able to send out an extensive range of leaflets and claim packs to customers.

BHF National Centre for Physical Activity and Health
Loughborough University
Loughborough
Leicestershire
LE11 3TU
Tel: 01509 223259
Fax: 01509 223972
Web: www.bhfactive.org.uk
The BHF National Centre for Physical Activity and Health has a website which is aimed at providing practical ideas and advice for professionals to promote physical activity. They also provide resources to support the promotion of physical activity.

British Association for Sexual and Relationship Therapy
PO Box 13686
London
SW20 9ZH
Tel (Admin only): 0208 543 2707
Web: www.basrt.org.uk
The Association holds a list of qualified practitioners and clinics providing sexual or relationship therapy in the UK. Please send a stamped addressed envelope for details or visit the website. There is no helpline available.

British Lung Foundation
73–75 Goswell Road
London
EC1V 7ER
Helpline: 08458 50 50 20
Fax: 020 7688 5556
Web: www.lunguk.org
The British Lung Foundation's Breathe Easy Club is the only support group
throughout the UK for people with any type of lung condition, ranging from
asthma and bronchitis to emphysema and lung cancer.

British Nutrition Foundation
High Holborn House
52–54 High Holborn
London
WC1V 6RQ
Tel: 020 7404 6504
Fax: 020 7404 6747
Web: www.nutrition.org.uk
The British Nutrition Foundation promotes the well-being of the population
by the impartial interpretation and effective dissemination of scientifically
based nutritional knowledge and advice. It works in partnership with academic
and research institutes, the food industry, educators and government.

British Snoring and Sleep Apnoea Association
Castle Court
41 London Road
Reigate
Surrey
RH2 9RJ
Tel (Helpline): 0800 085 1097
Tel (Administration): 01737 245 638
Web: www.britishsnoring.co.uk
To promote public awareness that habitual snoring and sleep apnoea are gen-
erally treatable complaints and that help is available.

British Thoracic Society
Web: www.brit-thoracic.org.uk
The British Thoracic Society is a professional organisation but their website
includes a Patient Information section which is intended to help patients, their
friends and relatives and anyone else who is interested in respiratory (lung)
diseases.

Carer's Allowance Unit
Department of Work and Pensions

Palatine House
Lancaster Road
Preston
Lancashire
PR1 1HB
Tel: 01253 856 123
Web: www.dwp.gov.uk
Carer's Allowance is a government benefit which can be claimed by carers
who are 16 or over and care for a disabled person for at least 35 hours per
week. The disabled person has to be in receipt of a qualifying benefit and the
carer's earnings are taken into account.

Carers – Government Information
Web: www.carers.gov.uk
The Carers website is published by the Department of Health and gives information on services and benefits related to carers. The site includes information,
facts and figures and links to related websites.

Carers UK
Ruth Pitter House
20–25 Glasshouse Yard
London
EC1A 4JT
Tel (CarersLine): 0808 808 7777
Tel (Office): 020 7490 8818
Fax: 020 7490 8824
Web: www.carersuk.org
Carers UK (formerly the Carers National Association) aims to help anyone
who is caring for a sick, disabled or elderly, frail friend or relative at home.

CLEANAIR Website
33 Stillness Road
London
SE23 1NG
Tel: 020 8690 4649
Web: www.ezme.com/cleanair
Web: www.geocities.com/bimanmullick/SmokeWeb/WHO-notepad.htm
CLEANAIR is an independent, voluntary and non-profit-making organisation
which has been engaged in drawing public attention to smoking and its effects
on health and the environment since 1972. Its main aim is to help create a
smoke-free society for all to share and enjoy.

Couples Counselling Network
Web: www.ukcouplescounselling.com

Couples Counselling Network provides well-qualified counsellors, who have specialist training and many years experience working with couples. All are carefully selected to work within the Network and all counsellors abide by the Code of Ethics of the British Association for Counselling (BACP) or United Kingdom Council for Psychotherapy (UKCP).

Crossroads Caring for Carers
Information and Communications Department 3rd Floor
49 Charles Street
Cardiff
CF10 2GD
Tel: 0845 450 0350
Fax: 029 2022 2311
Web: www.crossroads.org.uk
Crossroads is committed to providing practical support where it is most needed, in the home. Trained Carer Support Workers go into carers' homes to take over caring tasks, giving the carer an essential break and 'time to themselves'.

Extend (Exercise Training Ltd)
2 Place Farm
Wheathampstead
Hertfordshire
AL4 8SB
Tel: 01582 832760
Fax: 01582 832760
Web: www.extend.org.uk
EXTEND provides recreational movement to music for the over-sixties and for the less able of any age.

Food Standards Agency
Aviation House
125 Kingsway
London
WC2B 6NH
Tel: 020 7276 8000
Tel (to request booklets): 0845 606 0667
Tel: (Admin): 020 7276 8829
Fax: 020 7972 2340
Web: www.food.gov.uk
The Food Standards Agency was set up to protect people's health and the interests of consumers in relation to food.

Help the Aged
207–221 Pentonville Road

London
N1 9UZ
Tel (SeniorLine in England, Wales, Scotland): 0808 800 6565
Tel (SeniorLine in Northern Ireland): 0808 808 7575
Tel (SeniorLine Textphone): 0800 26 96 26
Tel (Office): 020 7278 1114
Fax: 020 7278 1116
Web: www.helptheaged.org.uk
Help the Aged provides practical support to help older people live independent lives, particularly those who are frail, isolated or poor. In addition to the charity's campaigning and fundraising activities, it provides direct services overseas and in the UK that support older people's independence.

Institute of Psychosexual Medicine
12 Chandos Street
Cavendish Square
London
W1G 9DR
Tel: 020 7580 0631
Web: www.ipm.org.uk
The IPM can provide a list of accredited doctors who accept psychosexual referrals. The list gives details of doctors and their clinics, both private and NHS throughout the United Kingdom.

National Federation of Shopmobility
The Hawkins Suite
Enham Place
Enham Alamein
Andover
Hants
SP11 6JS
Tel: 0845 644 2446
Fax: 0845 644 442
Web: www.justmobility.co.uk/shop
Shopmobility is a scheme which lends powered and manual wheelchairs and powered scooters to members of the public with limited mobility, to shop and use the leisure and commercial facilities of their town or city centre. The scheme operates in many towns and cities throughout the UK.

NHS Smoking Helpline
Tel: 0800 169 0 169
Web: www.givingupsmoking.co.uk
Commissioned by the Central Office of Information and funded by the Department of Health, this phoneline and website offers free information, advice and

support to people who are giving up smoking, and those who have given up smoking and do not want to start again. The service is also designed to support their friends and families, as well as health specialists.

Prescription Pricing Authority – Patient Services
Sandyford House
Archbold Terrace
Newcastle upon Tyne
NE2 1DB
Tel (Customer Enquiries): 0845 850 1166
Fax: 0191 203 5507
Web: www.ppa.org.uk
The Patient Services of the Prescription Pricing Authority provides income-related help with health costs.

QUIT
Ground Floor
211 Old Street
London
EC1V 9NR
Tel (Quitline): 0800 00 22 00
Tel (Admin): 020 7251 1551
Fax: 020 7251 1661
Web: www.quit.org.uk
QUIT is the UK's only charity whose main aim is to offer practical help to people who want to stop smoking. Quitting is not easy. QUIT does not lecture people but just gives down-to-earth help and advice about stopping for good.

Relate
Herbert Gray College
Little Church Street
Rugby
Warwickshire
CV21 3AP
Tel: 01788 573241
Fax: 01788 535007
Web: www.relate.org.uk
Relate is Britain's leading couple counselling agency. High-quality counselling, relationship education and training is provided to support couple and family relationships throughout life.

Sexual Dysfunction Association
Windmill Place Business Centre
2–4 Windmill Lane

Southall
Middlesex
UB2 4NJ
Helpline: 0870 7743571
Web: www.sda.uk.net
The Sexual Dysfunction Association is a charitable organisation which was set
up to help sufferers of impotence (erectile dysfunction) and their partners and
to raise awareness of the condition amongst both the public and the medical
profession.

Sleep Council
High Corn Mill
Chapel Hill
Skipton
North Yorkshire
BD23 1NL
Tel (Leaflet Requests): 0800 0187 4595 (24 hour answerphone)
Tel (Office): 0845 058 4595
Web: www.sleepcouncil.com
The Sleep Council is a non-profit-making generic organisation which aims to
promote the importance of a good night's sleep to health and well-being – and
the importance of a good bed, regularly replaced to achieving that good night's
sleep.

Tourism For All
C/O Vitalise
Shap Road Industrial Estate
Kendal
Cumbria
LA9 6NZ
Tel (Information): 0845 124 9971
Tel (Admin): 0845 124 9974
Tel (Reservations): 0845 124 9973
Fax: 01539 735567
Web: www.tourismforall.org.uk
Tourism for All (UK) incorporating Holiday Care is a national registered
charity and is a central source of information for older and disabled people
and their carers wishing to have a holiday break.

Index